# Editor's introduction

The Advanced Medicine Course offers an annual opportunity to survey those aspects of medical practice in the UK at the cutting edge of clinical science. For the course organiser, there is the added advantage of bringing a subjective eye to the course and to accentuate some areas of medicine which are particularly topical or fast moving.

In all aspects of medicine, it remains axiomatic that prevention of disease will always be superior to treatment of established disease. Sadly, if predictably, this more public health oriented approach does not always receive high profile in the medical and scientific press. However, the past year has been dominated by the latest results of the prevention of coronary artery disease and stroke through the lowering of cholesterol by statins. It was therefore timely for this volume to address in depth the current state of knowledge in cardiovascular prevention, including the most up-to-the-moment results of the Anglo-Scandinavian Cardiac Outcomes Trial (ASCOT) – the most cited clinical trial in *Lancet* 2003.

It is only in the past five years that many teaching hospitals in the UK have found that their budget for antiviral drugs now exceeds their antibiotic budget. The antiviral revolution, with effective therapy for chronic viral infections and specific therapy for acute respiratory viral infections, now demands a broader audience in general medicine. In future, the immune system will be harnessed to work in tandem with antiviral chemotherapy, and the first tentative steps to re-establishing immune control of Epstein-Barr virus lymphoproliferation are described here. The theme of infection and immunity is echoed in the Lumleian lecture, 'Immunology as taught by Darwin', and further by accounts of multidrug resistant tuberculosis and the current status of therapy of malaria.

In common with many physicians, I struggle with the diagnosis and management of psychosomatic disease. As so many of these presentations are gastrointestinal, this volume includes a detailed account of a rational approach to 'medically unexplained gastrointestinal conditions'; this may be of benefit far more widely across all aspects of clinical medicine. Similarly, this volume addresses the common diagnostic problems of management of headache, chronic obstructive pulmonary disease and renal disease.

The best practice in medicine is often achieved through cutting across traditional barriers of specialty and profession; surgeons and radiologists contributed their expertise to this volume so as to better understand their role in dealing with issues often considered to be strictly medical.

We are fortunate to have both breadth and depth in clinical medicine to draw upon in the UK, so as to present the very best of British medicine at the forefront of international developments. Considerable increase in investment will be required to maintain this critical mass, and we must not lose any opportunity to press for the maintenance of this important national resource.

JONATHAN WEBER
*November 2003*

# Horizons in Medicine

*number* **15**

Edited by

**Jonathan Weber**

*Chairman, Wright Fleming Institute, Imperial College London*

**Royal College of
Physicians of London**

Royal College of Physicians of London
11 St Andrews Place, London NW1 4LE

Registered Charity No. 210508

Copyright © 2003 Royal College of Physicians of London
ISBN 1 86016 196 0

Typeset by Dan-Set Graphics, Telford, Shropshire
Printed in Great Britain by The Lavenham Press Ltd, Sudbury, Suffolk

British Library Cataloguing in Publication Data
A catalogue record of this book is available from the British Library

# Contributors

SIMON ALLISON *Professor in Clinical Nutrition, University Hospital, Queen's Medical Centre, Nottingham NG7 2UH*

DAVID J P BARKER *Director, MRC Environment Epidemiology Unit, University of Southampton, Southampton General Hospital, Southampton SO16 6YD*

D GARETH BEEVERS *Professor of Medicine, University Department of Medicine, City Hospital NHS Trust, Dudley Road, Birmingham B18 7QH*

EDWINA A BROWN *Consultant Nephrologist, Charing Cross Hospital, Fulham Palace Road, London W6 8RF*

W RODNEY BURNHAM *Consultant Physician and Gastroenterologist, Barking, Havering and Redbridge Hospitals NHS Trust, Clinical Diagnostic Centre, Oldchurch Hospital, Waterloo Road, Romford, Essex RM7 0BE*

PETER M A CALVERLEY *Professor of Medicine, Pulmonary and Rehabilitation Research Group, Department of Medicine, University Hospital Aintree, Clinical Sciences Centre, Longmoor Lane, Liverpool L9 7AL*

JOHN C CHAMBERS *Cardiology Specialist Registrar, St Mary's Hospital, Norfolk Place, London W2 1NY*

DUNCAN CHURCHILL *Consultant Physician, Lawson Unit, Royal Sussex County Hospital, Eastern Road, Brighton BN2 5BE*

RICHARD J COKER *Senior Lecturer, ECOHOST, Department of Public Health and Policy, London School of Hygiene and Tropical Medicine, Keppel Street, London WC1E 7HT*

DOROTHY H CRAWFORD *Professor of Medical Microbiology and Head of School of Biomedical and Clinical Laboratory Sciences, Hugh Robson Building, University of Edinburgh, George Square, Edinburgh EH8 9XD*

GEORGE C EBERS *Action Research Professor of Clinical Neurology, Head of Department, Department of Clinical Neurology, University of Oxford, Radcliffe Infirmary, Woodstock Road, Oxford OX2 6HE*

MEGUID M EL NAHAS *Professor of Nephrology, Sheffield Kidney Institute, Sheffield Teaching Hospitals Trust, Northern General Campus, Herries Road, Sheffield S5 7AU*

**WLADYSLAW GEDROYC** *Consultant Radiologist, Interventional Magnetic Resonance Unit, St Mary's Hospital NHS Trust, Praed Street, London W2 1NY*

**SEBASTIAN L JOHNSTON** *Professor of Respiratory Medicine, National Heart and Lung Institute and Wright Fleming Institute of Infection and Immunity, Faculty of Medicine, Imperial College London, Norfolk Place, London W2 1PG*

**RAJU KAPOOR** *Consultant Neurologist, National Hospital for Neurology and Neurosurgery, Queen Square, London WC1N 3BG; Northwick Park Hospital, Watford Road, Harrow HA1 3UJ*

**JOHN R KIRWAN** *Consultant and Reader in Rheumatology, Head of Academic Rheumatology Unit, Department of Clinical Medicine, University of Bristol Division of Medicine, Bristol Royal Infirmary, Marlborough Street, Bristol BS2 8HW*

**JASPAL S KOONER** *Professor of Clinical Cardiology, National Heart and Lung Institute, Imperial College, Hammersmith Campus, Du Cane Road, London W12 0NN*

**PETER G KOPELMAN** *Professor of Clinical Medicine and Vice-Principal, Barts and The London, Queen Mary's School of Medicine and Dentistry, University of London, Turner Street, London E1 2AD*

**YING KUAN** *Specialist Registrar in Nephrology, Sheffield Kidney Institute, Sheffield Teaching Hospitals Trust, Northern General Campus, Herries Road, Sheffield S5 7AU*

**PATRICK MALLIA** *Clinical Research Fellow, National Heart and Lung Institute and Wright Fleming Institute of Infection and Immunity, Faculty of Medicine, Imperial College, Norfolk Place, London W2 1PG*

**ROBERT MARSTON** *Consultant Orthopaedic Surgeon, St Mary's Hospital, Praed Street, London W2 1NY; Honorary Senior Lecturer at Imperial College School of Medicine*

**PETER W MATHIESON** *Professor of Renal Medicine, University of Bristol; Honorary Consultant Nephrologist, North Bristol NHS Trust, Academic Renal Unit, Southmead Hospital, Bristol BS10 5NB*

**RAJUL PATEL** *Consultant Genito-Urinary Physician, Senior Lecturer, University of Southampton, Department of Genito-Urinary Medicine, Royal South Hants Hospital, St Mary's Road, Southampton SO14 0YG*

**RODNEY PHILLIPS** *Professor of Clinical Medicine; Chairman, The Peter Medawar Building for Pathogen Research, University of Oxford, South Parks Road, Oxford OX1 3SY*

**JONATHAN M RHODES** *Professor of Medicine, Department of Medicine, University of Liverpool, Duncan Building, Daulby Street, Liverpool L69 3GA*

**DAVID G I SCOTT** *Consultant Rheumatologist and Honorary Professor, University of East Anglia, Department of Rheumatology, Norfolk and Norwich University Hospital NHS Trust, Colney Lane, Norwich NR4 7UY*

**PETER SEVER** *Professor of Clinical Pharmacology and Therapeutics, Department of Clinical Pharmacology, Imperial College London, QEQM Wing, 10th Floor, St Mary's Hospital, South Wharf Road, London W2 1NY*

**JOHN STRADLING** *Consultant Physician, and Professor of Respiratory Medicine, University of Oxford, Oxford Centre for Respiratory Medicine, Churchill Hospital, Old Road, Headington, Oxford OX3 7LJ*

**MARK THURSZ** *Reader in Medicine, Faculty of Medicine, Imperial College, St Mary's Campus, Norfolk Place, London W2 1PG*

**ROLAND M VALORI** *Consultant Physician and Gastroenterologist, Gloucestershire Royal Hospital, Great Western Road, Gloucester GL1 3NN*

**JONATHAN WEBER** *Chairman, Wright Fleming Institute, Imperial College London, St Mary's Campus, Norfolk Place, London W2 1PG*

**PETER WINSTANLEY** *Professor of Clinical Pharmacology, Department of Pharmacology and Therapeutics, University of Liverpool, Liverpool L69 3GE*

# Contents

# Renal

# Chronic kidney failure: advances in understanding and treatment

Meguid El Nahas and Ying Kuan

## ☐ INTRODUCTION

An increasing number of patients worldwide suffer every year from end-stage renal failure (ESRF), possibly the direct consequence of the ageing of the population in developed countries and the worldwide explosion in the incidence of type 2 diabetes mellitus. In the UK, there are about 100 new cases of ESRF per million population each year compared with approximately 300 per million a year in the US where diabetic nephropathy is the most common cause (accounting for over 40% of cases).[1] In both countries the incidence of ESRF is three- to fourfold higher in the elderly than in younger patients.[1] It is predicted that the steady increase in the number of patients reaching ESRF and requiring dialysis will continue unabated for at least another decade.[2] The cost of renal replacement therapy is increasing in parallel: an estimated $17 billion in the US in 2000.[1]

ESRF is the direct consequence of progressive chronic kidney diseases (CKD). It has been estimated that approximately 10% of the US population may have some manifestation of kidney disease,[3] possibly reflecting the high prevalence of hypertension and diabetes and common renal involvement in these conditions.[3] In view of such a large number of patients with, or at risk of, CKD it is important to review the advances made over the last 25 years in the understanding of the pathophysiology and management of progressive kidney diseases. Before doing this, it is necessary to give a brief update on new classifications of CKD and risk factors associated with CKD.

## ☐ CLASSIFICATION

In a recent classification of CKD, the American National Kidney Foundation has renamed 'chronic renal failure' as 'chronic kidney failure' (CKF) to make it easier for nonspecialists to understand.[4] CKD has been divided into five stages (Table 1).

## ☐ RISK FACTORS

The three groups of risk factors for CKD concern:

☐ susceptibility

**Table 1** The five stages of chronic kidney disease.

| Stage | GFR | Other features |
|---|---|---|
| 1 | Normal | Some degree of renal involvement (eg haematuria or proteinuria) |
| 2 | 90–60 ml/min | |
| 3 | 59–30 ml/min | |
| 4 | 29–15 ml/min | |
| 5 | <15 ml/min | ESRF |
| | | RRT should be considered |

ESRF = end-stage renal failure; GFR = glomerular filtration rate; RRT = renal replacement therapy.

☐   initiation, and

☐   progression.

## Susceptibility factors

### Genetic background

A range of genetic polymorphisms has been associated with susceptibility to diabetic and nondiabetic nephropathies. Those involving the gene coding for the angiotensin-converting enzyme (ACE) have been the most studied and reported.[5]

### Race

African-Caribbeans in the UK and African-Americans in the US have a much higher prevalence of CKD than Caucasians. In the US, native and Hispanic Americans also have a higher incidence. This may reflect the high prevalence of type 2 diabetes in these populations. In the UK, Asians appear to have a higher incidence than Caucasians, in particular of diabetic nephropathy.

### Age

The incidence and prevalence of CKD are much higher in the elderly, possibly reflecting the high prevalence of hypertension, including renovascular hypertension, and type 2 diabetes in this age group.

### Gender

The ratio of men to women with ESRF is around 1.5:1, perhaps related to the greater susceptibility of men to some forms of renal diseases. It may also be because men often have a faster rate of progression of CKD, possibly due to the effect on the progression of CKD and the associated kidney scarring of the different endocrine milieu in men and women.

**Initiation factors**

*Systemic hypertension*

Both systolic and diastolic hypertension have been associated with a higher incidence of ESRF in the general population.[6]

*Proteinuria*

Studies in the US and Japan have shown that individuals with proteinuria/albuminuria have a much higher risk of developing ESRF.

*Hyperglycaemia*

The poor control of glycaemia in the years following diagnosis of diabetes mellitus is associated with a higher risk of developing diabetic nephropathy (microalbuminuria).

*Dyslipidaemia*

High serum triglyceride levels and, to a lesser extent, cholesterol have been associated with increased risk of development of ESRF.

*Smoking*

A growing body of evidence has linked heavy smoking to the development of diabetic and nondiabetic nephropathies.[7]

*Other possible factors*

It has been suggested that excessive alcohol consumption (>2 units/day) as well as recreational drug intake (opiates) are associated with a higher risk of developing ESRF, while excessive coffee drinking has been associated with raised blood pressure.

**Progression factors**

As with initiation of CKD, systemic hypertension, proteinuria, hyper-cholesterolaemia and smoking are the major risk factors for the progression of established diabetic and nondiabetic nephropathies.[5] In addition, hyperglycaemia is now known to be a significant risk factor for the progression of diabetic nephropathy. More recently, a link has been proposed between hyperuricaemia and CKF progression. In most nephropathies, the combination of more than one risk factor is a key determinant for the progression of the disease. Most significant is the presence of both systemic hypertension and heavy proteinuria.

☐ PATHOPHYSIOLOGY

Considerable advances have been made over the last 25 years in improving our understanding of the mechanisms underlying the progression of CKD and the associated kidney scarring.[8] In particular, research has clarified many of the effects of systemic hypertension and proteinuria on progressive CKD. This review will focus on the effects of hypertension and proteinuria on progressive kidney scarring.

Kidney scarring is characterised by the progressive depletion of resident kidney cells and their replacement by infiltrating inflammatory cells (inflammation) and ultimately by fibrous tissue (fibrosis) – thus explaining the progressive, and often relentless, decline in kidney function of patients with CKD. Both hypertension and proteinuria contribute to such progressive kidney scarring.

### Hypertension and scarring

Research, intensified since the late 1970s, has concluded that it is not solely the elevation of systemic blood pressure that initiates and accelerates kidney scarring but also the transmission to the kidney of systemic hypertension.[9] Animal experiments, based on micropuncture of the nephron, showed convincingly that loss of glomerular autoregulation leads to free transmission of systemic hypertension to the glomeruli, thus initiating glomerular hypertension. It is this combined elevation of systemic and glomerular hypertension that causes glomerulosclerosis. The elevation of glomerular capillary pressure damages the glomerular protective endothelial lining; this is followed by release by endothelial cells of pro-agreggant and pro-inflammatory mediators. These, in turn, attract platelets and inflammatory cells (lymphocytes and monocytes) into the glomerular capillaries and facilitate their adhesion to, and infiltration of, the glomeruli. Through the release of cytokines and growth factors, infiltrating monocytes interact with glomerular mesangial cells, stimulating their proliferation and the synthesis of collagenous extracellular matrix (ECM). Mesangial cells, the equivalent of vascular smooth muscle cells, are activated, then they proliferate and transform in response to stimulation and injury. They acquire a new phenotype reminiscent of their mesenchymal precursors and expressing characteristics of myofibroblasts, with excessive ECM production. The glomerular epithelial cells, podocytes (glomerular equivalent of vascular pericytes), are also affected because increased glomerular capillary pressure and hypertension lead to their stretching, resulting in areas of denuded glomerular basement membrane.[10] This facilitates the flux of macromolecules through the glomerular capillary wall and exacerbates proteinuria. Ultimately, injured endothelial, mesangial and epithelial cells die through apoptosis; they are replaced by fibroblastic cells releasing increasing amounts of ECM until the glomerulus becomes fibrosed and obsolescent, and filtration ceases.

In many respects, the stages of glomerulosclerosis bear marked similarities to those known to take place during the development of atherosclerosis. The endothelial, smooth muscle (mesangial) and pericyte (podocyte) response to injury is identical in vascular and glomerular capillary walls. This is why the term 'glomerulatherosis' was coined in the 1980s to describe these changes, glomerulosclerosis being a form of localised capillary atherosclerosis.

### Proteinuria

Excessive trafficking of circulating macromolecules, including albumin and proteins, through the glomeruli contributes to glomerulosclerosis.[11] These macromolecules are able to overload both mesangial and visceral epithelial (podocyte) cells, which may contribute to the dysfunction and subsequent apoptosis of these cells and their replacement by ECM.

More recently, research interest has focused on the effect of proteinuria on tubulo-interstitial scarring, which is also characterised by the replacement of tubule cells by inflammatory and fibroblastic cells. Ultimately, ECM accumulates and fibrous tissue replaces the normal tubulo-interstitial structure. Experiments have shown that proteinuria leads to the overload and activation of proximal tubular cells, which then release a variety of chemotactic, pro-inflammatory and profibrotic factors.[12] Interstitial inflammation is initiated, the influxing monocytes start to interact with interstitial fibroblasts which stimulates their proliferation and the synthesis of ECM. Increased synthesis and the associated decreased breakdown of ECM are features of progressive kidney scarring. Injured or overloaded tubule cells die through apoptosis and are replaced by the expanding pool of fibroblasts and their release product, ECM. Fibrosis ensues, and renal function ceases.

The progression of kidney scarring is therefore associated with hypertension- and proteinuria-induced kidney cell injury/activation, followed by micro-inflammation and ultimately fibrosis. Lipids and smoking are also likely to be involved. The prevention of CKF will therefore concentrate on the control of these four risk factors in an attempt to slow or even halt the progression of CKD.

## ☐ MANAGEMENT

### Hypertension

There is little doubt that control of systemic hypertension is the most important intervention to slow the progression of CKF.[13,14] In experimental models of CKD, the most effective agents are those able to reduce both systemic and glomerular hypertension, such as ACE inhibitors or angiotensin-receptor blockers (ARBs).[9] This has since been translated to the clinical arena,[15] although some doubt remains as to whether the therapeutic advantage of ACE inhibitors and ARBs in human nephropathies is independent of achieving better blood pressure control. Data in diabetic nephropathy would argue that the most important factor in slowing progression is optimal blood pressure control, more or less regardless of the antihypertensive agent used.[16]

### Proteinuria

Proteinuria is a key risk factor for the progression of CKD,[5,17] so it is imperative to reduce it to attempt to slow the progression. It is anticipated that if the level of proteinuria were less than 1 g/24 hours, the rate of decline of CKF would be considerably slowed down. The effective antihypertensive agents, ACE inhibitors and ARBs, have the added advantage of reducing proteinuria. They are therefore often used as first-line therapy for hypertensive/proteinuric patients with CKD (eg in diabetic and nondiabetic nephropathies).

Close monitoring of kidney function is required with these agents in patients with moderate to severe CKD as they can lead to further functional decline in susceptible individuals. Serum creatinine should be measured within a few days of initiating the treatment. An increment of up to 25% is expected and acceptable, but higher rises in serum creatinine reflect a drop in glomerular filtration rate by more than 25% and should lead to the discontinuation of the ACE inhibitor or ARB. Elderly patients and those with renovascular disease are particularly susceptible to the nephrotoxicity of these drugs and must be treated with caution.[18]

It has been consistently shown that to optimise the antihypertensive as well as the antiproteinuric effects of ACE inhibitors and ARBs, it is often necessary to combine them with dietary salt restriction and/or diuretic therapy.

The antiproteinuric effects of other antihypertensive agents are variable, with good effects reported in diabetic nephropathy with nondihydropyridine calcium antagonists such as diltiazem and verapamil, but little effect with agents such as amlodipine and nifedipine. The antiproteinuric effect of beta-blockers appears negligible. It has been suggested that the differential antiproteinuric and protective effects of antihypertensive agents in CKF, whilst apparent at high blood pressure (140/90 mmHg), may be less obvious when blood pressure is reduced below 125/75 mmHg.[9]

## The hypertension-proteinuria complex

More recent publications, standards and guidelines[4] have focused on the definition of optimal blood pressure control in patients with CKD. The consensus seems to be that in patients with no or minimal proteinuria (<1 g/day) a target blood pressure of 130/80 mmHg or below would slow the progression of CKD, but that a target of 125/75 mmHg or below would be more effective in diabetic nephropathy and in patients with proteinuria in excess of 1 g/day (Fig 1).[4]

These guidelines stress the importance of taking into consideration the level of proteinuria when treating systemic hypertension. The higher the proteinuria, the lower should be the target blood pressure. Treating hypertension alone is insufficient to slow the progression of CKD. It is essential to treat the hypertension-proteinuria complex. It is therefore advisable to reduce proteinuria to less than 1 g/day. Uptitration of ACE inhibitors, ARBs or their combination is justifiable if blood pressure target levels have been achieved but proteinuria remains elevated (Table 2).

## Other risk factors

### Hyperlipidaemia

Control of hyperlipidaemia is recommended in patients with CKD. Experimental evidence suggests that reduction in serum lipids slows the progression of CKD and the associated scarring process. Clinical confirmation is awaited, although a meta-analysis of published data is encouraging.

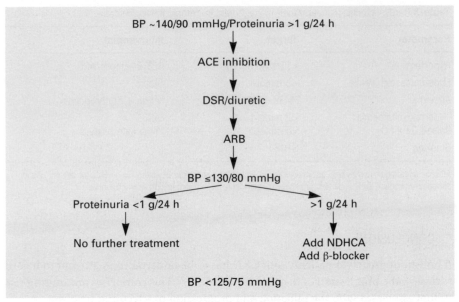

**Fig 1** Algorithm for control of the hypertension-proteinuria complex (ACE = angiotensin-converting enzyme; ARB = angiotensin- receptor blocker; BP = blood pressure; DSR = dietary salt restriction; NDHCA = nondihydropyridine calcium antagonist).

**Table 2** Management of chronic kidney failure: targets and interventions.

| Parameter | Target | Intervention |
|---|---|---|
| Blood pressure:<br>  proteinuria<br>  none or <1 g/day<br>  >1 g/day | <br><br>≤130/80 mmHg<br>≤125/75 mmHg | 1  ACE inhibitor<br>2  DSR/diuretic<br>3  ARB<br>4  NDHCA<br>5  Beta-blocker |
| Proteinuria | <1 g/day | As above |
| Hypercholesterolaemia | <5 mmol/l | Statin |
| Smoking | STOP | |

ACE = angiotensin-converting enzyme; ARB = angiotensin-receptor blocker; DSR = dietary salt restriction; NDHCA = nondihydropyridine calcium antagonist.

## Dyslipidaemia

Cardiovascular diseases are the major cause of morbidity and mortality in patients with CKD. It is therefore important to control dyslipidaemia to reduce the cardiovascular complications, as well as controlling the other conventional cardiovascular risk factors such as hypertension and smoking.[19] Liberal use of statins in patients with CKF both controls hypercholesterolaemia and reduces cardiovascular risk. Patients with CKD also have renal related cardiovascular risk factors such as anaemia and hyperphosphataemia; these warrant attention to avoid long-term cardiovascular complications (Table 3).

**Table 3** Cardiovascular risks and their management in chronic kidney disease.

| Parameter | Target | Intervention |
| --- | --- | --- |
| Hypertension | <130/80 mmHg | ACE inhibitors/ARB |
| Hypercholesterolaemia | <5 mmol/l | Statin |
| Anaemia | Ht 33–36% | iv Iron ± Erythropoietin |
| Hyperphosphataemia | <2 mmol/l | DPR |
| Raised Ca x PO$_4$ | <5 mmol/l$^2$ | Phosphate binders |
| Smoking | STOP | |

ACE = angiotensin-converting enzyme; ARB = angiotensin-receptor blocker; Ca × PO$_4$ = serum calcium × phosphate product; DPR = dietary phosphorus restriction; Ht = haematocrit; iv = intravenous.

## ☐ CONCLUSIONS

A holistic approach to patients with CKD has to be undertaken to attempt to halt or even slow the progression of their kidney failure.[20,21] This comprises minimising risk factors associated with the initiation and progression of CKD, and involves:

☐ strict and aggressive control of blood pressure and proteinuria (the hypertension-proteinuria complex)

☐ correction of metabolic abnormalities such as hyperglycaemia and dyslipidaemia associated with progressive kidney diseases, and

☐ minimising the cardiovascular risks associated with CKD.

Control of blood pressure, lipids, anaemia and hyperphosphataemia are key interventions. Cessation of smoking may benefit progression of CKF and is essential to minimise long-term cardiovascular diseases.

## REFERENCES

1  US Renal Data System. USRDS 2001 Annual data report. National Institutes of Health, National Institute of Diabetes and Digestive and Kidney Diseases, Bethesda, MD. Incidence and prevalence of ESRD. *Am J Kidney Dis* 2001;**38**(Suppl 3):S37–52.

2  Xue JL, Ma JZ, Louis TA, Collins AJ. Forecast of the number of patients with end-stage renal disease in the United States to the year 2010. *J Am Soc Nephrol* 2001;**12**:2753–8.

3  Coresh J, Wei GL, McQuillan G, Brancati FL *et al.* Prevalence of high blood pressure and elevated serum creatinine level in the United States: findings from the third National Health and Nutrition Examination Survey (1988-1994). *Arch Intern Med* 2001;**161**:1207–16.

4  K/DOQI clinical practice guidelines for chronic kidney disease: evaluation, classification, and stratification. Kidney Disease Outcome Quality Initiative. National Kidney Foundation (NKF) Kidney Disease Outcome Quality Initiative (K/DOQI) Advisory Board. *Am J Kidney Dis* 2002;**39**(2 Suppl 2):S1–246.

5  Locatelli F, Del Vecchio L. Natural history and factors affecting the progression of chronic renal failure. In: El Nahas AM, Anderson S, Harris KP (eds). *Mechanisms and management of progressive renal failure*. London: Oxford University Press, 2000:20–79.

6  Klag M, Whelton PK, Randall BL, Neaton JD *et al.* Blood pressure and end-stage renal disease in men. *N Engl J Med* 1996;**334**:13–8.

7   Orth SR. Smoking and the kidney. *J Am Soc Nephrol* 2002;**13**:1663–72.

8   Fogo AB. Progression and potential regression of glomerulosclerosis. *Kidney Int* 2001; **59**:804–19.

9   Dworkin LD, Weir MR. Hypertension in renal parenchymal disease: In: El Nahas AM, Anderson S, Harris KP (eds). *Mechanisms and management of progressive renal failure.* London: Oxford University Press, 2000:173–210.

10  Kriz W, Lemley KV. The role of the podocyte in glomerulosclerosis. Review. *Curr Opin Nephrol Hypertens* 1999;**8**:489–97.

11  Remuzzi G, Bertani T. Pathophysiology of progressive nephropathies. Review. *N Engl J Med* 1998;**339**:1448–56.

12  Jernigan SM, Eddy AA. Experimental insights into the mechanisms of tubulointerstitial scarring. In: El Nahas AM, Anderson S, Harris KP (eds). *Mechanisms and management of progressive renal failure.* London: Oxford University Press, 2000:104–45.

13  Coles GA, El Nahas AM. Clinical interventions in chronic renal failure. In: El Nahas AM, Anderson S, Harris KP (eds). *Mechanisms and management of progressive renal failure.* London: Oxford University Press, 2000:401–23.

14  Adamczak M, Zeir M, Dikow R, Ritz E. Kidney and hypertension. Review. *Kidney Int Suppl* 2002:62–7.

15  Ruggenenti P, Perna A, Remuzzi G, Gruppo Italiano di Studi Epidemiologici in Nefrologia. ACE inhibitors to prevent end-stage renal disease: when to start and why possibly never to stop: a post hoc analysis of the REIN trial results. Ramipril Efficacy in Nephropathy. *J Am Soc Nephrol* 2001;**12**:2832–7.

16  Hovind P, Rossing P, Tarnow L, Smidt UM, Parving HH. Remission and regression in the nephropathy of type 1 diabetes when blood pressure is controlled aggressively. *Kidney Int* 2001;**60**:277–83.

17  Jafar TH, Stark PC, Schmid CH, Landa M *et al.* Proteinuria as a modifiable risk factor for the progression of non-diabetic renal disease. *Kidney Int* 2001;**60**:1131–40.

18  Tamimi N, El Nahas AM. Angiotensin-converting enzyme inhibition: facts and fiction. Review. *Nephron* 2000;**84**:299–304.

19  Levey AS, Beto JA, Coronado BE, Eknoyan G *et al.* Controlling the epidemic of cardiovascular disease in chronic renal disease: what do we know? What do we need to learn? Where do we go from here? National Kidney Foundation Task Force on Cardiovascular Disease. *Am J Kidney Dis* 1998;**32**:853–905.

20  Hebert LA, Wilmer WA, Falkenhain ME, Ladson-Wofford SE *et al.* Renoprotection: one or many therapies? Review. *Kidney Int* 2001;**59**:1211–26.

21  Pereira BJ. Optimization of pre-ESRD care: the key to improved dialysis outcome. *Kidney Int* 2000;**57**:351–65.

# Treatment of glomerulonephritis

Peter Mathieson

## ☐ INTRODUCTION

The term glomerulonephritis (GN) covers a group of conditions in which there is inflammation in the glomerulus, either occurring as a primary glomerular disease or as part of a systemic disorder. In considering the treatment of this group of conditions, this review will:

- ☐ discuss those forms of therapy that may be useful, irrespective of the GN subtype, including antihypertensives, antiproteinuric drugs, cholesterol lowering drugs and anticoagulants

- ☐ describe the hierarchical approach to systemic immunosuppression often applied to GN

- ☐ emphasise that many treatments used in an attempt to influence the natural history of GN are empirical, not evidence-based, and to consider some of the reasons

- ☐ illustrate that rational treatment *is* available for certain rare forms of GN, and that lessons learned from these conditions have been applied to GN more widely, and

- ☐ highlight some areas of optimism for improved therapies in the future.

## ☐ BACKGROUND

### Classification

GN may occur as a primary disorder limited to the kidney, as part of various systemic illnesses (such as lupus or vasculitis) or as a complication of infections, tumours or drugs. In these latter situations GN is classified as 'secondary' and the treatment and prognosis depend entirely upon the underlying cause. For example, most drug-induced GN will improve once the offending agent is withdrawn, and the prognosis of tumour-associated GN generally relates to the prognosis of the tumour itself. For these reasons, in diagnosing GN it is important for the physician to consider carefully whether there is evidence from the history and/or examination of any such underlying cause. Secondary GN will not be considered further in this review except to state that many of the treatments outlined below can be useful in those patients with secondary GN in whom the underlying cause cannot be removed (eg untreatable tumours).

In patients in whom no underlying cause or systemic illness can be identified, the GN is considered 'primary' and will be the focus of this article.

## Diagnosis

Diagnosis of GN, particularly its subdivision into various categories, depends upon clinical features, laboratory data and ultimately histological analysis – and therefore requires renal biopsy in specialist centres. Table 1 lists the accepted histological entities. The terminology is complex and daunting, but its significance is overrated as it merely describes histological pattern recognition. Detailed consideration of clinical presentation, diagnosis and pathogenesis are beyond the scope of this article but have recently been reviewed elsewhere.[1]

**Table 1** Primary glomerulonephritis (GN) subtypes.

- Antiglomerular basement membrane disease
- Idiopathic rapidly progressive GN (renal-limited vasculitis)
- Minimal change nephropathy
- Focal segmental glomerulosclerosis
- Membranous nephropathy
- Immunoglobulin A nephropathy (Berger's disease)
- Mesangiocapillary GN (membranoproliferative GN)

## The case for treatment

GN is associated with considerable morbidity and mortality. Symptoms can be severe and disabling, especially when there is heavy proteinuria as in the nephrotic syndrome.[2] It is often associated with hypertension and/or hyperlipidaemia with their attendant cardiovascular risk. GN is an important cause of end-stage renal failure which is associated with major morbidity and mortality and consumes a disproportionate amount of health resources. Therefore, the case for treating GN is strong. The aims of treatment are:

☐ symptom relief

☐ modification of cardiovascular risk, and

☐ reduction of rate of progressive loss of excretory renal function.

## ☐ TREATMENT OF GLOMERULONEPHRITIS

### General treatments, irrespective of subtype

Symptomatic treatments are often effective, for example:

☐ oedema can be reduced by salt restriction and diuretics

☐ hypercholesterolaemia is common and should be treated with a statin if dietary measures alone are ineffective

☐   because of a predisposition to infection, there should be a low threshold for systemic antibiotics

☐   there is a prothrombotic state, so disproportionate limb swelling, breathlessness, chest pain or haemoptysis should lead to the suspicion of thromboembolism and the need for systemic anticoagulation (eg warfarin).

In patients with nephrotic syndrome, there is a particular risk of renal vein thrombosis (RVT). This may be silent or cause flank pain, macroscopic haematuria or deterioration in excretory renal function as well as pulmonary embolism. Risk/benefit analyses favour prophylactic anticoagulation if the serum albumin is below 20 g/l, especially in patients with membranous nephropathy in whom the risk of RVT is particularly high.

GN is frequently associated with hypertension, and it is well established that good blood pressure control improves the prognosis. In recent years, interest has focused on drugs blocking the renin-angiotensin cascade and there is accumulating evidence that drugs such as angiotensin-converting enzyme (ACE) inhibitors may have beneficial effects over and above their efficacy as antihypertensive agents.[3] ACE inhibitors, and probably also angiotensin-receptor antagonists, can markedly reduce proteinuria. This can have useful symptomatic benefit in patients with severe nephrotic syndrome and may also directly contribute to improving the prognosis.

Reduction of proteinuria can also be achieved using non-steroidal anti-inflammatory drugs, although usually at the expense of a fall in glomerular filtration rate. If nephrotic syndrome is life-threatening, drastic measures to reduce proteinuria can include renal embolisation or even bilateral nephrectomy. Renal infarction invariably leads to acute renal failure, and should not be undertaken unless (as with bilateral nephrectomy) patient and physician are prepared to sacrifice excretory renal function. There are anecdotal reports of partial recovery of renal function without recurrence of severe nephrotic syndrome in patients treated by bilateral renal embolisation.

Before taking such drastic measures and committing the patient to the need for renal replacement therapy, it is important to remember that many types of GN can recur in renal transplants.

## The hierarchical approach to systemic immunosuppression

If symptomatic treatments are ineffective and/or deemed insufficient, for example in severe nephrotic syndrome or when excretory renal function shows progressive deterioration, intervention with more aggressive forms of therapy will be required. In the belief that immunological mechanisms underlie most forms of GN, this will usually take the form of systemic immunosuppression. It is essential to balance the potential toxicities of such therapy against the dangers posed by GN, and to ensure that the consequences of the treatment are not worse than the condition. This has led to the evolution of a hierarchical approach to the treatment of GN, similar to that used in other inflammatory disorders (eg rheumatoid arthritis). The choice of agents is influenced by clinical severity/urgency, glomerular morphology and (sometimes) by evidence although, as outlined below, there are few robust clinical trials on which to base treatment choices.

First-line therapy is usually with corticosteroids. Second-line agents, often given with corticosteroids, include calcineurin antagonists (cyclosporin and tacrolimus), alkylating agents (usually cyclophosphamide or chlorambucil) and antimetabolites (eg methotrexate, azathioprine). If these fail, various experimental or salvage therapies may be tried, including plasma exchange, novel immunosuppressive agents such as mycophenolate mofetil and sirolimus, and monoclonal antibodies directed against individual cell types or cytokines.

### The lack of evidence base for treatment

The literature on the treatment of the various GN subtypes has recently been extensively reviewed in an attempt to produce evidence-based guidelines.[4] Unfortunately, this review reported that there is 'limited evidence found on which to develop recommendations', 'clear and precise therapeutic approaches ... (are) ... often lacking', studies showed 'absence of uniformity' and interpretations were 'prone to serious errors'. [4]

There are few examples in GN of robust evidence derived from large, prospective, randomised controlled trials. Possible reasons include:

☐   the relative rarity of the condition

☐   heterogeneity of clinical conditions and therapeutic approaches, and

☐   firmly-held opinions amongst nephrologists which may limit enthusiasm for randomisation.

However, empirical therapy has proved effective in some forms of GN. This, together with cautious interpretation of the literature, allowing for its limitations, enable some firm recommendations to be made. These will be outlined in the next section.

### *Antiglomerular basement membrane disease*

Truly rational therapy (ie based on an understanding of pathogenesis) is available for the rare form of GN associated with antibodies to glomerular basement membrane (GBM), usually referred to as antiGBM disease or Goodpasture's disease. (This should be distinguished from Goodpasture's *syndrome* which is the pulmonary-renal syndrome of alveolar haemorrhage and necrotising GN. Although antiGBM disease is one cause of Goodpasture's syndrome, it is not numerically the most important since systemic vasculitis accounts for most patients presenting with the pulmonary-renal syndrome.)

In antiGBM disease, a pathogenic immunoglobulin G (IgG) autoantibody binds to the GBM and incites marked local inflammation. Typically, this presents as rapidly progressive GN (RPGN) where renal function can be lost rapidly over days or weeks. The aim of therapy is to:

☐ remove preformed antibody from the circulation by plasma exchange

☐ suppress inflammation due to deposited antibody with high-dose corticosteroids

☐ limit further autoantibody synthesis with cyclophosphamide.

This treatment approach is undoubtedly effective at altering the natural history of the condition, but the main determinant of outcome is the extent of tissue damage at diagnosis. Early diagnosis and aggressive treatment are essential if renal function is to be preserved.

*Systemic vasculitis*

A treatment approach similar to that used in antiGBM disease was adopted some years ago for another aggressive form of GN associated with small-vessel systemic vasculitis (SSV). Originally empirical, the treatment was given a quasi-rational basis with the description of autoantibodies (antineutrophil cytoplasm antibodies (ANCA)) in patients with SSV. These antibodies are not of proven pathogenic potential but provide a helpful diagnostic test and can be used in monitoring response to treatment.[5] The entity previously known as idiopathic RPGN is usually also associated with ANCA and is now regarded as a renal-limited vasculitis. Steroids and cyclophosphamide are effective in ANCA-associated GN if started early, but until recently the role of additional plasma exchange was more controversial. A series of multinational clinical trials in Europe in recent years examined the treatment of SSV.[6] The most recent of these provided an evidence base for plasma exchange, showing that patients with advanced renal impairment were more likely to recover renal function if they received plasma exchange.[7]

*Minimal change nephropathy*

Most patients with minimal change nephropathy (MCN) usually respond to corticosteroids, although relapse is common when the steroid dose is reduced and many patients will remain steroid-dependent. In the paediatric literature this condition is known as steroid-sensitive nephrotic syndrome; it accounts for most of the children presenting with nephrotic syndrome, so steroid therapy will often be initiated without a renal biopsy to prove the diagnosis. A Cochrane review of corticosteroid therapy for nephrotic syndrome in children provides advice on choice of agent, duration of therapy etc.[8] For adults with MCN, a suggested treatment schedule is shown in Fig 1.

*Second-line treatment.*   Second-line agents are used if:

☐ initial steroid treatment fails

☐ there are frequent relapses and/or relapse at a high dose of steroid, or

☐ there is steroid-dependency at an unacceptably high maintenance dose.

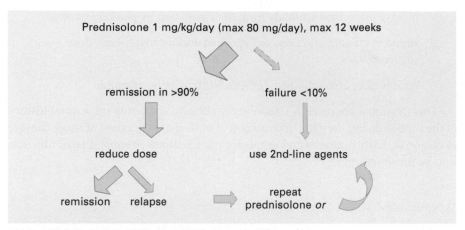

**Fig 1** Treatment schedule for minimal change nephropathy.

Cyclophosphamide 1.5–2 mg/kg/day for 8–12 weeks is successful in some cases. Blood counts must be monitored frequently and the dose reduced or stopped if leucopenia develops. Cyclosporin is effective in some steroid-resistant or steroid-dependent patients at a dose of 3–5 mg/kg/day, adjusted according to drug blood levels. An alternative is tacrolimus, starting at 0.15 mg/kg/day and similarly adjusted according to blood levels. Unfortunately, patients treated with cyclosporin and tacrolimus tend to relapse when these agents are stopped. The potential nephrotoxicity of these drugs makes them unattractive agents for the long-term treatment of a form of renal disease which does not usually pose a threat to long-term kidney function. Levamisole (2.5 mg/kg on alternate days in children and (this author's practice) 1.25 mg/kg/day in adults) is useful in maintenance of remission and allows some patients to reduce steroid maintenance doses. There are some encouraging recent reports of success with mycophenolate mofetil.

### Focal segmental glomerulosclerosis

The treatment approach in focal segmental glomerulosclerosis (FSGS) is similar to that in MCN but the outcomes are poorer and in a significant proportion of patients there is a risk of deterioration of excretory renal function. A suggested protocol is shown in Fig 2. In all patients receiving high-dose corticosteroids, routine prescription of gastric protection with a proton pump inhibitor and bone prophylaxis with an oral biphosphonate is common practice.

### Membranous nephropathy

The subtype of GN in which it is most important to exclude an underlying cause (as discussed above) is membranous nephropathy since identical clinical and histological features can occur as a direct complication of drug therapy or malignancy. In nephrotic syndrome due to primary membranous GN, there is about a 25% chance of spontaneous remission. Many nephrologists would therefore

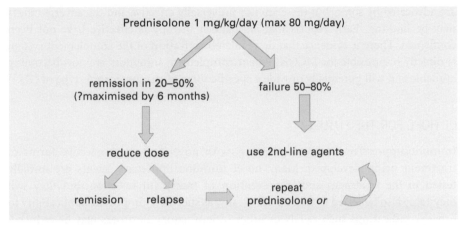

**Fig 2** Suggested treatment protocol for nephrotic focal segmental glomerulosclerosis.

initially use symptomatic treatments alone, possibly including warfarin as outlined earlier, and reserve immunosuppressive therapy for the subset of patients (25–30% in most series) in whom excretory renal function begins to decline. For such patients, corticosteroids alone are ineffective and various combinations of second-line agents have been tested. Clinical trials in Italy have supported using a combination of corticosteroids and chlorambucil, given in a complex schedule of alternating monthly cycles for a total of six months.[9] A Canadian group has reported that treatment with cyclosporin for a year can have sustained benefits in many patients.[10] In the UK, a current prospective trial is comparing these two treatment approaches with supportive therapy alone.[11]

### Immunoglobulin A nephropathy (Berger's disease)

The natural history of IgA nephropathy is also variable and many patients have an excellent long-term prognosis without specific therapy. Heavy proteinuria and/or declining excretory renal function are the most reliable adverse prognostic indicators. Success has been reported in high-risk patients with high-dose corticosteroids.[12] A more innocuous treatment is with fish oils, but there is conflicting literature on its effectiveness.

There is accumulating evidence that IgA nephropathy is due to a primary abnormality of glycosylation of the IgA molecule rather than being an autoimmune disease. It is hoped that in the future a more selective method of tackling the abnormal IgA biosynthesis will be developed to replace non-specific immunosuppressive or anti-inflammatory treatments.[13]

### Mesangiocapillary glomerulonephritis

There are no proven treatments for mesangiocapillary glomerulonephritis (MCGN) (also known as membranoproliferative GN). High-dose alternate-day corticosteroids are advocated by some, but these are not universally effective and the adverse effects may be limiting. Early reports that antiplatelet therapy is effective have not been confirmed. There is evidence that dysregulated activation of the complement system is directly responsible for MCGN. Potent complement inhibitors are now becoming available and will potentially provide a specific form of therapy for this type of GN.[14]

## □ HOPE FOR THE FUTURE?

Immunosuppressive therapy is evolving, with novel and more selective forms of treatment being developed. Many novel immunosuppressive agents are initially tested in the treatment and/or prevention of transplant rejection, but they will inevitably also be tested in GN. Paradoxically, as specificity improves, applicability to broader indications such as GN or other inflammatory disorders may be reduced. Improved understanding of the pathogenesis of GN is essential if more specific forms of therapy are to be developed. Examples include:

□ the realisation that primary abnormalities of IgA underlie IgA nephropathy

□ the dissection of the abnormalities of complement regulation that underlie various forms of MCGN

□ the increasing appreciation in recent years of the key role of the glomerular epithelial cell or podocyte in MCN and probably also in FSGS.[15] Corticosteroids have direct effects on podocytes and may exert some or all of their therapeutic effects in these diseases on the podocyte rather than on the immune system.

Detailed dissection of the pathogenesis of GN and modes of action of existing and novel therapies holds considerable promise for the development of new treatments. However, adequate testing of treatments for GN will depend on large-scale clinical trials. Nephrologists must overcome any reluctance to participate in such trials if the current lack of evidence base is to be tackled.

## □ CONCLUSIONS

In many patients with GN, supportive treatments aimed at oedema, hypertension, hyperlipidaemia and the prothrombotic state can provide symptomatic relief and/or improvement in the long-term prognosis. Therapy aimed at modifying the underlying GN itself is not currently usually evidence-based, although many forms of treatment are effective when used in an empirical and hierarchical manner. Real improvements in future will depend in equal measure upon three factors:

1   Improved understanding of pathogenetic mechanisms.

2   Development of novel forms of specific therapies.

3   Formal testing of treatment approaches in rigorous large-scale prospective clinical trials.

# REFERENCES

1   Macanovic M, Mathieson PW. Glomerulonephritis. In: Savage CO, Gaskin G (eds). *Renal disorders. Medicine* 2003;**31**:36–42.

2   Bernard D. Extrarenal complications of the nephrotic syndrome. *Kidney Int* 1988;**33**: 1184–202.

3   Ruggenenti P, Perna A, Gherardi G, Gaspari F *et al.* Renal function and requirement for dialysis in chronic nephropathy patients on long-term ramipril. Gruppo Italiano di Studi Epidemiologici in Nefrologia (GISEN). Ramipril Efficacy in Nephropathy. *Lancet* 1998;**352**: 1252–6.

4   Evidence-based guidelines for the management of glomerulonephritis. *Kidney Int* 1999; **55**(Suppl 70):S1–S62.

5   Kamesh L, Harper L, Savage CO. ANCA-positive vasculitis. Review. *J Am Soc Nephrol* 2002;**13**: 1953–60.

6   http://www.vasculitis.org.uk

7   Gaskin G, Jayne DR. Adjunctive plasma exchange is superior to methylprednisolone in acute renal failure due to ANCA-associated glomerulonephritis. *J Am Soc Nephrol* 2002;**13**:2A.

8   Hodson EM, Knight JF, Willis NS, Craig JC. Corticosteroid therapy for nephrotic syndrome in children (Cochrane Review). In: *The Cochrane Library,* Issue 2, 2003. Oxford: Update Software. http://www.cochrane.org/cochrane/revabstr/ab001533.htm

9   Ponticelli C, Zucchelli P, Passerini P, Cesana B *et al.* A 10-year follow-up of a randomized study with methylprednisolone and chlorambucil in membranous nephropathy. *Kidney Int* 1995; **48**:1600–4.

10   Cattran DC, Greenwood C, Ritchie S, Bernstein K *et al.* A controlled trial of cyclosporine in patients with progressive membranous nephropathy. Canadian Glomerulonephritis Study Group. *Kidney Int* 1995;**47**:1130–5.

11   Mathieson PW. Membranous nephropathy. *Br J Renal Med* 2002;**7**:17–20.

12   Pozzi C, Bolasco PG, Fogazzi GB, Andrulli S *et al.* Corticosteroids in IgA nephropathy: a randomised controlled trial. *Lancet* 1999;**353**:883–7.

13   Feehally J, Allen AC. Structural features of IgA molecules which contribute to IgA nephropathy. Review. *J Nephrol* 1999;**12**:59–65.

14   Mathieson PW. Is complement a target for therapy in renal disease? Review. *Kidney Int* 1998;**54**:1429–36.

15   Mathieson PW. Role of the podocyte in glomerular injury. *Hong Kong J Nephrol* 2001;**3**:51–6.

# Selection of dialysis modality

Edwina Brown

## ☐ INTRODUCTION

The aim of renal replacement therapy (RRT) is not simply correction of blood abnormalities and maintenance of fluid balance. Patients can live on RRT for decades so the aim is for them to live as normal a life as possible. It is therefore important that they use a mode of RRT that they tolerate well and will comply with, that provides physical well-being, and allows social and employment rehabilitation.

## ☐ TREATMENT MODALITIES

The many current treatment modalities for end-stage renal disease (ESRD) are listed in Table 1.

**Table 1** Treatment modalities for end-stage renal disease.

| Dialysis modality | |
|---|---|
| Haemodialysis | • Centre<br>• Satellite<br>• Home |
| Peritoneal dialysis | • Continuous ambulatory<br>• Automated |
| Transplantation | • Cadaver<br>• Living donor (related or unrelated) |
| Conservative management | • Best supportive care |

There has been no randomised study (and never will be), but evidence from various national registries shows that patient survival is the same whether patients start on haemodialysis (HD) or peritoneal dialysis (PD).[1] Selection of dialysis modality for an individual patient should be based on medical indications and which mode will provide optimal quality of life (QoL) for that patient. Selection for transplantation will not be discussed in this chapter. Transplantation is not an option for the increasing number of elderly patients starting on dialysis, and patients who are suitable will usually spend some time on dialysis before receiving their transplant. Finally, not all patients want dialysis, and some have too many comorbidities to cope with dialysis; the option of conservative management, or best supportive care, should therefore also be considered.

For patients who can use any modality, the choice of HD or PD will depend on individual patient preference, nephrologist bias and local resources. This is reflected in the percentage of use of different modalities in different countries (eg approximately 20% of patients start PD in USA, 40% in UK and 90% in Hong Kong), and even in different hospitals (35% new patients start PD in one London hospital compared with 10% in another three miles away).

## ☐ MEDICAL INDICATIONS FOR DIALYSIS MODALITY

Patients starting on dialysis will usually have some residual renal function, a virgin peritoneal cavity (unless they have had prior abdominal surgery) and untouched arm blood vessels for fistula formation (though some will have had multiple forearm venous access and/or atherosclerotic arteries). This of course changes during a patient's time on dialysis, which can last for over 20 years. The medical indications for HD and PD, shown in Table 2, will vary during life on dialysis. Thus, patients starting on PD may not get enough dialysis when they have lost all their residual renal function. Similarly, though less common, patients on HD may have to switch to PD if they no longer have any vascular access.

**Table 2** Medical indications for dialysis modality.

|  | Haemodialysis | Peritoneal dialysis |
|---|---|---|
| **Indications** | • Obese/large patient<br>• Unable to do PD<br>• Unable to provide adequate dialysis or ultrafiltration on PD | • No vascular access<br>• Poor cardiac function with hypotension |
| **Contraindications** | • Difficult or no vascular access<br>• Poor cardiac function | • Previous pelvic intraperitoneal surgery<br>• Presence of colostomy, ileostomy, ileal conduit<br>• Recurrent hernias<br>• Unable to learn technique unless carer available |

PD = peritoneal dialysis.

## ☐ WHAT DETERMINES SURVIVAL ON DIALYSIS?

Survival on dialysis is not dependent on modality but is determined by age and comorbidity. Figure 1 shows similar survival on HD and PD using data from the Canadian renal registry corrected for age and comorbidity.[1] This is true even for the elderly; in the North Thames Dialysis Study of patients starting dialysis over 70 years old, survival at one year was 77% for HD and 76% for PD.[2] In a study of 292 patients starting dialysis over four years at Lister Hospital, Stevenage, Chandna *et al*[3] showed that survival on dialysis is determined primarily by age, comorbidity and functional status, as measured by the Karnofsky performance score (Fig 2).

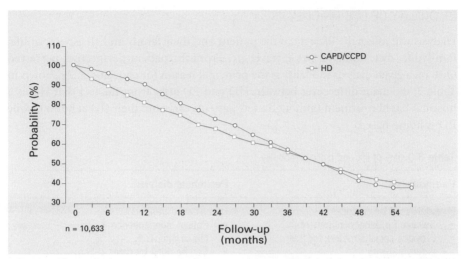

**Fig 1** Comparison of peritoneal dialysis and haemodialysis (HD) mortality (Canadian registry data 1994–97) (CAPD = continuous ambulatory peritoneal dialysis; CCPD = continuous cyclical peritoneal dialysis).[1]

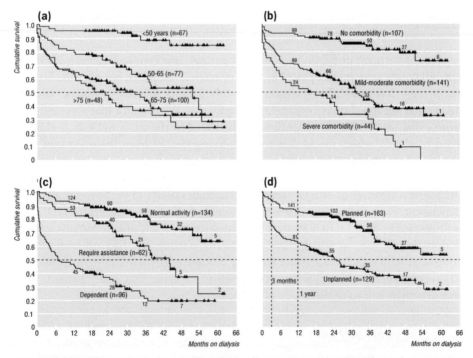

**Fig 2** Kaplan-Meier survival curves: **(a)** effect of age on survival; **(b)** effect of comorbidity (comorbidity severity score: 1–4, mild-moderate comorbidity; 5–8, severe comorbidity); **(c)** survival in three groups defined by Karnofsky performance scale; **(d)** difference in survival between planned and unplanned presentation for dialysis. Each step represents one death, and each triangle denotes survivor at latest follow-up. Numbers above curves are patients remaining in analysis at each time point.[3]

## □ QUALITY OF LIFE ON DIALYSIS

Dialysis will affect the lifestyle of the patient and their family and all aspects of life: family life, diet, holidays, work, travel etc. From the patient perspective, perceived QoL on a given dialysis modality is the principal reason for choosing it. As shown in Table 3, the main differences between HD and PD arise from the fact that HD is a hospital-based treatment (although a few patients carry out their HD at home) while PD is home-based.

**Table 3** Quality of life and dialysis modality.

| Haemodialysis | Peritoneal dialysis |
| --- | --- |
| Hospital-based treatment:<br>• Suitable for dependent patients<br>• Provides social structure for frail elderly patients<br>• Transport can be a problem<br>• Interferes with work | Home-based treatment:<br>• Patient independence<br>• Fits in with work<br>• Can be done by carer at home<br>• Fewer visits to hospital |
| Increased hospitalisation for vascular access problems | |
| Difficult to travel for holiday or work | Easier to travel and go on holiday |

One of the main problems with HD is the travel time involved. Historically in the UK, HD units were mostly placed in tertiary referral hospitals, but over the last few years there has been an expansion of satellite units in local hospitals, thereby decreasing the travel time for patients. Despite this, the distance that a patient lives from a dialysis unit influences choice, as illustrated by the study of Little *et al* in the West Midlands[4] which found that patients living further from the main unit were more likely to choose PD.

The main limitation of PD is that the treatment has to be carried out either by the patients themselves or by a carer (some families prefer to perform the PD for a dependent relative rather than have thrice weekly visits to the hospital for HD). This is illustrated by the CHOICE study, a large multicentre study of new patients starting dialysis in the US, in which 52% of patients starting PD had no comorbidity compared with only 30% starting HD (Fig 3).[5] Strikingly, 22% of patients starting PD were graded as having severe comorbidity, implying that many patients with comorbidities still want this mode of dialysis.

## □ ELDERLY ON DIALYSIS

Patients starting on dialysis are becoming older. As shown in the study by Little *et al* (Fig 4),[4] most patients are over 60 years old when they start on dialysis. The North Thames Dialysis Study, a prospective study specifically examining outcomes and QoL in the over-70s, found that the outcomes on HD and PD were similar and depended on age and the number of comorbidities.[6] Overall annual mortality rate

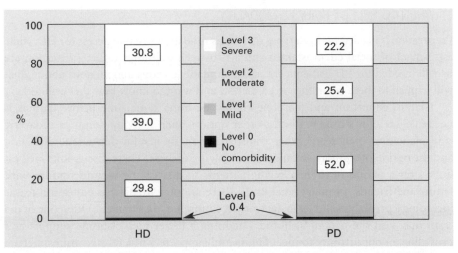

**Fig 3** Influence of comorbidity on selection of dialysis modality: comparison between patients starting on peritoneal dialysis (PD) and haemodialysis (HD).[5]

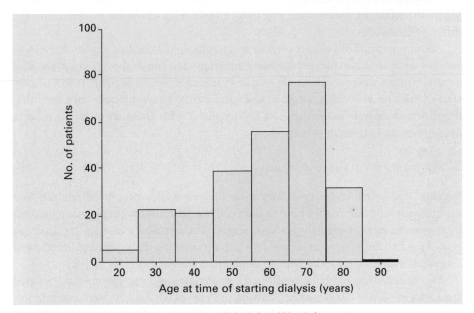

**Fig 4** Age distribution of patients starting on dialysis in a UK unit.[4]

was 25%, comparing favourably with younger patients. A third of patients were not hospitalised over a 12-month period. QoL was measured by Short Form-36 (SF-36): although physical scores were lower than in elderly comparison groups, mental scores were similar.

There is therefore no evidence that dialysis should be restricted amongst the elderly. As survival is independent of modality in the elderly, as in other age groups,[2] selection depends on medical and QoL issues.

## ☐ WHEN TO SELECT DIALYSIS MODALITY

Preparation is needed for both types of dialysis modality: vascular access for HD, while assessment of social circumstances and a two-week wait after catheter insertion are usually needed for PD. Patients are understandably curious and anxious about what will happen to them when they need dialysis and want to know how they will feel.

Dialysis education and planning should be done some time before dialysis is needed. This allows time to discuss other options such as living donor or cadaveric transplantation, pancreatic-renal transplantation in insulin-dependent diabetics, and the option of supportive care and not having dialysis. These discussions are best done over a period of time, allowing patients to discuss the various options with family and friends. In many renal units, there are now predialysis education teams including a predialysis nurse, social worker, counsellor, dietitian etc. Often one of the team may visit the patient at home, obtaining a better idea of home support and providing an opportunity to meet family and supporters in a relaxed atmosphere.

Another method of education is to organise group sessions, with the added advantage of patients meeting others with similar problems and able to give each other mutual support. It also provides an opportunity for patients already on dialysis to talk to predialysis patients and give them a better idea of what is involved with the different modalities.

About one-third of patients present to a nephrologist needing urgent dialysis, so are not able to have the predialysis education described above. They are also generally much sicker and less able to take in information. Such patients will usually start directly on HD using temporary venous access. However, once they are fitter, the different dialysis modalities can be discussed with them in order to make a decision about long-term management.

## ☐ IMPORTANCE OF EARLY REFERRAL

Patients cope better and survive longer on dialysis if they have been referred to a nephrologist long before they have to start dialysis. In addition, predialysis education is an essential part of predialysis management. The retrospective study by Chandna et al[3] found an 86% one-year survival for patients starting dialysis as a planned event compared with 63% for those with an unplanned presentation (Fig 5).

This observation has been confirmed by a recent large study from the US Renal Data System of over 2,000 patients starting dialysis, of whom 32% were late referrals (less than four months before needing dialysis).[7] They had 65%, 57% and 22% higher mortality risks than early referral patients at six months, one year and two years, respectively. Other differences found for late referral patients were that they were less likely to be on erythropoietin, to have had an angiotensin-converting enzyme inhibitor predialysis or to have had vascular access before starting dialysis. They had also seen a dietitian less frequently and had more abnormal blood results and less good blood pressure control. As a result, more were anaemic, had a low plasma albumin and needed insertion of a central venous dialysis catheter to start HD.

The two major complications of central venous catheters are infection and venous occlusion. Septicaemia from central line infections can have life-threatening

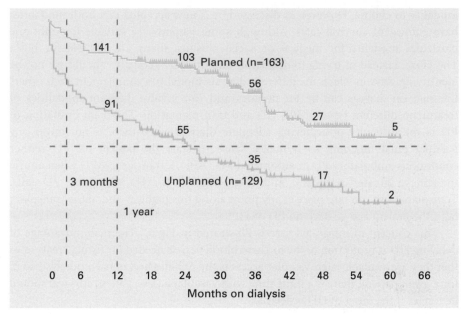

**Fig 5** Effect of planned and unplanned presentation to nephrologist on survival in dialysis.[3]

complications such as endocarditis and discitis with epidural abscesses. Central venous occlusion can also exclude future vascular access formation in that arm.

This and other studies have shown that a smaller proportion of late referral patients eventually use PD. Once patients have been started on HD as an emergency, they are less likely to change modality. The costs of PD are less than HD, so this has major resource implications. The advantages of early referral to a nephrologist are summarised in Table 4.

**Table 4** Advantages of early referral to a nephrologist.

---

- Mortality and morbidity increase when patient referred to renal unit <3 months before starting dialysis
- Neck lines usually used for urgent dialysis, with increased infection risk
- Patients requiring urgent dialysis are often sicker, with more complications or comorbidities
- If there is less time for patient education, there is increased risk of noncompliance and poor psychosocial adjustment
- Less likely that patient will end on PD, with resource implications

---

PD = peritoneal dialysis.

## ☐ CONCEPT OF INTEGRATED CARE

Much of the dialysis literature is based on trying to prove that PD or HD is a better modality, and the aim of predialysis education is to enable patients to decide which modality to choose. However, as discussed, it is now accepted that both modalities have equivalent survival rates. Although some patients are suitable for only one particular modality for medical or social reasons, many are suitable for both. Therefore, instead of trying to decide on one or other modality, should we not be identifying ways in which the different dialysis modalities complement each other? Lifespan on dialysis can be for decades and can involve different modalities of treatment: different types of PD, HD and transplantation. The main limitation of PD is the difficulty of achieving adequate dialysis when there is no longer any residual renal function, so it makes sense to start the patient on PD (either continuous ambulatory PD or automated PD (APD)), transfer to APD when anuric to achieve greater adequacy, and then transfer to HD when the PD fails. Transplantation can take place at any point along this pathway and, if the transplant fails, the patient can go back on PD or HD.

This concept of integrated care is illustrated in Fig 6.[8] The main advantage of delaying HD is protection of the forearm blood vessels needed for fistula creation so that they are available later. Vascular access is the Achilles heel of haemodialysis so if, for a given patient, there is a finite time with vascular access, patient survival should be longer if the onset of HD is delayed.

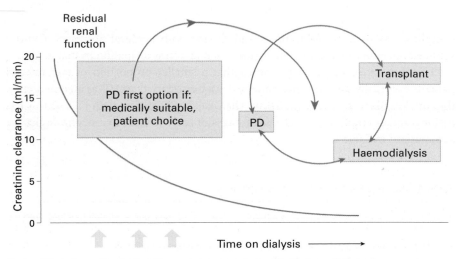

**Fig 6** Integrated end-stage renal disease care. Use of different modalities during lifetime with renal failure (PD = peritoneal dialysis).[8]

### Case history illustrating advantages of integrated care

A 35-year-old man with polycystic kidneys started HD in 1988 using a Cimino fistula in his left arm. One year later, he had a successful renal transplant. Ten years later he developed chronic rejection and renal function deteriorated. He was reluctant to contemplate PD at this stage and wanted to restart dialysis using HD.

Unfortunately, three attempts at creating vascular access failed and in 1999 he started APD as he had no other option. He found that he liked the independence of PD and refused further attempts at vascular access formation. In 2002, he became increasingly tired and lost weight due to underdialysis, having now lost all residual renal function from his transplant kidney. Changes were made to his PD regimen to improve dialysis adequacy and a further attempt at vascular access (a thigh graft) was attempted but again failed. Currently, he continues on PD, better dialysed, feeling better, and hoping for another renal transplant.

*Comment*

PD was not as successful in 1988 as it is now, so most patients started on HD. This patient's successful fistula clotted shortly after transplantation (a common occurrence). PD after transplantation utilises the residual renal function that can persist for some time even when immunosuppression (as in this case) is withdrawn. However, now that this residual renal function has been lost, he is getting barely enough dialysis from PD, but is unable to be established back on HD as all attempts at creating further vascular access have failed. His life expectancy is therefore severely shortened, unless he can be successfully transplanted.

## □ CONSERVATIVE MANAGEMENT

With the increasing age, comorbidity and number of patients with ESRD, there is debate within the renal community about the suitability of all patients being offered dialysis.[9,10] Not all patients want dialysis or indeed will benefit from this procedure. Dialysis is not a panacea and will not ameliorate the many other comorbid conditions that are found in the increasingly elderly population of patients presenting with ESRD. This is another advantage of early referral – it gives an opportunity to discuss the options for such patients. Some may decide on a trial of dialysis (which will usually be HD in these circumstances), but others will decide that dialysis is not for them. This decision, of course, belongs to the patient, if mentally competent, not to the family or doctor.

Patients who are not mentally competent are more difficult to manage. This situation is also easier if the patient is referred early because it is difficult to know how much confusion will be reversible if a patient is severely uraemic. If a patient is mentally incompetent, for whatever reason (psychiatric, dementia, learning problems), the decision about whether dialysis is appropriate has to be made carefully and will depend on whether the patient will be able to cope with the rigours of dialysis. Although the doctor looking after the patient ultimately makes this decision, it has to be made with the help of the multidisciplinary team.

The decision not to dialyse does not mean no care. The patient should be offered supportive care for their renal disease, including treatment of anaemia with erythropoietin which can greatly improve their QoL. Symptoms due to fluid overload can be treated with diuretics (often in large dosages) and appropriate palliative care should be available at the end of life.

## REFERENCES

1   Fenton SS, Schaubel DE, Desmeules M, Morrison HI *et al.* Hemodialysis versus peritoneal dialysis: a comparison of adjusted mortality rates. *Am J Kidney Dis* 1997;30:334–42.

2   Harris SA, Lamping DL, Brown EA, Constantinovici N. Clinical outcomes and quality of life in elderly patients on peritoneal dialysis versus hemodialysis. *Perit Dial Int* 2002;22:463–70.

3   Chandna SM, Schulz J, Lawrence C, Greenwood RN, Farrington K. Is there a rationale for rationing chronic dialysis? A hospital based cohort study of factors affecting survival and morbidity. *BMJ* 1999;318:217–23.

4   Little J, Irwin A, Marshall T, Rayner H, Smith S. Predicting a patient's choice of dialysis modality: experience in a United Kingdom renal department. *Am J Kidney Dis* 2001;37:981–6.

5   Miskulin DC, Meyer KB, Athienites NV, Martin AA *et al.* Comorbidity and other factors associated with modality selection in incident dialysis patients: the CHOICE study. Choices for Healthy Outcomes in Caring for End-Stage Renal Disease. *Am J Kidney Dis* 2002;39:324–6.

6   Lamping DL, Constantinovici N, Roderick P, Normand C *et al.* Clinical outcomes, quality of life, and costs in the North Thames Dialysis Study of elderly people on dialysis: a prospective cohort study. *Lancet* 2000;356:1543–50.

7   Stack AG. Impact of timing of nephrology referral and pre-ESRD care on mortality risk among new ESRD patients in the United States. *Am J Kidney Dis* 2003;41:310–8.

8   Gokal R. Taking peritoneal dialysis beyond the year 2000. *Perit Dial Int* 1999;19(Suppl 3): S35–42.

9   Moss AH. Controversies in nephrology: too many patients who are too sick to benefit start chronic dialysis. Nephrologists need to learn to 'just say no'. *Am J Kidney Dis* 2003;41:723–7.

10  Levinsky NG. Controversies in nephrology: too many patients who are too sick to benefit start chronic dialysis. Nephrologists need to learn to 'just say no'. Con. *Am J Kidney Dis* 2003; 41:728–32.

# ☐ RENAL SELF ASSESSMENT QUESTIONS

**Chronic kidney failure: advances in understanding and treatment**

1   The following are risk factors for renal disease progression:
   (a)   Smoking
   (b)   Gout
   (c)   Hypercholesterolaemia
   (d)   Proteinuria
   (e)   Systemic hypertension

2   In renal scarring:
   (a)   There is associated loss of glomerular autoregulation
   (b)   Mesangial cells proliferate and transform into fibroblasts
   (c)   Podocytes are unaffected
   (d)   A major mechanism is proteinuria, leading to activation of distal tubular cells
   (e)   Hypertension potentiates the action of proteinuria

3   In managing hypertension:
   (a)   Blood pressure below 140/90 mmHg offers sufficient protection for both diabetic and nondiabetic nephropathies
   (b)   There is clear evidence that angiotensin-converting enzyme (ACE) inhibitors offer renoprotective actions independent of blood pressure control
   (c)   Diuretics potentiate antihypertensive action of ACE inhibitors
   (d)   Salt restriction is of no benefit
   (e)   Dihydropyridine calcium-channel blockers have effective antiproteinuric effects

4   Dyslipidaemia in chronic kidney disease (CKD) patients:
   (a)   Is characterised by low triglyceride levels
   (b)   Is best treated by fibrates
   (c)   May accelerate progression of kidney disease
   (d)   Is a risk for cardiovascular morbidity and mortality
   (e)   Should be treated with a target cholesterol of less than 6.5 mmol/l

5   In the approach to treating patients with CKD:
   (a)   Treatment of hyperphosphataemia is important
   (b)   Anaemia of renal disease can be treated effectively by oral iron supplementation
   (c)   Low dietary protein intake (<40 g/kg/day) is of proven benefit in delaying renal disease progression
   (d)   A target proteinuria of below 1 g/day is desirable
   (e)   ACE inhibitors are beneficial but may require care in the elderly

**Treatment of glomerulonephritis**

1   Glomerulonephritis (GN):
(a)   Describes inflammation in the interstitial compartment of the kidney
(b)   Typically causes albuminuria
(c)   Is numerically the most important cause of macroscopic haematuria
(d)   May be a primary renal disorder or part of a systemic illness
(e)   Treatment is firmly evidence-based

2   Diagnosis of GN:
(a)   Rarely requires renal biopsy
(b)   Shows different histology in 'primary' and 'secondary' cases
(c)   Includes different histological patterns with different typical clinical presentations
(d)   Typically carries a grim prognosis for excretory renal function
(e)   Accounts for around 10% of cases of end-stage renal failure in the UK

3   Hypertension in patients with GN:
(a)   Carries independent prognostic significance
(b)   Is treated with angiotensin-converting enzyme inhibitors as agents of first choice
(c)   May undergo 'malignant' transformation
(d)   Resolves after renal transplantation
(e)   Accounts for about 40% of cases of so-called 'essential' hypertension

4   Immunosuppression for GN:
(a)   Is used in a hierarchical approach
(b)   Is typically very effective in mesangiocapillary GN
(c)   Has been extensively studied in randomised clinical trials
(d)   Is designed on a rational basis in antiglomerular basement membrane disease
(e)   Predisposes to opportunistic infection

5   Prognosis in GN:
(a)   Is better in minimal change nephropathy than in focal segmental glomerulosclerosis
(b)   Is worse in patients with heavy proteinuria
(c)   Is worse in male patients
(d)   Is improved by effective blood pressure control
(e)   Is improved by warfarin in patients with membranous nephropathy

**Selection of dialysis modality**

1   A 35-year-old man with severe renal failure should start on haemodialysis (HD) because:
(a)   He has an ileal conduit

   (b)   His job involves travelling
   (c)   Survival is better than if he started on peritoneal dialysis (PD)
   (d)   He is diabetic
   (e)   He is severely overweight

2    A 81-year-old man with rheumatoid arthritis and ischaemic heart disease (IHD) is referred to a renal clinic because a routine blood test shows a plasma creatinine of 185 μmol/l. Renal ultrasound shows two small kidneys. Despite good blood pressure control, his renal function declines. After 18 months his plasma creatinine is 350 μmol/l and haemoglobin (Hb) 9.2 g/dl. He is started on erythropoietin. Six months later his Hb has risen to 11.5 g/dl and plasma creatinine to 456 μmol/l. Discussions are started about the need for dialysis. Factors predicting a poor outcome on dialysis are:
   (a)   Presence of small kidneys
   (b)   Age
   (c)   He has IHD
   (d)   The development of anaemia
   (e)   Rate of decline of renal function

3    Early referral of patients with renal failure results in improved survival on dialysis because:
   (a)   Patients are less likely to start on HD with neck lines
   (b)   More patients go on to PD
   (c)   More patients are on erythropoietin
   (d)   Patients are more likely to be transplanted
   (e)   Blood pressure control is better

# International Health

# The emerging threat of multidrug resistant tuberculosis

Richard Coker

## □ INTRODUCTION

Over about the past decade the spectre of multidrug resistant tuberculosis (MDRTB) and the challenges and uncertainties associated with it have caused concern at the highest national and international policy making levels. MDRTB is high on the public health policy agenda, a challenge to clinical management and a threat to public health.

In the early 1990s the World Health Organization (WHO) drew public attention to the inadequacies of global tuberculosis (TB) control efforts, describing the situation as an 'emergency'. In 1998, five years after New York effectively responded to its predominantly home-grown epidemic of MDRTB, three international organisations, Médecins sans Frontières (MSF), Medical Emergency Relief International (MERLIN) and the Public Health Research Institute (PHRI), invoked the name of another pathogen when they described the spread of MDRTB in Russia as 'ebola with wings'. This captured an image that was also taken up, and subsequently built upon, by the WHO in a report in 1999, *The global impact of drug-resistant tuberculosis*, highlighting both the global nature of the epidemic and the potential for international spread.[1] With approximately two million people crossing international borders every day and mass movements of people because of economic woes or conflict, it is argued that transnational movements of diseases, including MDRTB, may threaten us all and challenge clinicians worldwide.

This chapter describes some of the challenges, many of them formidable, facing those involved in countering the threat posed by MDRTB.

## □ DEVELOPMENT OF MULTIDRUG RESISTANT TUBERCULOSIS

MDRTB, TB resulting from organisms resistant to at least isoniazid and rifampicin, develops through selection pressures. The bacterial population in cavitary pulmonary disease may be $10^7$–$10^9$ organisms, and spontaneous mutations leading to drug resistance occur with a frequency of one in $10^6$–$10^8$ replications depending on the drug. Therefore, in any cavitary population there are likely to be a few organisms resistant to single anti-TB drugs. Thus, exposure to one drug gives a selective advantage to only a small number of organisms; subsequent exposure to a second drug will again selectively advantage those few organisms resistant to both the first drug and the second – hence the development of MDRTB. Primary drug resistance occurs when a patient who has previously not received treatment develops disease with an organism that is already resistant, an indication of past programmatic frailties (ie inappropriate treatment, poor drug supplies and transmission in institutions). Acquired drug resistance, that is resistance developing in a patient who has received or is receiving treatment, suggests contemporary programme weaknesses.

## □ GLOBAL EPIDEMIOLOGY OF MULTIDRUG RESISTANT TUBERCULOSIS

Much of our understanding of the global epidemiology of MDRTB is based upon data collated from surveys and national surveillance programmes and analysed by WHO and the International Union Against Tuberculosis and Lung Disease (IUATLD) in collaboration.[2] The prevalence of MDRTB in most Western European countries is low (about 1% of all TB cases) but in some countries, notably in Central and Eastern Europe, high levels have been described. Of concern in understanding the global picture, however, is the paucity of data on MDRTB from much of the world including much of Europe and Asia. In Russia, for example, data from only two of 89 regions (or oblasts), Ivanovo Oblast and Tomsk Oblast, are available for global survey (Fig 1). Consequently, sizeable gaps remain in our understanding of the global distribution of cases, detailed systematic determinations of temporal trends remain patchy and the magnitude of the global burden of disease due to MDRTB is uncertain.

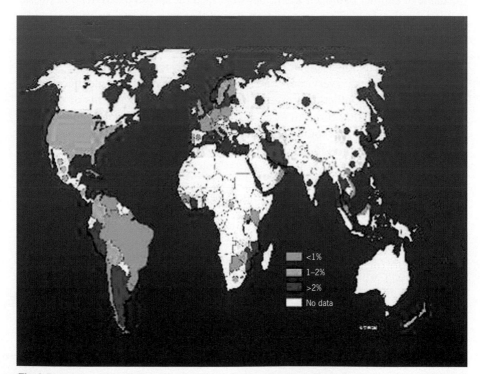

**Fig 1** Prevalence of multidrug resistant tuberculosis among new tuberculosis cases in countries and regions surveyed 1994–1999.[2]

These gaps notwithstanding, estimates of the global burden have been made. One estimate, based on data from 64 countries, is that the annual incidence of MDRTB is 273,000 cases – a fraction of the estimate of eight million annual incident cases of TB worldwide.

## ☐ TREATMENT

### First-line drugs

Why is MDRTB a feared scourge? Clinical responses to treatment of MDRTB with standard first-line drug regimens have been poor, with cure rates of 5–60%. In a study from a prison in Baku, Azerbaijan, for example, treatment was successful in only 54% of patients. Treatment failure was associated with several factors,[3] including:

☐  the breadth of the spectrum of drug resistance of isolates

☐  positive sputum microscopy at the end of the initial treatment period

☐  cavitary disease, and

☐  poor treatment compliance.

Both the Baku study and a subsequent multisite study showed that:

an approximately linear increase in the likelihood of treatment failures was observed as the number of drugs to which the strains were resistant increased.[4]

This multisite study reported relative risks of treatment failure and death in patients with MDRTB and in those with drug-sensitive strains of 15.4 and 3.73, respectively.

### Second-line drugs

Until recently there were few reports from low-income countries on treatment of MDRTB with second-line drugs. However, such approaches to treatment have now been reported in these countries, notably Peru,, though there were high treatment failure rates in proven MDRTB cases.[5,6] With second-line drugs, treatment success in MDRTB varies, with 45% to more than 80% of patients cured (or probably cured). However, length of follow-up and survival analysis in most of these studies were relatively short (or unclear), and both the long-term implications of treatment for individuals and the public health impact of these interventions remain somewhat uncertain.

These issues are important when considering resource allocations.[7] Moreover, because clinical trials have yet to determine the most effective clinical approaches to management of MDRTB, treatment strategies still largely depend on professional experience and on drawing inferences from case series and cohort studies. Several of these reports suggest that poor clinical condition prior to treatment initiation and resistance to a large number of drugs are associated with poor outcomes.[5,6]

Furthermore, survival may be poor in those patients in whom sputum sterilisation is not achieved.

One of the challenges facing clinicians, therefore, is to decide what regimen is most effective for any given patient. Broadly, two approaches are taken:

1    Standardised treatment approach.

2    Individualised treatment regimens.

### Standardised treatment approach

The first strategy is based on an assessment of the background prevalence of drug resistance and an assumption that chronic patients are likely to have strains of similar pattern. However, much of this approach rests, first, on considerable uncertainty about epidemiological patterns of resistance to second-line drugs and, secondly, on assumptions that resistance to second-line drugs that have not been widely used is unlikely to be a significant factor in determining MDRTB treatment regimens.

The so-called standardised treatment approach that includes second-line drugs is usually given over a period of 18 months to two years. The National TB Control Programme of Peru adopted this approach, using a regimen comprising kanamycin, ciprofloxacin, ethionamide, pyrazinamide and ethambutol.[5]

### Individualised treatment regimens

The alternative strategy, which is more usually adopted in resource-rich settings, is to use individualised treatment regimens. An assessment of the likely sensitivity is made on the basis of previous regimens used and a determination of first- and second-line drug resistance patterns through drug-susceptibility testing derived from patient specimens. Regimens therefore vary for each patient depending on clinical history and sensitivity patterns of isolates. Delays in the determination of sensitivity patterns (usually about two months) cause possible delay in the initiation of definitive regimens; clearly, once they are known, they must be acted upon promptly and appropriately if clinical benefit is to be maximised.

### □ CHALLENGES

### Appropriate treatment

Choice of appropriate treatment is an important determinant of more favourable outcomes. If patients receive treatment early to which the organism is subsequently shown to be sensitive, the treatment is more likely to be successful. One of the challenges facing those charged with managing MDRTB is, therefore, whether rapid diagnostics using amplification techniques to determine rifampicin resistance (as a potential marker for MDRTB) early after presentation are an effective (and cost-effective) clinical tool, such that treatment for individuals might be more appropriately tailored and outcomes improved.

### Public health impact

A further important challenge is to answer the question whether such an approach, in public health terms, will impact on efforts to control the public health threat of MDRTB. The outcomes of most importance to the individual and his treating physician are reduction in morbidity and improving survival, but reducing transmission is of critical importance for those charged with protecting public health.

### New drugs

Few drugs with effective antimycobacterial properties have been developed recently. The therapeutic armamentarium to combat MDRTB is largely made up of drugs developed many decades ago, many of which have become almost obsolete because of their relatively poor activity and potent toxicity. Restricting the widespread use of the few newer antimicrobials that have antimycobacterial activity has also been a substantial challenge, and one that has not been met. The widespread use of quinolones, for example, means that their effectiveness as antiTB agents may already be becoming diminished.

## ☐ CO-INFECTION WITH HIV

An important, perhaps the *most* important, prognostic determinant of success in the treatment of MDRTB is the presence of HIV co-infection. Clinical outcomes may be poor. In the mid-1990s, Turett[8] showed that if MDRTB associated with advanced HIV disease was treated with antiTB drugs to which the organism was unlikely to be sensitive, mortality rates approaching 100% were likely within two months. If, however, a regimen was used to which organisms were likely to be sensitive, one-year survival was about 60%. More recently, Drobniewski[9] showed that immuno-compromised individuals in the UK with MDRTB are nine times more likely to die than nonimmunocompromised patients. Other studies support the view that early institution of appropriate treatment may extend survival even if individuals are HIV-positive. Some studies suggest that management at specialised centres appears to confer prognostic benefits for patients co-infected with HIV and MDRTB.

## ☐ COST

### Low-income countries

Many experts have argued that treatment of MDRTB in low-income countries is an inefficient use of limited resources. It is certainly considerably more expensive than treating drug-sensitive disease. Indeed, some have suggested that treating the global burden of MDRTB may cost as much as treating all the remaining drug-sensitive cases worldwide. There has also been much debate about whether relatively resource-poor countries, where much of the burden of MDRTB falls, could afford to manage such cases.

Until recently, the response to the epidemic of MDRTB in New York was held up as an example of the potential costs that might be incurred to address MDRTB adequately in some settings. Reports of the $1 billion expended to support TB control efforts in the early 1990s in that city (much of it spent on restructuring health services) have led many to consider that the management of MDRTB is beyond the resources of lower-income nations but, at the same time, have offered a glimpse of the possible. A more recent estimate in London is that the cost of treating a patient with MDRTB is about £60,000 – ten times that of drug-sensitive disease.

However, a recent cost-effectiveness analysis of a treatment programme in Peru of patients with MDRTB found that cases can be treated under a standardised treatment approach for as little as approximately $2,400 per case.[5] This important study showed that such an approach is potentially feasible in some low-income settings. Clearly, however, the organisational capacity, and the political, patient and professional commitment demonstrated in Peru may not be replicated in other areas. How it could be developed elsewhere would be an important lesson.

**The Green Light Committee**

One considerable advance in the promotion of treatment strategies to combat MDRTB has been the effectiveness of the Green Light Committee. This multi-institutional partnership has been charged with negotiating lower prices for second-line drugs to combat MDRTB and with facilitating access to these drugs at negotiated prices for programmes deemed to adhere to internationally accepted control practices. Substantial price reductions have been achieved for a raft of second-line drugs; over the past couple of years estimated drug costs for an 18-month course of treatment have fallen from approximately $5,000 to $1,800. However, whilst this clearly favours middle-income countries with strong 'directly observed treatment – short course' programmes, these prices are likely to be beyond the reach of many low-income countries.

## ☐ TRANSMISSION DYNAMICS

Critical to informing policy making and the allocation of resources to managing MDRTB is an understanding of the transmission dynamics of MDRTB and the balance between individual needs and public health protection. If epidemics of MDRTB are self-limiting even if treatment strategies are not adopted, policy makers may prefer to allocate scarce resources to individual and public health interventions that provide greater returns on their investment. The ethical and cultural frameworks by which such questions are considered are important.[7]

## ☐ INFECTIOUS RISK

One of the most significant challenges in the control of MDRTB is understanding more about the relative infectiousness of both resistant and drug-sensitive strains of *Mycobacterium tuberculosis*, using this understanding to tailor control policies more effectively.

Somewhat conflicting epidemiological evidence suggesting that MDRTB strains are less or more infectious comes from a variety of sources. In some settings, cases of MDRTB appear to cluster less than drug-sensitive strains, for example, and molecular fingerprinting to identify clustering has, in some studies, suggested a reduced propensity to cluster. Other epidemiological studies, including longitudinal studies, have suggested higher cluster rates with MDRTB. It remains uncertain whether these patterns result from differences in transmissibility, pathogenicity (or a mixture of both) of MDRTB strains compared with drug-sensitive strains or from variations in the effectiveness of control programmes causing distortions in rates.

## ☐ CONCLUSIONS

### Size and impact of MDRTB

The challenges posed by MDRTB are substantial. There is considerable uncertainty about the size of the problem and the potential impact of another epidemic, HIV, in parts of the world reporting high prevalence rates of MDRTB. Most notable, and perhaps most worrying, is the situation in some states of the former Soviet Union (FSU). Together with huge political, economic, social and cultural changes, many FSU countries have healthcare and social welfare infrastructures that have crumbled or are fractured almost beyond repair and ill-equipped to respond to these new threats. With regional borders shifting with the enlargement of the European Union, other international borders remaining porous, conflicts and other causes of social turmoil precipitating mass migrations, it seems sensible that nation states of the affluent West should remain focused on supporting efforts to address MDRTB globally – out of self-interest, if not for humanitarian reasons.

### Focus of support

It remains uncertain where this support should be focused. Some would argue that the urgency of the task means that programmes should be initiated now, drawing on what evidence exists to support practical approaches. Although the evidence base upon which programmes may be founded may not be as robust as some purists might wish, they believe that the unfolding humanitarian disaster demands action now rather than later. Others argue that to adopt approaches that have not been subjected to robust critical analysis from a public health perspective may result in inefficient, indeed counterproductive, outcomes. At the heart of this challenge is considerable uncertainty about the transmission dynamics of MDRTB strains and the most appropriate practical ways to enhance control efforts.

### Development of drug resistance

Other issues challenge MDRTB control. Foremost are approaches to prevent the development of drug resistance in patients by ensuring treatment is appropriate and that systems are in place to support adherence. Moreover, prevention of spread through those with disease is a major challenge, particularly in settings which rely on institutionalisation of patients and vulnerable groups such as many countries of the FSU. Spread of MDRTB amongst those infected with HIV within prisons, shelters for the homeless and hospitals has been documented in recent years. It is likely to become a substantial threat to public health in some parts of the world over the next decade as epidemics of HIV and MDRTB collide. Evidence in support of preventive therapy is almost non-existent – a challenge that will assume considerably greater importance as the epidemics of MDRTB and HIV collide in parts of the FSU. New, highly effective drugs for *M. tuberculosis* remain elusive.

### Ethical and legal dilemmas

Another challenge concerns the ethical and legal dilemmas of managing patients who either decline treatment or are untreatable but threaten the public health.[10] If effective treatment for many individuals with MDRTB remains illusory, do these patients face a disease career that parallels disease in the pre-chemotherapeutic era, with about 30% of cases remaining smear-positive and infectious? What policies will be developed to respond to these populations?

### Public health challenges

The public health challenges raised by the spectre of MDRTB are manifold. They range from the epidemiological to the diagnostic, from the economic to the legal, and from the institutional to the social. In facing these challenges and contemplating remedies, we should perhaps reflect on the insight of René and Jean Dubos:

> Tuberculosis is a social disease, and presents problems that transcend the conventional medical approach.[11]

The fact that MDRTB is a man-made phenomenon does not diminish the authority of those words.

*Note:* a fuller version of this paper is under consideration by *Tropical Medicine & International Health*.

## REFERENCES

1   Farmer P, Becerra M, Kim JY (eds). *The global impact of drug-resistant tuberculosis.* Boston, MA: Harvard Medical School, Open Society Institute, 1999.
2   World Health Organization. *Anti-tuberculosis drug resistance in the world.* Second report. Report No. WHO/CDS/TB/2000.278. Geneva: WHO, 2000.
3   Coninx R, Mathieu C, Debacker M, Mirzoev F *et al.* First-line tuberculosis therapy and drug-resistant *Mycobacterium tuberculosis* in prisons. *Lancet* 1999;**353**:969–73.
4   Espinal MA, Kim SJ, Suarez PG, Kam KM *et al.* Standard short-course chemotherapy for drug-resistant tuberculosis: treatment outcomes in 6 countries. *JAMA* 2000;**283**:2537–45.
5   Suarez PG, Floyd K, Portocarrero J, Alarcon E *et al.* Feasibility and cost-effectiveness of standardised second-line drug treatment for chronic tuberculosis patients: a national cohort study in Peru. *Lancet* 2002;**359**:1980–9.
6   Mitnick C, Bayona J, Palacios E, Shin S *et al.* Community-based therapy for multidrug-resistant tuberculosis in Lima, Peru. *N Engl J Med* 2003;**348**:119–28.

7    Coker R. Should tuberculosis programmes invest in second-line treatments for multidrug-resistant tuberculosis (MDR-TB)? *Int J Tuberc Lung Dis* 2002;**6**:649–50.

8    Turett GS, Telzak EE, Torian LV, Blum S *et al.* Improved outcomes for patients with multidrug-resistant tuberculosis. *Clin Infect Dis* 1995;**21**:1238–44.

9    Drobniewski F, Eltringham I, Graham C, Magee JG *et al.* A national study of clinical and laboratory factors affecting the survival of patients with multiple drug resistant tuberculosis in the UK. *Thorax* 2002;**57**:810–6.

10   Coker R. Just coercion? Detention of nonadherent tuberculosis patients. Review. *Ann N Y Acad Sci* 2001;**953**:216–23.

11   Dubos R, Dubos J. *The white plague: tuberculosis, man, and society.* Boston: Little, Brown, 1952.

# Malaria for the physician

Peter Winstanley

## ☐ INTRODUCTION

Unlike HIV disease or tuberculosis (TB), both of which are also major threats to public health throughout the tropics, uncomplicated malaria (of whatever species) is relatively cheaply and rapidly cured, usually in outpatients. However, in common with HIV and TB (but to varying degrees) control of malaria is threatened by inadequate resources and drug resistance. Worldwide, Africa carries the greatest burden of malaria mortality and morbidity; by no coincidence, Africa is also the most resource-limited.

The World Health Organization (WHO) (through its Roll Back Malaria (RBM) programme) aims to halve malaria mortality by 2010. The control of both mortality and morbidity hinges on the best use of sparse resources. This review will focus on the control of falciparum malaria in Africa. Some of the main modalities available include:

☐ Prevention of infection by the use of insecticide dipped bednets.

☐ Intermittent presumptive treatment (IPT) for certain targeted subgroups (pregnant women, especially primigravidae, and perhaps also infants).

☐ Case management of uncomplicated disease.

☐ Improved management of severe malaria syndromes.

These options will be considered and an attempt made to highlight the main challenges involved in implementing these strategies within a public health system on a shoestring.

## ☐ BACKGROUND

Four species of malaria parasite cause disease in humans but *Plasmodium falciparum* causes the most problems in terms of prevalence, virulence and drug resistance. The pathogenicity of this parasite is thought to result from its rapid rate of asexual reproduction in the host and its ability to sequester in small blood vessels. The burden of falciparum malaria is mainly carried by tropical Africa, where almost everyone becomes infected during childhood. Most mortality/morbidity is seen in children under the age of five years and pregnant women (most conspicuously primigravidae). Most children gradually develop 'partial immunity' which protects them from severe disease, but a small proportion – although a numerically huge group – develop severe malaria which kills about a million people (mainly children) annually.[1]

In tropical countries, people with uncomplicated falciparum malaria are normally treated as outpatients – indeed, many do not seek professional healthcare but self-medicate using drugs bought at local shops. Treatment is with antipyretics (paracetamol or aspirin) plus inexpensive oral antiparasitic drugs. Patients with severe malaria need (but often do not get) expert supportive care plus parenteral formulations of effective antimalarial drugs (usually quinine or an artemisinin). When the patient's condition improves this is often followed by oral administration of an antimalarial drug.

## ☐ PREVENTION OF DISEASE

### Insecticide treated bednets

Bednets have been used for a long time – Herodotus mentions their use in the Nile delta in the fourth century BC – but dipping them in insecticide has given them extra benefit. The value of insecticide treated bednets (ITBN) was shown in the Gambia during the 1980s and in Kilifi (Kenya) during the 1990s. In both instances, introduction of ITBN led to significant reductions in childhood mortality and life-threatening malaria among children aged 1–59 months.[2] More recently, a large series of studies in Kisumu (Kenya) has shown that using ITBN reduces childhood mortality/morbidity, has a major positive impact on pregnant women, and even protects people who do not sleep under ITBN but sleep within a certain distance of the nets.

These results are remarkably encouraging, but were obtained by a research group with adequate funding. The key to making ITBN help public health will be the exploration of their use under 'real world' circumstances in which there are small budgets and little manpower. The main challenge for the coming few years will be the implementation and maintenance of bednet programmes within public health systems on a shoestring.

### Targeted chemoprophylaxis and intermittent presumptive treatment

Travellers to malarious areas are encouraged to use effective chemoprophylaxis. They are exposed to risk from the drug for a limited period of time and, crucially, can easily afford the intervention. In contrast, if people who live in areas of intense transmission were to take long-term chemoprophylaxis, they would be exposed to a cumulative risk of adverse drug reactions (ADR). Perhaps more importantly, few people (or health services) could afford such a general measure. However, it is possible to target groups at high risk, namely pregnant women (especially those in their first or second pregnancy) and perhaps also young children.

#### *Pregnancy*

In areas of endemic transmission, malaria in pregnancy (especially primigravidae) is associated with severe maternal anaemia and low birth weight babies.[3] Chloroquine prophylaxis has been used in the past and still has utility in some parts of Africa, but resistance to this drug is now widespread and there is a switch to sulfadoxine-pyrimethamine (SP). IPT with SP once in both the second and the third trimesters[4] has a high protective efficacy against parasitaemia and anaemia in HIV-negative women. HIV-positive women may require a monthly SP regimen, but even this proves cost-effective. The two-dose and monthly SP strategies cost US$11 and $14, respectively, well within the range considered cost-effective.

The main challenge here is the identification of practicable drugs that are not threatened by resistance.

### Infants

Clinical malaria and severe anaemia are major causes of hospital admission and death among infants in many malaria-endemic settings. Recently, IPT with SP examined in this setting has shown good protective efficacy against both clinical malaria and severe anaemia.[5] This is a new approach to malaria control and has great potential. WHO is planning studies to examine its cost-effectiveness in areas with different patterns of malaria endemicity.

### Intermittent presumptive treatment with sulfadoxine-pyrimethamine

Critical to the IPT use of SP are:

- [ ] effectiveness

- [ ] the large therapeutic range of both component drugs

- [ ] a good safety profile, and

- [ ] its very low cost.

Slow elimination might be added as another critical feature of SP (see below), but this is less clear. It is unknown whether IPT/SP works by providing chemo-prophylaxis or by intermittent reduction of parasitosis. Allergy to sulphonamides (especially among HIV-positive people) is a major theoretical risk, but does not seem to be a real concern for its widespread deployment. Furthermore, although it is an antifolate drug, SP does not *seem* to be associated with an increased risk of birth defects (although the evidence of SP safety in pregnancy is not extensive or sufficiently robust to permit strong statements). The major problem is drug resistance, especially in East Africa (see below). It seems likely that chlorproguanil-dapsone (CPG-DDS) (Lapdap™; GlaxoSmithKline) will be licensed later in 2003, and the utility of this inexpensive drug for IPT remains to be studied. (This drug was developed by GlaxoSmithKline, WHO Special Programme for Research and Training in tropical diseases (TDR), UK Government Department for International Development (DFID) and the University of Liverpool.)

### ☐ CASE MANAGEMENT OF UNCOMPLICATED MALARIA

Symptomatic patients self-select and present themselves for treatment, making this the simplest means of malaria control. First-line treatment is often obtained from local retail outlets because people have little time or money and the local shop is both quick and inexpensive. This may prove satisfactory in a proportion of patients, but there are problems:

☐ People are often seeking *symptomatic* treatment for themselves or their children, and may have little concept of the fundamental differences between antipyretic drugs such as paracetamol and antiparasitic medicines. Some vulnerable patients (especially young children) may not receive prompt antiparasitic drugs.

☐ Drugs are often sold under proprietary names, so people may buy the same generic drug under different names, with the risk of exceeding the recommended maximum dose of drugs with small therapeutic indices.

☐ The dispenser is usually untrained and cannot give reliable advice.[6]

☐ Given that patients are usually poor, antimalarial drug doses may be unacceptably low.

Probably about 50% of people invest their scarce funds (bus fares and prescription charges) and time off work to obtain antimalarial treatment and advice from the formal health sector. Most African countries now have national malaria control programmes (NMCP) which publish guidelines on antimalarial drug policy – but NMCP managers have few drug choices.

### Chloroquine and amodiaquine

Chloroquine remains the first-line treatment for uncomplicated falciparum malaria in much of Africa, even in areas of high-level resistance. It is cheap, safe and well tolerated, but its failure to eliminate parasitaemia may eventually lead to the development of profound anaemia. Amodiaquine, a close congener of chloroquine, may still be useful in some circumstances where established resistance precludes the use of chloroquine for uncomplicated malaria. Amodiaquine is also of use in combination with other drugs.[7]

### Sulfadoxine-pyrimethamine

A decision to replace chloroquine as first-line treatment for falciparum malaria will soon have to be made in much of Africa. The switch to SP has already been made in many countries. This drug has the great advantages of being a single-dose treatment and inexpensive. However, resistance to SP is predicted to develop within a few years, facilitated by its slow elimination from the body. Malawi, the first to switch to SP has evidence of worsening SP resistance,[8] but the process has not been as rapid as was feared and many lives have been saved by the timely change in national policy in 1993. Nevertheless, although the drug still works, there is little doubt that the situation is worsening: for example, the SP failure rate in Muheza (Tanzania) has now reached alarming levels.[9] Thus, a burning question is what drug (or drugs) comes next? Worryingly for public health in Africa, there is no easy answer.

## Chlorproguanil-dapsone

As stated above, CPG-DDS is likely to be licensed during 2003. Daily CPG-DDS for three days (CPG 2.0 mg/kg and DDS 2.5 mg/kg daily) is an effective treatment for uncomplicated falciparum malaria in African children,[10] and seems to be well tolerated. It will cost less than US 50 cents for a three-day adult treatment course in the public sector.

There is evidence that SP treatment of parasite strains with *dhfr* mutations at positions 108, 51 and 59 often results in clinical failure; in contrast, the risk of clinical failure seems lower with CPG-DDS.[8,9] It is also probable that CPG-DDS exerts a smaller degree of 'selection pressure for resistance' than SP.[11] All this sounds good, but there are some caveats.

### Effectiveness

CPG-DDS is efficacious in the clinical trial setting but is eliminated rapidly from the body,[12,13] and poor compliance might have a major impact on outcome. There is thus a need to examine the 'real world' effectiveness of the drug.

### Safety

The safety of CPG-DDS will be judged by national regulatory authorities (including the British Medicines Control Agency). It is, however, characteristic of such dossiers that they contain data on 2,000–3,000 people, whereas life-threatening ADRs often have a prevalence around 1:5,000 or 1:10,000. It will not be possible to assume that the safety profile of CPG-DDS is fully understood until there are post-marketing surveillance data.

### Selection of drug resistance

The available evidence suggests that CPG-DDS selects resistance less readily that SP. However, it needs to be seen whether resistance is selected when the drug is in widespread use in the 'real world' when the ideal regimen may not be followed. The possibility is being studied that combining CPG-DDS with an artemisinin drug will reduce the rate of drug resistance.

Assuming that CPG-DDS is given regulatory approval, there is probably a need for a Phase 4 programme to examine these issues before considering the large-scale adoption of CPG-DDS into malaria control programmes.

## Quinine

Quinine is an effective replacement for chloroquine and a drug of choice for non-immune patients with falciparum malaria. However, it has the disadvantage that it must be taken three times a day for seven days, tastes bitter and predictably causes unpleasant symptoms at normal therapeutic dose. Therefore, compliance is a major problem. In those parts of South-East Asia where parasite sensitivity to quinine is declining, and where few alternatives are available, cure rates are improved if the drug is combined with tetracycline or clindamycin.

### Mefloquine

Given as a single dose (or in divided doses 6–8 hours apart to reduce the risk of vomiting), mefloquine was initially highly effective against multiresistant strains of falciparum malaria worldwide. However, in some areas, notably the border regions of Thailand, mefloquine resistance has developed rapidly and a combination of mefloquine with artesunate is currently used. The relatively high cost of mefloquine limits its usefulness in Africa.

### Atovaquone-proguanil

Atovaquone-proguanil is an effective and well-tolerated drug, but its price puts it out of reach for most people in Africa.

### Artemisinin 'combination therapy'

If treatment is with two (or more) drugs, the chance of a mutant emerging resistant to both drugs can be calculated from the product of the individual per-parasite mutation rates (assuming that the resistance mutations are not 'linked'). The artemisinin derivatives reduce the parasite biomass by around 4-logs for each asexual cycle, making them the most rapidly efficacious antimalarial drugs in use.[14] This has a major theoretical role when artemisinin derivatives are combined with another antimalarial drug in that the parasite population available to develop mutations to the second drug is reduced by several log-orders. When mefloquine was used in combination with artemisinin drugs in Thailand, the rate of development of mefloquine resistance was reduced.[15] The WHO-RBM programme recommends artemisinin 'combination therapy' (ACT) as part of the 'ideal' strategy for malaria control in Africa, but there are practical concerns:

1   ACT will be relatively expensive. There is only one fixed-ratio combination, lumefantrine with artemether (Coartem; Riamet), which will be available at about US$ 2.50 per adult treatment course. This price is generous and courageous of the manufacturer (in Switzerland, Riamet is selling at SFr 78.50 (US$ 57.00) for a three-day adult course) and a singular success for the WHO–RBM negotiators. However, there are still problems:

   ☐   US$ 2.50 is still too expensive for generalised use of this combination as first-line treatment by most African nations.

   ☐   There is concern that the concessionary price may prove to be unstable (it represents an awesome commitment by the manufacturer) unless the new Global Fund can contribute large revenue costs. Work has started on the development of a chlorproguanil-dapsone-artesunate (CDA) triple combination tablet by a public-private partnership that involves the Medicine for Malaria Venture. The real cost of CDA will probably be much less than that of lumefantrine-artemether, but its development is likely to take another two years.

2    ACT has been shown to work in Thailand, but it is not clear whether it will work in a real-world African setting, and the ongoing hospital-based clinical trials will probably offer only supportive evidence. The large-scale population based trials planned for Tanzania and Mozambique should provide definitive answers but will take several years to complete.

3    A great deal of operational work will be needed to ensure smooth translation of ACT from policy into implementation. The complicated dosage regimen of Coartem (twice daily for three days) poses a challenge in this regard.

4    ACT probably offers advantage over 'monotherapy' treatments, but faces major deployment and financial hurdles.

Of course, any new initiative is surrounded by doubt and beset by practical difficulty. The above concerns are **not** reasons to set ACT aside, but need to be seriously addressed.

## ☐ WHAT HAPPENS WHEN A FIRST-LINE DRUG FAILS?

Life-threatening malaria can evolve within a day of the first symptom, so that even if an effective drug is available for uncomplicated disease the patient may still develop life-threatening illness before treatment can be given. The empirical prediction that the use of an ineffective first-line drug would carry an increased risk of deterioration to severe malaria seems to be true.[16] The population at most risk from severe malaria worldwide are the under-fives in sub-Saharan Africa, the two main syndromes of concern being cerebral malaria and severe anaemia. Falciparum malaria can cause many other life-threatening syndromes, but these lie beyond the scope of this chapter (there is an excellent WHO summary of severe and complicated malaria[17]).

## ☐ SEVERE MALARIA SYNDROMES

### Cerebral malaria

Unlike the other species of malaria parasite, *P. falciparum* can cause acute life-threatening encephalopathy loosely referred to as 'cerebral malaria'. The diagnostic feature is unrousable coma, seizures being common (especially in children). Unrousable coma can of course be multifactorial, including hypoglycaemia, recent (or ongoing) seizure, severe acidosis and the prior use of sedative antiepileptic drugs at high dose. Thus, although sequestration of parasites in the cerebral microcirculation is considered to be the prime cause of 'cerebral malaria', the clinical case definition is not homogeneous and is associated with a wide variety of prognoses. When faced with an unconscious patient in whom falciparum malaria is suspected, the basic principles of management can be summarised as shown in Table 1.

**Table 1** Basic principles of management of the unconscious patient with suspected falciparum malaria.

- Treatment should be started immediately the diagnosis is suspected
- A drug regimen should be chosen appropriate for the known local pattern of drug resistance; quinine and the artemisinin-derivatives are the preferred drugs for severe malaria
- Dosage should be calculated according to the patient's body weight, rather than estimated
- The antimalarial drug should be given parenterally where possible
- If quinine is used, a loading dose should be given unless the patient has received parenteral quinine/quinidine or oral halofantrine within the previous 24 hours
- Therapeutic response should be monitored frequently by:
  - clinical assessment
  - examination of blood films
  - measurement of blood glucose, temperature, pulse, blood pressure
- Antimalarial drugs should be given orally as soon as patients are able to swallow and retain tablets

## Quinine

Quinine has a narrow therapeutic range, and doses should always be adjusted for body weight, with an initial loading dose divided between two or more sites to achieve therapeutic concentrations more rapidly. This practice is mainly based on sound pharmacokinetic data and empirical medical practice. If patients develop severe malaria following mefloquine treatment, a full dose of quinine should be given (there is no evidence that mefloquine and quinine in combination are cardiotoxic).

Quinine must never be given as a bolus intravenous (iv) injection because there is a high risk of serious ADRs, including shock and arrhythmia. The preferred route of administration is slow, constant-rate infusion of the drug diluted in crystalloid solution. If neither infusion pump nor burette is available, the drug may be added to iv fluid in the bag.[18] This may be difficult in young children because of the need for caution with fluid volumes. If iv administration is impossible, identical doses of quinine may be given intramuscularly.[19] Coagulopathy is a relative contraindication to this route, but quinine is absorbed reliably even in the sickest patients. The dose should be diluted with water (up to 1:5 v:v) for injections because undiluted quinine dihydrochloride 300 mg/ml has a pH of 2 and is painful.

### Maintenance quinine

Maintenance doses of quinine are usually given every eight hours, but 12-hourly maintenance is effective in African children.[20] Maintenance courses are usually shorter in semi-immune African patients (5 days being standard in many countries), and combination with antibiotics or sulphonamide-pyrimethamine is not usual. In South-East Asia, quinine (combined with tetracycline or clindamycin) is given for seven days – shorter courses are associated with recrudescences. This difference between practice in Africa and Asia reflects the degrees of immunity to malaria in the two populations.

*Monitoring*

Frequent blood glucose measurements are mandatory for patients on parenteral quinine because of the risk of drug-induced hypoglycaemia. Clinical judgement should be used about the frequency of measurement which will vary between cases. If possible, blood films should be examined six-hourly and a quantitative parasite count performed. Parasite counts often remain unchanged, but they may rise during the first 18–24 hours of treatment with quinine; this is not reliable evidence for drug failure. After 24 hours of treatment, counts usually fall in a log-normal manner and asexual parasitaemia should disappear within five days. Gametocytes may persist, but they are non-pathogenic and of no clinical import, although of some public health relevance. A rising or unchanging parasite count after 24 hours of quinine treatment may indicate drug resistance; this is particularly likely in infections acquired in South-East Asia.

## Artemisinins

There is a rapid reduction in total body parasite load with the artemisinin drugs, so a better clinical outcome than with quinine might be predicted. Disappointingly, in a large meta-analysis[21] there were no statistically significant differences between artemether and quinine in case fatality, coma recovery, fever clearance times or the development of neurological sequelae. However, combined 'adverse outcome' (death or sequelae) was significantly less frequent in the artemether group, and subgroup analyses suggested that artemether was significantly more effective than quinine in reducing mortality in adults and in all Asian patients. This might have been due to the greater prevalence of quinine resistance in Asia.

Artemether is usually dispensed in 1 ml ampoules containing 80 mg artemether in peanut oil. An initial loading dose is recommended, followed by once-daily administration of the maintenance dose for at least three days or until an oral formulation of an artemisinin or another antimalarial drug can be taken by mouth.

Currently, only artesunate is available for iv administration.[22] A loading dose of artesunate is given by iv bolus injection followed by a maintenance dose at 12 and 24 hours, then daily to complete seven days of treatment.

Suppositories of artemisinin and artesunate have proved effective in adults and children with cerebral and other forms of severe malaria in China and South-East Asia. Although plasma concentration profiles are more erratic than with iv administration, inadequate absorption is unusual. This is a particularly promising route of administration in patients with moderately severe malaria at the most peripheral level of the health service, and trials are being conducted by the WHO.

## Supportive care

The choice and correct use of antiparasitic drugs are important but patients also need expert supportive care.[16] Detailed consideration of such intensive care management lies outside the scope of the present article, but it includes the management of:

☐   hypoglycaemia and acidosis

☐   seizures

☐   brain swelling

☐   coagulopathy

☐   renal failure, and

☐   pulmonary oedema.

## ☐ CONCLUSIONS

*P. falciparum* remains an immense threat to public health in Africa where drug resistance now threatens a major increase in mortality and morbidity. The main ways in which it may be possible to control this problem are with ITBNs, IPT for pregnant women (perhaps also for infants), improved case management of uncomplicated disease and improved management of severe malaria syndromes. All these strategies are faced by major challenges:

☐   ITBNs work in the research setting. They now have to be made effective and sustainable in the real world – on a shoestring budget.

☐   Drugs for both uncomplicated malaria and IPT need to be effective in a real world setting rather than simply in clinical trials, also safe, inexpensive and not prone to selection of resistance. ACT is likely to be the preferred option of WHO, but it faces hurdles including the practicalities of implementation, sustainable finance and safety. The role of new monotherapy drugs (including CPG-DDS) is yet to be defined.

☐   Antimalarial drugs for severe malaria syndromes (mainly quinine and the artemisinins) are not currently threatened by drug resistance in Africa. The key to reducing mortality and morbidity in this setting is optimisation of practical supportive care measures, including the use of blood transfusion.

To hold our ground against malaria there will need to be continued collaboration between scientists, the pharmaceutical industry and public health workers.

## REFERENCES

1   Snow RW, Craig MH, Deichmann U, Marsh K. Estimating mortality, morbidity and disability due to malaria among Africa's non-pregnant population. *Bull WHO* 1999;77:624–40.
2   Nevill CG, Some ES, Mung'ala VO, Mutemi W *et al.* Insecticide-treated bednets reduce mortality and severe morbidity from malaria among children on the Kenyan coast. *Trop Med Int Health* 1996;1:139–46.
3   Brabin BJ, Hakimi M, Pelletier D. An analysis of anemia and pregnancy-related maternal mortality. Review. *J Nutr* 2001;131(2S-2):604–14S; discussion 614–5S.
4   Shulman CE, Dorman EK, Cutts F, Kawuondo K *et al.* Intermittent sulphadoxine-pyrimethamine to prevent severe anaemia secondary to malaria in pregnancy: a randomised placebo-controlled trial. *Lancet* 1999;353:632–6.

5    Schellenberg D, Menendez C, Kahigwa E, Aponte J *et al.* Intermittent treatment for malaria and anaemia control at time of routine vaccinations in Tanzanian infants: a randomised, placebo-controlled trial. *Lancet* 2001;**357**:1471–7.

6    Marsh VM, Mutemi WM, Muturi J, Haaland A *et al.* Changing home treatment of childhood fevers by training shop keepers in rural Kenya. *Trop Med Int Health* 1999;**4**:383–9.

7    Staedke SG, Kamya MR, Dorsey G, Gasasira A *et al.* Amodiaquine, sulfadoxine/pyrimethamine, and combination therapy for treatment of uncomplicated falciparum malaria in Kampala, Uganda: a randomised trial. *Lancet* 2001;**358**:368–74.

8    Kublin JG, Dzinjalamala FK, Kamwendo DD, Malkin EM *et al.* Molecular markers for failure of sulfadoxine-pyrimethamine and chlorproguanil-dapsone treatment of *Plasmodium falciparum* malaria. *J Infect Dis* 2002;**185**:380–8.

9    Mutabingwa TK, Kilama E, Winstanley P, Watkins W. Treatment and re-treatment of *Plasmodium falciparum* infections with pyrimethamine-sulfadoxine (PSD): a study to predict the useful therapeutic life of PSD as therapy for non-severe falciparum malaria in east Africa. *Lancet* 2001;**358**:1218–23.

10   Amukoye E, Winstanley PA, Watkins WM, Snow RW *et al.* Chlorproguanil-dapsone: an effective treatment for uncomplicated falciparum malaria. *Antimicrob Agents Chemother* 1997;**41**:2261–4.

11   Nzila AM, Nduati E, Mberu EK, Hopkins Sibley C *et al.* Molecular evidence of greater selective pressure for drug resistance exerted by the long-acting antifolate pyrimethamine/sulfadoxine compared with the shorter-acting chlorproguanil/dapsone on Kenyan *Plasmodium falciparum*. *J Infect Dis* 2000;**181**:2023–8.

12   Winstanley PA, Watkins W, Muhia D, Szwandt S *et al.* Chlorproguanil/dapsone for uncomplicated *Plasmodium falciparum* malaria in young children: pharmacokinetics and therapeutic range. *Trans R Soc Trop Med Hyg* 1997;**91**:322–7.

13   Ward SA, Manyando C, Horton J, Stubbs T, Winstanley PA. *The pharmacokinetics of Lapdap in man.* American Society of Tropical Medicine and Hygiene, 50th Annual Meeting, Atlanta, 11–15 November 2001 (abstract 576).

14   White NJ. Delaying antimalarial drug resistance with combination chemotherapy. *Parasitologia* 1999;**41**:301–8.

15   Nosten F, van Vugt M, Price R, Luxemburger C *et al.* Effects of artesunate-mefloquine combination on incidence of *Plasmodium falciparum* malaria and mefloquine resistance in western Thailand: a prospective study. *Lancet* 2000;**356**:297–302.

16   Trape JF, Pison G, Preziosi MP, Enel C *et al.* Impact of chloroquine resistance on malaria mortality. *C R Acad Sci III* 1998;**321**:689–97.

17   Severe falciparum malaria. World Health Organization, Communicable Diseases Cluster. Review. *Trans R Soc Trop Med Hyg* 2000;**94**(Suppl 1):S1–90.

18   Winstanley PA, Mberu EK, Watkins WM, Murphy SA *et al.* Towards optimum regimens of parenteral quinine for young African children with cerebral malaria: unbound quinine concentrations following a simple loading dose regimen. *Trans R Soc Trop Med Hyg* 1994;**88**:577–80.

19   Winstanley P, Newton C, Watkins W, Mberu E *et al.* Towards optimal regimens of parenteral quinine for young African children with cerebral malaria: the importance of unbound quinine concentration. *Trans R Soc Trop Med Hyg* 1993;**87**:201–6.

20   Pasvol G, Newton CR, Winstanley PA, Watkins WM *et al.* Quinine treatment of severe falciparum malaria in African children: a randomized comparison of three regimens. *Am J Trop Med Hyg* 1991;**45**:702–13.

21   Artemether-quinine meta-analysis study group. A meta-analysis of trials comparing artemether with quinine in the treatment of severe falciparum malaria using individual patient data. Final report, July 99 (unpublished).

22   Newton P, Suputtamongkol Y, Teja-Isavadharm P, Pukrittayakamee S *et al.* Antimalarial bioavailability and disposition of artesunate in acute falciparum malaria. *Antimicrob Agents Chemother* 2000;**44**:972–7.

23   Nosten F, van Vugt M, White NJ. Intrarectal artemisinin derivatives. Review. *Med Trop (Mars)* 1998;**58**(3 Suppl):63–4.

## ☐ INTERNATIONAL HEALTH SELF ASSESSMENT QUESTIONS

**The emerging threat of multidrug resistant tuberculosis**

1   Multidrug resistant tuberculosis (MDRTB):
   (a)   Is TB resistant to at least two first-line antiTB drugs
   (b)   Can be treated successfully, the possibility of cure being closely related to the number of drugs to which the strain is resistant
   (c)   Treatment is highly effective with second-line drugs with outcomes similar to treatment of drug-sensitive disease with first-line drugs
   (d)   Treatment success is only marginally affected by coexistent HIV infection
   (e)   Primary drug resistance indicates past programme weaknesses

2   MDRTB:
   (a)   Surveillance is good and there is a good understanding of its global epidemiology
   (b)   Treatment is beyond the public purse of all but the most affluent countries
   (c)   Treatment costs have fallen because costs of second-line drugs have fallen
   (d)   Control programmes should be initiated as priority before other TB programme weaknesses are addressed
   (e)   Strains are clearly more infectious than drug-sensitive strains

3   MDRTB:
   (a)   Has been termed 'Ebola with wings'
   (b)   Results from selective advantage of resistant strains to first-line drugs
   (c)   Acquired drug resistance always suggests poor patient compliance with treatment
   (d)   Is a particular challenge in some countries of Eastern Europe
   (e)   Is a man-made public health challenge

**Malaria for the physician**

1   In African countries the mortality/morbidity in endemic populations due to falciparum malaria is commonly controlled by:
   (a)   Chemoprophylaxis
   (b)   Insecticide impregnated nets
   (c)   Vaccination
   (d)   Drainage of standing water
   (e)   Case management of uncomplicated disease

2   The following are appropriate drugs for case management of uncomplicated falciparum malaria throughout Africa:
   (a)   Tetracycline
   (b)   Sulfadoxine-pyrimethamine
   (c)   Artemether-lumefantrine

   (d)   Co-trimoxazole
   (e)   Amodiaquine

3   In the management of cerebral malaria in Africa, quinine:
   (a)   Remains a drug of first choice
   (b)   May be given on suspicion of the diagnosis
   (c)   Should never be given as a bolus injection
   (d)   May be given intramuscularly
   (e)   May be given by nasogastric tube

# Neurology

# Multiple sclerosis

George Ebers

## □ INTRODUCTION

Multiple sclerosis (MS) was first recognised as a clinical pathological entity in the 19th century, but examples in the medical literature indicate that the disease existed considerably earlier. An unequivocal case was described in the early 19th century by Ollivier.[1] Many 'modern' diseases are recognisable in the 17th and 18th century texts of Morgagni and Willis, but not MS. Pushing things back further is impeded by the several hundred years of 'dark ages' during which few detailed medical accounts survive.

One broad exception to this general paucity of information comes from the legends and lives of saints. The story of the 8th century patron saint of Oxford may be relevant. Legend has it that St Frideswide was an attractive nun whose virtue was pursued by Algar, a local king. Allegedly while in hot pursuit, he was struck blind, which must have dampened his ability to find her if not his ardour. In a most Christian manner, while hiding in a nunnery from his presumably unwanted advances, she generously prayed for him and his sight returned. Although the miracle to which credit was assigned must figure in the differential diagnosis, this may well have been an early example of optic neuritis. The story is outlined in the Burne-Jones window at Christ Church. Interestingly, St Frideswide's subsequent miracles favoured neurological therapeutics, with both remitting blindness and paraplegia a recurrent theme.

## □ CURRENT BELIEFS

It is widely believed that MS is a primary demyelinating disease which affects only European populations and has a predilection for women over men of approximately 2:1. It is also generally thought to be a primary autoimmune disease, the target being central nervous system myelin and, more specifically, myelin basic protein (MBP). There appears to be a genetic background to the disease, exemplified by the presence of HLA DRB1501 in twice as many cases as in controls. Many smaller genetic effects may also be present.

A large environmental effect is inferred from the usual discordance of monozygotic twins and the striking differences in incidence among similar gene pools depending on their place of habitation, usually thought to be connected to endemic viral flora. It has been believed for some time that disability results from the succession of serial exacerbations of the disease and that cases without these exacerbations (primary progressive) constitute some kind of different entity. For many, magnetic resonance image (MRI) lesions 'are the disease'. It is widely believed that these are excellent surrogate markers, the suppression of which should lead to a major impact on the disease. Finally, there appears to be a consensus that immunosuppression and beta interferon (IFN) spectacularly suppress MRI activity, which should translate into the prevention of long-term disability. It is possible that many of these statements will prove to be incorrect.

## ☐ MULTIPLE SCLEROSIS AS A PRIMARY DEMYELINATING DISEASE

There are reasons to be at least somewhat sceptical of the concept that MS is a *primary* demyelinating disease. None is conclusive, but final accounting of MS will have to take these findings into consideration. Animal models of experimental allergic encephalitis (EAE) have been influential in our thinking about the disease; they can be induced with a variety of nervous system components, usually in the presence of non-specific stimulators of the immune system such as complete Freund's adjuvant. From a more practical standpoint, several hundred unrelated compounds appear to suppress EAE, none of which has led to useful therapy in MS.

More troublesome is the observation that antigen-specific cells reactive to MBP are not more common in MS than in stroke and are certainly present in HLA DRB1501-negative normals. Furthermore, the presence of retinal lesions and uveitis in MS are not easily explained on the basis of myelin specificity. It has become increasingly clear that demyelination is only relative and that axonal loss, which is selective and tends to affect small corticospinal tract axons early,[2] may occur independent of demyelination and not as a direct result. Long-term follow-up of patients treated with IFN show that 'plaques' (ie MRI T2 signal by MRI scanning) may be nearly completely suppressed yet have no impact on the gradual atrophy of the brain which occurs in this disease (Fig 1).[3] Indeed, MRI identified markers to date indicate that they are possibly the most expensively misleading surrogate markers in medical history, although there will be additional chapters in this story.

Finally, study of other diseases in which the primary process was thought to be demyelinative has revealed evidence warranting reconsideration. For example, in adrenoleukodystrophy, there are mutations in an ABC transporter gene active in peroxisomes, leading in many cases to an intensive inflammatory demyelination. However, presymptomatic men and carriers show axonal abnormalities before demyelination. This and similar, but less clear, findings in some forms of Charcot-Marie-Tooth disease lend support to the possibility that inflammatory demyelination could be a secondary process in MS. At present, a reasonable hypothesis is that there is a disruption in the axonal-glial interactions necessary for reciprocal function and maintenance.

## ☐ NON-INVASIVE IMAGING AS AN AID TO DIAGNOSIS

The diagnosis of MS has been greatly aided by non-invasive imaging, particularly MRI. It is not easy to determine if this has improved diagnostic accuracy, and no

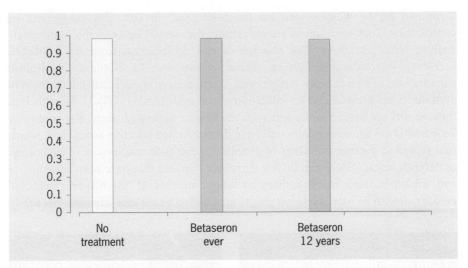

**Fig 1** Brain atrophy over 12 years in multiple sclerosis.

evidence that it has done so in specialist centres. Using standard clinical criteria and prolonged follow-up, diagnostic accuracy in excess of 95% has been recorded.[4] MRI provides a quick, non-invasive means of excluding structural lesions of many kinds, although there is still occasional confusion in the case of degenerative disorders.

There has been considerable pressure to use MRI scanning to identify the occurrence of new lesions in patients with monosymptomatic disease such as optic neuritis which often develops into MS. This pressure seems to derive partly from industry and industry-funded investigators who have, perhaps unknowingly, followed the blueprint of stock analysts. These have advised that the general fiscal health of companies manufacturing therapies said to be disease-modifying will be improved by:

☐   increasing the number of patients diagnosed

☐   making the diagnosis earlier so that patients would be on therapy longer, and

☐   tacitly obviating the recognition by patients and their physicians that they might do well without therapy, and thus claim credit for what is the natural history of the disease.

The uncritical acceptance of these dictats under the guise of patient interest has provided yet another shameful chapter in a desperate disease which engenders such intense desire to find effective treatment that experienced judgement can be clouded.

Counter-intuitively, in a paradox which may well be the main contribution of MRI scanning so far, the correlation of T2 'spots' or plaques with disability outcome has been disappointing. The oft repeated mantra that 'MRI is the disease' is unsupportably well into its second decade. In no case has a confirmed correlation value exceeded 0.25; thus, much less than 10% of the variance in disability can be accounted for by what is seen on the MRI scan. In fact, this exaggerates its contribution. Such correlations are univariate; they would be lower if a multivariate analysis were performed. The absence of this information from the published literature warrants investigation. Serial claims for T2 burden, gadolinium enhancement, T1 black holes, atrophy and magnetisation transfer still fall far short of even the most liberal criteria for validation of surrogate markers (Fig 2). Nevertheless, these results are entirely consistent with the known neuropathology. Key studies by Ferguson *et al*[2] and Evangelou *et al*[5] have demonstrated selective axonal loss, which may represent the core pathology of disability rather than much more obvious areas of demyelination. There can be few surrogate markers that have been as seductive and whose shortcomings have been so long concealed. If 'the emperor's clothes' analogy were to be used, axon loss might turn out to be the real 'invisible thread'.

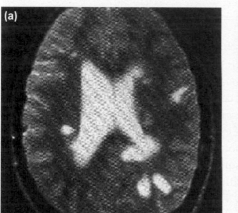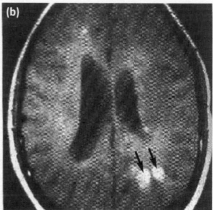

**Fig 2** Gadolinium enhancement of multiple sclerosis lesions: **(a)** multiple hyperintense lesions are present on axial T2-weighted image; **(b)** gadolinium-enhanced T1-weighted image shows enhancement of acute plaques (arrowed).

## ☐ NATURAL HISTORY OF MULTIPLE SCLEROSIS

A brief summary of the natural course of the disease from onset to walking with a cane is illustrated in Table 1. The median times to disability measures are surprisingly good for many patients, although there is considerable interindividual variability. At least 50% of patients will remain ambulatory at 15 years. Survival curves of patients with many relapses who become progressive, those with single attacks who become progressive, and those with no attacks but who begin with progression show a 6–8 year difference in time from onset to cane for the last group who progress more quickly. However, there are no differences if the same curves are calculated from the time of onset of progression. Thus, for the total population, the number of attacks preceding the onset of the progressive phase appears to have no influence on long-term outcome. This has implications for the selection of outcome measures in the disease, sample size calculations and the interpretation of results of clinical trials which demonstrate that relapses, but not progression, are suppressed.

**Table 1** Natural history of multiple sclerosis: median times to disability.

| | EDSS | |
| --- | --- | --- |
| Disability | Relapsing remitting (years) | Primary progressive (years) |
| Cane | 6–15 | 6–8 |
| Wheelchair | 7–20 | 7–12 |
| Bedridden | 8–25 | 8–15 |

EDSS = expanded disability status scale.

In the London, Ontario, natural history database comprising about 25,000 patient-years of essentially untreated follow-up, there was no correlation between the total number of relapses and outcome – despite the number of relapses in the first year associating with outcome. The explanation for this paradox appears to lie in the indirect way in which early relapses associate with long-term outcome. The largest prognostic factor by far in this disease is the development of a progressive course.

## ☐ MULTIPLE SCLEROSIS AND IMMUNOSUPPRESSION

If response to immunosuppression were the best evidence that MS is an autoimmune disease, the case would be weaker than it is. Marginal to no efficacy for relapse-free progressive disability has characterised studies of cyclophosphamide, ciclosporin, azathioprine, methotrexate, campath 1, cladribine, anti-CD4, mitoxantrone and even bone marrow transplantation.

A weak argument for proof of principle can still be made on clinical or MRI surrogates, but in this author's opinion it is not yet evidence-based therapy. The ethics of continued studies of potentially hazardous drugs aimed non-specifically at suppressing the immune system should be debated. Such trials surely must include a consent form because of the relatively unsuccessful context in which these studies can be placed. The evidence is increasingly strong that these drugs are ineffective in preventing disease progression.

## ☐ LONG-TERM TREATMENT WITH INTERFERON

Steve Karlik and George Rice, in London, Ontario, evaluated the long-term effects of IFN therapy in 43 patients enrolled in the original pivotal trial of beta IFN in 1999. Important among some surprising findings was the observation that changes in most MRI measures used for outcomes in clinical trials are clearly driven by a minority of patients since many patients had little or no change from the treatment. After 12 years, patients receiving no treatment had a 20% increase in T2 burden (increased signal on T2-weighted images), whereas scans of patients receiving IFN were better in terms of T2 burden than at base line (Fig 3). If it had been suggested in 1989 that a treatment was available which would completely suppress T2 lesions,

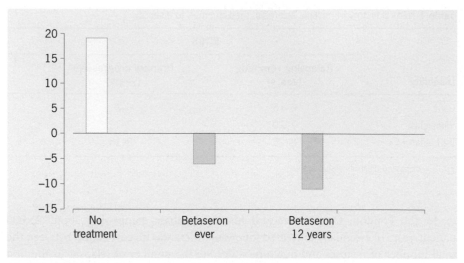

**Fig 3** Change in T2 burden over 12 years in multiple sclerosis.

most observers would have said that MS was now treatable. However, at 12 years the evolution of brain atrophy continued unabated in patients and controls, highlighting questions about the relationship between plaques and disability (Fig 1).

## □ PATHOGENESIS

### Twin studies

The evidence remains overwhelming that susceptibility to MS, like so many other disorders, is determined by a combination of genes and environment. A systematic twin study in Canada of 319 pairs found 27% concordance in monozygotic twins and 4.1% in dizygotics. Concordance was somewhat higher in dizygotic twins than in siblings, probably independent of ascertainment, implying a possible modest effect of birth timing. Phenotype and age of onset were also correlated in identical twins compared with siblings, and it was found that concordance develops a narrow time-window.

### Familial occurrence

The familial recurrence of MS in Canada is 20–25%. The environmental component does not appear to be transmissible. Definitive studies of adoptees, half-siblings, conjugal cases and offspring of consanguineous marriages all indicate that familial risk is determined by genes and that population risk is determined by environment.[6]

### Environment

It is widely believed that environmental factors in MS have something to do with specific or ubiquitous viruses more operative in northern climates. In my view, this is unlikely. Upper respiratory tract infections appear to be more common in the winter (Shakespeare's poem 'Winter' notes how 'coughing drowns the parson's saw'). It is not clear how this would relate to a major environmental factor in MS, which must occur at an early age based on migration studies. The latter implies an association with the development or maturation process in the neurosystem and/or immune system.

### Migration data

The well-known migration data in MS indicating that risk is acquired by place of residence before age 15 have been extended in Australia. Although the essential results have been confirmed, these data indicate that the effect may continue into adulthood. The size of the environmental factor acting early in life is large and probably related directly or indirectly to climate. A sixfold difference in MS and prevalence is well documented between Tasmania and Queensland. No genetic reason can be discerned for this.

### Genes

There is a clear association with genes within the major histocompatibility complex (MHC) and increasing evidence that two or more genes may interact to produce susceptibility. Recent data[6,7] seem to suggest that the responsible allele near the class 2 locus is not HLA DRB1501 since sib pairs lacking this allele are as likely to share each of the haplotypes as those who have it. Some investigators insist that linkages and associations have been found outside the MHC, but data show only 1/20 of associations are confirmed. Bias of some kind must be operative, since the published aggregation of $p$ values favours a lengthy list of plausible candidates.

Different tactics warrant exploration. One is the collection of families in which MS has a high recurrence risk – ideally, families with Mendelian inheritance, but no such family has been unequivocally shown to exist. We have identified a single pedigree with 19 affected members in whom the disease appears to segregate as an autosomal dominant, but proof requires linkage studies and identification of a specific gene.

### ☐ DRUG THERAPY

Further discussion of the merits and demerits of so-called disease-modifying drugs (IFNs and glatiramer acetate) is beyond the scope of this review. There is overwhelming evidence that type 1 IFNs suppress some MRI measures and clinical attacks by a third, but no therapy has been shown to reduce the rate of progression significantly.

### ☐ PRACTICAL MANAGEMENT

The value of the practical management of patients continues to be understudied. A number of drugs unambiguously improve symptoms, and several developments along these lines should be noted:

- *Neurogenic pain*: gabapentin has proved useful for the treatment for neurogenic pain which affects nearly half of MS patients at some point.

- *Spasticity* is usually controllable with a variety of medications including Lioresal (baclofen), and in severe cases more aggressive measures. Botulinum toxin injection, intrathecal Lioresal by pump injection infusion and even myelotomy can be necessary.

- *Depression* is common in MS and is effectively managed with selective serotonin reuptake inhibitors.

- *Fatigue* unrelated to depression is also common and responds in a significant number of patients to amantadine or, more recently, modafinil.

- *Bladder problems*: the key to managing bladder disturbances is to identify the bladder abnormality. The most common situation is when a hyperactive bladder struggles to empty against outflow resistance produced by true spasticity of the striated muscle round the bladder neck.

- *Impotence* responds well to sildenafil in 50% of MS patients so affected.

## ☐ CONCLUSIONS

MS is certainly one of the more challenging diseases to understand and manage.[8] It is useful to remember that average disease duration exceeds that of the professional life of most neurologists. Management can be viewed in terms of short-term reduction of symptoms and long-term management of the underlying disease process. The introduction of disease-modifying drugs has certainly boosted the spirits of patients and their families, but it is unclear whether or not there is a significant impact on the long-term course. In the meantime, progress in the field might be helped by using St Frideswide rather than Algar as a role model.

## REFERENCES

1   Paty DW, Ebers GC (eds). *Multiple sclerosis*, Ch 1. Philadelphia: FA Davis, 1998.
2   Ferguson B, Matyszak MK, Esiri MM, Perry VH. Axonal damage in acute multiple sclerosis lesions. *Brain* 1997;**120**:393–9.
3   Karlik S, Kirk S, Nicolle E, Kremenchutzky M, Rice GP. Evidence for very long-term MRI efficacy of interferon beta 1B in relapsing remitting MS patients. *Mult Scler* 2001;**7**(Suppl 1): S52.
4   Cottrell DA, Kremenchutzky M, Rice GP, Koopman WJ *et al*. The natural history of multiple sclerosis: a geographically based study: 5. The clinical features and natural history of primary progressive multiple sclerosis. *Brain* 1999;**122**:625–39.
5   Evangelou N, Konz D, Esiri MM, Smith S *et al*. Regional axonal loss in the corpus callosum correlates with cerebral white matter lesion volume and distribution in multiple sclerosis. *Brain* 2000;**123**:1845–9.
6   Herrera B, Ebers GC. Progress in deciphering the genetics of multiple sclerosis. Review. *Curr Opin Neurol* 2003;**16**:253–8.
7   Ligers A, Dyment DA, Willer CJ, Sadovnick AD *et al*. Evidence of linkage with HLA-DR in DRB1*15-negative families with multiple sclerosis. *Am J Hum Genet* 2001;**69**:900–3.
8   Compston A, Coles A. Multiple sclerosis. *Lancet* 2002;**359**:1221–31.

# Investigation and management of headache

Raju Kapoor

## ☐ INTRODUCTION

Most people experience headaches from time to time, but up to 5% of all adults have a troublesome headache on most days[1] and 12–15% of the UK population have migraine attacks. Headaches account for about 30% of outpatient referrals to neurologists and have many causes (Table 1). Although people with headache often worry about serious conditions, in reality almost all headaches are primary and their management depends more on proper clinical recognition than on detailed investigation. The definitions of 'primary' headaches continue to be debated but, with the recent advances in understanding the pathophysiology of headache, it is becoming clearer how investigations should be undertaken when a secondary cause is suspected.

**Table 1** Some causes of headache.

| Primary | Secondary |
| --- | --- |
| Tension type headache | Systemic or intracranial infection |
| Migraine | Intracranial tumour |
| Cluster headache | Subarachnoid haemorrhage |
| Chronic paroxysmal hemicrania | Head trauma |
| | Vasculitis |
| | Benign intracranial hypertension |
| | Low cerebrospinal fluid volume |

## ☐ THE PRIMARY HEADACHES (Table 2)

### Tension type headache and migraine

In 1962, tension headache was defined as:

> an ache or sensation of tightness, pressure, or constriction, widely varied in frequency and duration, long-lasting, commonly occipital, and associated with contraction of skeletal muscles, usually as part of the individual's reaction during life stress.[2]

Stress was considered to lead to abnormal contraction of the pericranial muscles, and hence to ischaemia which ultimately led to pain. This mechanism, based on research by Wolff and colleagues in the 1940s and 1950s, was later questioned when

**Table 2** Brief summary of the International Headache Society criteria for the common primary headaches, 1988.

| | |
|---|---|
| Migraine | • Headache lasting 4–72 hours<br>• Nausea/vomiting and/or sensitivity to light and sound<br>• Two of the following:<br>  – unilateral pain<br>  – pulsating pain<br>  – moderate/severe intensity<br>  – aggravation by routine physical activity<br>• With or without aura: reversible neurological dysfunction lasting less than 60 min, followed by headache within 60 min |
| Tension type headache | • At least two of the following:<br>  – pressing/tightening (non-pulsating) pain<br>  – mild or moderate intensity<br>  – bilateral location<br>  – no aggravation by routine physical activity<br>• With or without disorder of pericranial muscles<br>• No vomiting<br>• Nausea or light or sound sensitivity allowed in chronic tension type<br>• Light or sound sensitivity in episodic tension type |
| Cluster headache | • Severe unilateral (supra)orbital or temporal pain lasting 15–180 min<br>• Frequency from one every other day to eight a day<br>• Associated with one of the following:<br>  – conjunctival injection<br>  – lacrimation<br>  – eyelid oedema<br>  – meiosis<br>  – ptosis<br>  – nasal congestion<br>  – rhinorrhoea<br>  – forehead/facial sweating<br>• Episodic and chronic subtypes |

*Note*: these definitions require that there is no reasonable suspicion of a secondary cause.

it was found that pericranial muscle contraction is not always associated with the site or time of the pain. It was also difficult to decide whether psychological features such as depression and anxiety, which can be identified readily in people with tension headache, are the cause or the result of the headache. When the definition of tension headache was reviewed by the International Headache Society in 1988[3] muscle contraction and psychological mechanisms were no longer presumed to be causal.

Considerable uncertainty therefore surrounds the nature of what is now termed 'tension type' headache. Its definition simply refers to a rather bland, frequent headache. In contrast, migraine is a distinct clinical phenotype in which there are clear episodes of headache, exacerbated by effort, associated with nausea, photo- and phonophobia and sometimes with an aura.[3] In reality, this separation between migraine/episodic headache and tension type/frequent headache can seem artificial because many people who have frequent headaches have symptoms more typical of migraine.[4] In some cases, the two kinds of headaches may simply co-exist, whereas other people experience increasingly frequent migraine attacks which eventually convert into a near-daily headache, either spontaneously or, more usually, through the overuse of analgesics.

This clinical overlap between chronic migraine and chronic tension type headache has led to the suggestion that these two disorders are simply different aspects of a single biological continuum. They can share features, including:

☐ pericranial muscle overactivity

☐ biochemical markers, including low platelet serotonin levels

☐ high serum calcitonin gene-related peptide levels in some cases, and

☐ analgesic overuse, commonly found in both disorders.

However, migraine is more common in women, and many people with a mixture of headaches can distinguish attacks of migraine from those of tension type pain, regarding them as distinct subjective experiences.

### Chronic daily headache

Close observation of the population with chronic daily headache has revealed additional subtypes including:

☐ *hemicrania continua* (see below) and

☐ *new daily persistent headache*,[5] a bland, unremitting headache building up over the course of only a few days, commonly after a viral infection or head trauma, which resists treatment and spontaneously fades after a few years.

### Short-lived unilateral headache

There is also considerable clinical heterogeneity within the short-lived, unilateral headaches:[6]

☐ *Cluster headache* is the best known example; attacks of severe unilateral orbital or frontal pain are associated with ipsilateral autonomic features, including ptosis, pupil constriction, conjunctival injection and nasal stuffiness. Attacks may recur with clock-like precision for weeks or months.

☐ Similar symptoms occur in *chronic paroxysmal hemicrania* which, unlike cluster headache, reliably responds to indomethacin.

☐ *Hemicrania continua* is a milder, chronic unilateral headache with discrete exacerbations which may be associated with autonomic features; it also responds to indomethacin.

☐ At the other end of the spectrum, *short-lasting, unilateral neuralgiform headache with conjunctival injection and tearing* (SUNCT) consists of attacks of pain which last only for seconds and, unlike trigeminal neuralgia, are associated with autonomic features. SUNCT responds poorly to treatment, although success has been reported with lamotrigine.

# ☐ PATHOPHYSIOLOGY OF THE PRIMARY HEADACHES (Fig 1)

## The role of the nucleus caudalis neurones

The short-lived unilateral headaches have been called trigeminal autonomic cephalgias (TACs) because of their clinical features.[6] Cranial pain is known to be

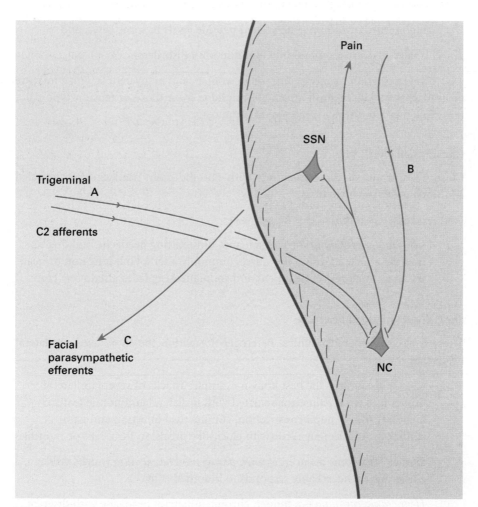

**Fig 1** Headache mechanisms and pain pathways. Numerous afferents (A), from trigeminal vascular endings and from trigeminal and C2 myofascial receptors, converge on the neurones of the trigeminal nucleus caudalis (NC). The activity of the NC neurones is also modulated by descending pathways (B). In some primary headaches, collaterals of the ascending NC axons can activate the premotor parasympathetic neurones of the facial nerve within the superior salivatory nucleus (SSN), leading to clinical autonomic features ipsilateral to the headache (C).

signalled in general by the activation of the neurones of the nucleus caudalis (NC) of the trigeminal nerve and their rostral axonal projections to the thalamus. In the TACs the activity of these NC neurones also propagates into branches of their axons which excite the parasympathetic portion of the facial nerve, giving rise to autonomic features. This mechanism explains the clinical features of the TACs. In addition, the activation of facial parasympathetic nerve terminals releases vasoactive intestinal peptide, whose circulating levels rise during attacks of pain.

As with all the primary headaches, however, the basic pathophysiological question is how and why the NC neurones and central pain pathway become activated in the first place (Fig 1).[7] A number of inputs are known to converge on these neurones, including afferents from the large intracranial arteries and veins, and from pericranial muscles. Vascular pain endings are overactive in migraine and in some patients with chronic tension type headache, which may drive the activity of the NC neurones. Afferent inputs from contracted pericranial muscles may have the same effect in some people with tension type headache. It has been suggested that the nature of the afferent stimulation could dictate the subjective character of the pain, whether throbbing (ie vascular) in migraine or pressing/aching (ie mechanical) in tension type headache. Electrophysiological techniques have shown that individual NC neurones receive convergent inputs from the trigeminal nerve and upper cervical roots. This synaptic convergence may explain the radiation into the head of pain arising from structures in the upper cervical spine; it is also consistent with the therapeutic efficacy of C2 nerve blocks in some primary headaches.

Headache is, therefore, pain mediated by the trigeminal NC neurones and may be driven by overactivity of muscle, vascular or upper cervical pain afferents. Alternatively, afferent pain traffic may be relatively normal and the NC neurones may be activated by descending pathways which modulate the pain system. In monkeys, for example, the firing rates of NC neurones to a given afferent input can be made to vary according to the animal's attentional state or by behavioural conditioning. Some of the descending modulatory pathways arise ultimately in the limbic system, so affective state could theoretically lead to central pain sensitisation in a manner reminiscent of the situation in patients who have tension type headache with little pericranial muscle contraction.

## Migraine

There is also evidence for central modulation in migraine. Functional imaging studies have shown increased activation of the periaqueductal grey, a key site for pain modulation, both during migraine attacks and after the attacks have been terminated by sumatriptan.[8] Similarly, activation of the ipsilateral hypothalamus has been observed in attacks of cluster headache induced by nitroglycerin.[9] It is possible that periodic overactivity within these sites may give rise to the episodic occurrence of migraine and cluster headache.

Neuronal dysfunction during attacks of migraine is now known to be widespread; this, rather than primary vascular pathology, is the basis of the disorder. Migraine is an all-or-none phenomenon which, once initiated, continues through a sequence of phases until its termination. The headache itself is superimposed on a number of symptoms, indicating alterations of mood, sleep, hunger and perception, which imply considerable dysfunction of the basal forebrain and brain stem. In addition, the migraine aura may consist of a visual disturbance which expands across the visual field over several minutes and can be mapped to dysfunction spreading across the visual cortex at the rate of 1–2 mm/min. The visual aura can progress to involve sensation or speech, implying that the dysfunction can cross over vascular territories – indeed, such slowly spreading dysfunction has been demonstrated in positron emission tomographic and functional magnetic resonance imaging (MRI) studies of people during attacks of migraine.

Recent experimental work in animals suggests that cortical spreading depression of this kind can lead to the release of vasoactive compounds such as nitric oxide (NO), which can activate trigeminovascular afferents and thereby trigger the onset of headache.[10] However, there is an opposing view that spreading depression and headache may simply occur in parallel during migraine attacks. Whatever its mode of action, NO may have a general role in the primary headaches, since NO donors such as glyceryl trinitrate can induce delayed headaches in patients with migraine and in some with chronic tension type headache.

Most recently, the idea that migraine is primarily a neuronal disorder has received support from the identification of missense mutations of the P/Q calcium channel gene in patients with hemiplegic migraine.[11] Deletion mutations of the same gene occur in some patients with episodic cerebellar ataxia. Migraine may, therefore, overlap with neurological conditions associated with channelopathies.

## ☐ MANAGEMENT OF PRIMARY HEADACHES

It is likely that the management of the primary headaches[1] will improve as the result of better understanding of their basic mechanisms. However, specific treatment will depend on a precise clinical diagnosis; to some extent, this is already the case. In general, management is escalated through a series of steps, beginning with general advice about how to identify and avoid triggering factors such as sleep deprivation, hypoglycaemia and food additives. Acute management of headache episodes begins with over-the-counter analgesics, but may need more specific agents such as the triptans for migraine and cluster headache. Currently, there is great interest in developing drugs which could inhibit cortical spreading depression, including NO and glutamate antagonists.

Preventive treatment also depends on diagnosis. Some TACs respond dramatically to indomethacin, while chronic daily headache associated with analgesic overuse responds well to analgesic withdrawal and detoxification. Antidepressants are more successful in chronic daily headache, as are pizotifen, beta-blockers and anticonvulsants in migraine, but there is a degree of overlap. There is also increasing interest in calcium-channel modulating drugs, including flunarizine, in situations in which a channelopathy appears to be implicated.

Failure to respond to appropriate treatment should prompt a review of the diagnosis, the dose and duration of drug treatment, and compliance.

## ☐ INVESTIGATION OF HEADACHE

There is a consensus that stable, chronic headache without associated neurological features is associated with a serious imaging abnormality in less than 0.5% of cases, similar to the percentage found in asymptomatic people.[12] The imaging abnormalities identified in a small proportion of such patients may be found by chance and may not be the cause of the headache. This needs to be borne in mind when imaging is arranged with the aim of providing reassurance. There are insufficient comparative studies to know whether such imaging should be by computed tomography (CT) or MRI, and whether contrast should be routinely considered. Indeed, the choice of the appropriate investigation of headache is becoming increasingly complicated and needs to be guided clinically, as illustrated by some specific pathologies.

### Cerebral tumours

Cerebral tumours now tend to present early with what appear to be tension type headaches or migraine. Only the presence of either rapid deterioration or associated neurological symptoms or signs may suggest the need to investigate further.[13] Fewer than 20% have a classical tumour headache, with early morning exacerbation and nausea. CT is generally sufficient to image tumours above the tentorium, but posterior fossa lesions are likely to be better visualised using MRI. Most tumours produce headaches which gradually become worse, but abrupt onset headaches can occur with either colloid cysts of the third ventricle which block cerebrospinal fluid (CSF) circulation, or periventricular epidermoid cysts which may burst to give episodes of chemical meningitis.

### Sudden-onset headache

Approximately 25% of sudden onset (less than one minute) severe headache is caused by subarachnoid haemorrhage (SAH), and half the patients with SAH have additional neurological features. There is often great concern that the diagnosis may be missed, partly because retrospective studies suggested that a substantial minority of patients with SAH had previously experienced abrupt 'sentinel' headaches typical of small warning leaks. However, prospective work has shown that few patients with SAH have sentinel headaches[14] and that their prognosis is similar to that of patients without such warning leaks. SAH seems to be effectively excluded by a normal CT brain scan and CSF examination. These investigations become less useful as time passes, becoming normal after 2–3 weeks. MR angiography (Fig 2) is proving useful in identifying intracranial aneurysms in patients who present late.

### Cerebral sinus thrombosis

Relatively sudden headaches can also arise in cerebral sinus thrombosis; MRI or MR venography may be required if the diagnosis is suspected. Sudden, unilateral head or neck pain should also raise the suspicion of arterial dissection which can occur

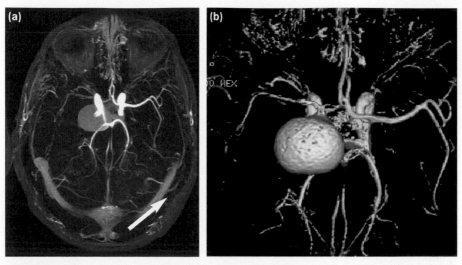

**Fig 2 (a)** Magnetic resonance angiogram, showing an aneurysm of the middle cerebral artery (arrowed); **(b)** the aneurysm is seen more clearly in a 3-D remodel of the original data (images reproduced courtesy of the Queen Square Imaging Centre).

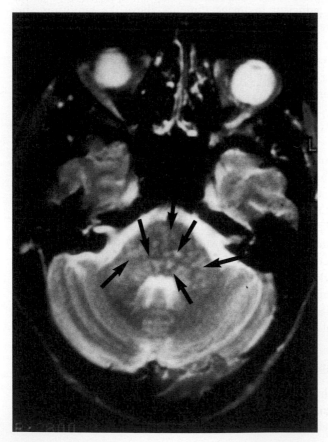

**Fig 3** T2 weighted magnetic resonance image scan of a patient with headaches and primary angiitis of the central nervous system, showing small scattered brainstem lesions (arrowed). Vasculitis can be associated with a wide variety of imaging abnormalities.

without prior trauma. The headache may precede stroke by an average of 15 hours (vertebral dissection) to four days (carotid dissection). Diagnosis may depend on appropriate imaging, particularly MR angiography.

### Cerebral vasculitis

A diagnosis of cerebral vasculitis is sometimes suspected in patients with chronic, unremitting headache since the associated neurological features can be subtle. The incidence of isolated primary headache is higher in systemic lupus erythematosus. The headache is often migrainous, which in itself does not suggest central nervous system (CNS) vasculitis. There are no systemic inflammatory markers in CNS primary angiitis, but the headache is associated with an abnormal MRI scan (Fig 3) and/or abnormal CSF. For this reason, lumbar puncture is sometimes carried out in patients with refractory chronic daily headache and normal imaging. Angiography, which shows segmental narrowing of the intracranial arteries, is diagnostic but is seldom required.

Such segmental arterial narrowing has also been described in patients suffering phenotypically from chronic daily headache, migraine or coital cephalgia, and it has been suggested that such patients may have a particularly benign angiitis. An alternative view is that the arterial narrowing results from activation of the trigeminal innervation of the intracranial arteries that occurs in migraine attacks.

### Altered cerebrospinal fluid pressure

Headache arising from benign intracranial hypertension is well recognised, but more recently a group of patients with spontaneous low volume/pressure headache has also been recognised.[15] These patients generally develop a lumbar CSF leak, sometimes following relatively minor trauma, which gives rise to a headache like the one after lumbar puncture. The CSF pressure is usually below 50 mm, but the diagnosis can be made non-invasively by enhanced MRI which shows striking meningeal enhancement (Fig 4, overleaf). The response to intravenous caffeine or oral theophylline is usually good, and it is rarely necessary to identify or apply a blood patch to the site of the CSF leak.

### □ CONCLUSIONS

The great majority of headaches are primary, so it is becoming increasingly important to be aware of their different subtypes in order to provide effective management. Proper investigation of headache depends on an awareness of many relatively rare but potentially serious conditions.

### REFERENCES

1   Steiner TJ, MacGregor EA, Davies PT. *Guidelines for all doctors in the management and diagnosis of migraine and tension-type headache*, 2nd edn, 2001. *URL*: http://www.bash.org.uk
2   *Ad hoc committee on Classification of Headache of the NIH. JAMA* 1962;**179**:717–8.

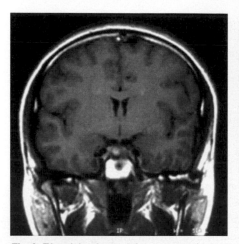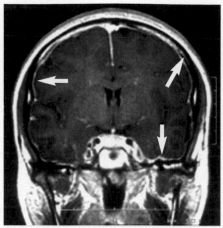

**Fig 4.** T1 weighted magnetic resonance image scan of a patient with severe orthostatic headaches following a bout of unaccustomed exercise: (a) unenhanced; (b) showing marked meningeal contrast enhancement (arrowed).

3   Classification and diagnostic criteria for headache disorders, cranial neuralgias and facial pain. Headache Classification Committee of the International Headache Society. *Cephalalgia* 1988;8(Suppl 7):1–96.

4   Silberstein SD, Lipton RB, Sliwinski M. Classification of daily and near-daily headaches: field trial of revised HIS criteria. *Neurology* 1996;47:871–5.

5   Vanast WJ. New daily persistent headaches: definition of a benign disorder. *Headache* 1986;26:318–20.

6   Goadsby PJ, Lipton RB. A review of paroxysmal hemicranias, SUNCT syndrome and other short-lasting headaches with autonomic feature, including new cases. *Brain* 1997;120:193–209.

7   Olesen J. Clinical and pathophysiological observations in migraine and tension-type headache explained by integration of vascular, supraspinal and myofascial inputs. Review. *Pain* 1991;46:125–32.

8   Weiller C, May A, Limmroth V, Juptner M *et al.* Brain stem activation in spontaneous human migraine attacks. *Nature Med* 1995;1:658–60.

9   May A, Bahra A, Buchel C, Frackowiack RS, Goadsby PJ. Hypothalamic activation in cluster headache attacks. *Lancet* 1998;352:275–8.

10  Iadecola C. From CSD to headache: a long and winding road. *Nature Med* 2002;8:110–2.

11  Ophoff RA, Terwindt GM, Vergouwe MN, van Eijk R *et al.* Familial hemiplegic migraine and episodic ataxia type-2 are caused by mutations in the Ca2+ channel gene CACNL1A4. *Cell* 1996;87:543–52.

12  Frischberg BM, Rosenberg JH, Matchar DB, McCrory DC *et al.* Evidence-based guidelines in the primary care setting: neuroimaging in patients with nonacute headaches. *URL:* http://www.aan.com/public/practiceguidelines

13  Forsyth PA, Posner JB. Headaches in patients with brain tumors: a study of 111 patients. *Neurology* 1993;43:1678–83.

14  Linn FH, Wijdicks EF, van der Graaf Y, Weerdesteyn-van Vliet FA *et al.* Prospective study of sentinel headache in aneurysmal subarachnoid haemorrhage. *Lancet* 1994;344:590–3.

15  Mokri B, Piepgras DG, Miller GM. Syndrome of orthostatic headaches and diffuse pachymeningeal gadolinium enhancement. *Mayo Clin Proc* 1997;72:400–13.

## ☐ NEUROLOGY SELF ASSESSMENT QUESTIONS

**Multiple sclerosis**

1   Magnetic resonance imaging (MRI) in multiple sclerosis (MS):
(a)   Has greatly improved diagnostic accuracy
(b)   Is highly correlated with neurological disability
(c)   Is highly predictive of the development of long-term disability
(d)   Should be used as a primary outcome measure in clinical trials
(e)   Is an unvalidated surrogate marker

2   MS prognosis:
(a)   Is characterised by median time to cane of 15 years
(b)   Is characterised by median time to partly bedridden status of 20 years
(c)   Is not associated with the number of relapses during the illness
(d)   Is associated with the number of relapses in the first 1–2 years of disease
(e)   Strongly correlates with an element of atrophy as measured by MRI

3   Long-term treatment of MS with interferon:
(a)   Has been shown to prevent or slow the need for cane requirement
(b)   Suppresses relapses by a third
(c)   Suppression of relapses in MRI 'spots' may not translate into suppression of atrophy
(d)   Long-term data on treatment outcomes are insufficient
(e)   Is ineffective in the secondary progressive phase of the disease

**Investigation and management of headache**

1   Chronic daily headache:
(a)   Affects 5% of adults
(b)   Is commonly associated with serious pathology
(c)   Can be linked to analgesic overuse
(d)   Does not respond to amitriptyline
(e)   Can respond to sodium valproate

2   Migraine:
(a)   Is also known as cluster headache
(b)   Is caused by cerebral vasoconstriction
(c)   Is associated with cortical spreading depression
(d)   Responds reliably to antidepressants
(e)   Can be treated with anticonvulsants

3   Tumour headaches:
(a)   Are often associated with other neurological symptoms and signs
(b)   Tend to become gradually more severe

(c)   Are usually worse in the morning and associated with nausea at presentation
(d)   Are never sudden in onset
(e)   Can mimic tension type headache or migraine

# Nutrition and Patients:
# a Doctor's Responsibility

# Why the metabolic syndrome?

Peter Kopelman

## ☐ INTRODUCTION

Obesity is now so common worldwide that it is beginning to replace undernutrition and infectious diseases as the most significant contributor to ill health. In 1980, 6% of men and 8% of women in the UK were obese; in 2000, the respective figures had increased to 21% and 21.4%. About 55% of the adult population is overweight or obese. Since 1980, self-reported energy intake has changed little, but changes in diet to a lower proportion of energy from carbohydrates and a higher proportion from fats have occurred, making it easier to eat an energy dense diet.[1] These changes, coupled with a marked decline in physical activity, increase the risk of obesity. Major advances in the understanding of overweight and obesity confirm that they constitute an important medical condition.

Many health problems are caused or exacerbated by obesity, both independently and in association with other diseases.[1] In particular, it is associated with the development of type 2 diabetes mellitus, coronary heart disease, increased incidence of certain forms of cancer, obstructive sleep apnoea, and osteoarthritis of large and small joints. The Build and Blood Pressure Study[2] has shown that the adverse effects of excess weight tend to be delayed, sometimes for 10 years or longer. Life insurance data and epidemiological studies confirm that increasing degrees of overweight and obesity are important predictors of decreased longevity.[3] Despite this evidence, many clinicians continue to consider obesity to be a self-inflicted condition of little medical significance.

Obesity can no longer be regarded simply as a cosmetic problem affecting certain individuals but must be considered an epidemic requiring effective measures for its prevention and management. This chapter will detail the pathophysiology of a number of important medical problems that constitute the metabolic syndrome, emphasising the importance of early intervention in the management of those overweight or obese who are at risk.

## ☐ CLINICAL PROBLEMS CAUSED BY OVERWEIGHT AND OBESITY

Increasing body fatness is accompanied by profound changes in physiological function which are, to a certain extent, dependent on the regional location of adipose tissue. This review focuses on the intra-abdominal visceral deposition of adipose tissue that characterises upper body obesity and is a major contributor to the development of:

☐   hypertension

☐   elevated plasma insulin concentrations and insulin resistance

☐   hyperglycaemia, and

☐   hyperlipidaemia.

The alterations in metabolic and physiological functions that follow an increase in adipose tissue mass are predictable when considered in the context of normal homeostasis. The intimate relationship between increasing fatness and type 2 diabetes has led some to coin the terms 'diabesity' or 'obesity dependent diabetes'. Several conditions particularly associated with obesity will be considered:

☐   The metabolic syndrome.

☐   Type 2 diabetes mellitus.

☐   Hepatic function.

☐   Haemostasis.

### The metabolic syndrome

In 1988 Reaven coined the term 'syndrome X' to refer to the clustering of (abdominal) obesity, hypertriglyceridaemia, reduced levels of high-density lipoprotein (HDL) cholesterol, hyperinsulinaemia, glucose intolerance and hypertension.[3] Further metabolic alterations have now been added, including increased atherogenic small, dense low-density lipoprotein (LDL) particles, elevated apolipoprotein B (apoB) concentrations and raised plasminogen activator inhibitor-1 (PAI-1). The syndrome is now referred to as the metabolic syndrome or insulin resistance syndrome, the latter identifying the likely pivotal biochemical abnormality. Reaven[3] estimated that the prevalence of insulin resistance within the sedentary adult population of North America is approximately 25% and closely linked to central (visceral) obesity. Several cohort studies have confirmed that upper body (visceral) obesity is associated with greater cardiovascular morbidity and mortality than obesity itself.[4]

### Type 2 diabetes mellitus

Obesity is characterised by elevated fasting plasma insulin and an exaggerated insulin response to an oral glucose load.[5] Overall fatness and distribution of body fat influence glucose metabolism through independent but additive mechanisms. Increasing central obesity is accompanied by a progressive increase in the glucose and insulin response to an oral glucose challenge, with a positive correlation between increasing upper body (central) obesity and measures of insulin resistance. Post-hepatic insulin delivery is increased in upper body obesity, leading to more marked peripheral insulin concentrations, in turn leading to peripheral insulin resistance. Figure 1 illustrates the key role of insulin within the liver and skeletal muscle in glucose metabolism.

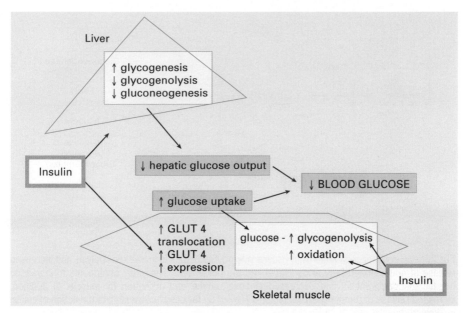

**Fig 1** The key role played by insulin within the liver and skeletal muscle in glucose metabolism. Insulin increases glycogenesis in the liver, decreases glycogenolysis and suppresses gluconeogenesis. In skeletal muscle, insulin enhances glucose uptake and utilisation by increasing glucose transporter 4 (GLUT4) transporter translocation and expression, and increases glucose utilisation.

The responsiveness to hormones that regulate lipolysis varies in different fat depots and according to fat distribution.[6] In both men and women, the lipolytic response to noradrenaline is more marked in abdominal than gluteal or femoral adipose tissue. Cortisol may also contribute to this enhanced lipolysis by further inhibiting the antilipolytic effect of insulin.

## Free fatty acids

These factors contribute to an exaggerated release of free fatty acids (FFAs) from abdominal adipocytes into the portal system.[6] FFAs have a deleterious effect on insulin uptake by the liver and contribute to the increased hepatic gluconeogenesis and hepatic glucose release in upper body obesity. Insulin insensitivity is not confined to adipocytes, the process being accentuated by skeletal muscle insulin resistance (Fig 2).

The elevation in plasma FFA concentration, particularly postprandially when it is usually suppressed by insulin, leads to inappropriate maintenance of glucose production and impairment of hepatic glucose utilisation (impaired glucose tolerance). Reduced hepatic clearance of insulin leads to increased peripheral (systemic) insulin concentrations and to a further downregulation of insulin receptors.

In the initial phases of this process, the pancreas can respond by maintaining a state of compensatory hyperinsulinaemia, preventing gross decompensation of glucose tolerance (Fig 3). However, with ever-increasing plasma FFA concentrations

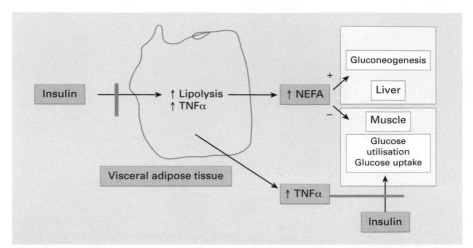

**Fig 2** Insulin resistance in abdominal visceral adipocytes results in increased lipolysis and increased release of nonesterified fatty acids (NEFA) into the portal vein. The latter contributes to increased hepatic gluconeogenesis and decreased glucose uptake and utilisation by muscle. In addition, increased release of tumour necrosis factor α (TNFα) by fat cells further inhibits the action of insulin in skeletal muscle.

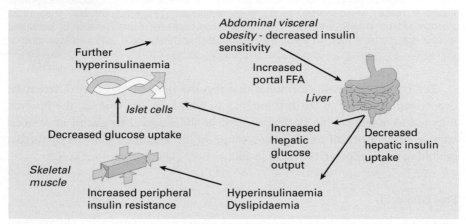

**Fig 3** The combination of factors described in Figs 1 and 2 lead to a vicious cycle of events with increasing insulin resistance and a compensatory release of additional insulin from the pancreatic islet cells. Increased share of free fatty acids (FFA) into the portal vein results in decreased hepatic clearance of insulin and continuing hepatic gluconeogenesis. These, in turn, lead to systemic hyperinsulinaemia and increased hepatic glucose output.

in the insulin-resistant individual, this state of compensatory hyperinsulinaemia cannot continue to be maintained and hyperglycaemia prevails.

## Abnormal lipid profile

Hyperinsulinaemia and insulin resistance are both significant correlates of a dyslipoproteinaemic state and contribute to the characteristic alterations of plasma lipid profile associated with obesity:

- [ ] elevated fasting plasma triglyceride concentration

- [ ] reduced HDL cholesterol

- [ ] marginal elevations of cholesterol and LDL cholesterol concentrations, and

- [ ] increased number of apoB-carrying lipoproteins.

This abnormal lipid profile in obese subjects may be associated with abnormalities in liver function, characterised by elevations in gamma-glutamyl transferase, alanine transaminase (ALT) and aspartate transaminase (AST).

## Hepatic function

### Nonalcoholic steatohepatitis

An emerging clinical problem among obese subjects, particularly those with central obesity, is nonalcoholic steatohepatitis (NASH): 40% of patients with NASH are overweight or obese, 20% have type 2 diabetes and 20% are hyperlipidaemic.[7] The development of the characteristic pathological changes within the liver is intimately related to the various clinical and biological markers of the metabolic syndrome:

- [ ] body mass index (BMI)

- [ ] waist circumference

- [ ] hyperinsulinaemia

- [ ] hypertriglyceridaemia, and

- [ ] impaired glucose tolerance.

*Diagnosis.* The diagnosis of NASH rests on characteristic histological features that include substantial fatty infiltration, inflammation, necrosis and fibrosis in the absence of alcohol. In NASH, the ratio of serum ALT to AST is always greater than 1, whereas in alcoholic liver disease it is almost always below 1.[8] Histological evidence of fibrosis and/or cirrhosis is seen in up to 50% of patients. Most patients who initially show fibrosis develop cirrhosis after 10 years; it has been suggested that 'cryptogenic cirrhosis' represents 'burnt out' NASH. A liver biopsy is necessary for the diagnosis and is important for therapeutic and prognostic reasons. Ultrasound scanning of the liver is not sufficiently sensitive to be diagnostic.

*Causes.* The causative factors inducing necrosis, inflammation and fibrosis within the liver include:

- [ ] oxidative stress and subsequent lipid peroxidation

- [ ] factors associated with abnormal cytokine production, and

- [ ] factors associated with disordered fat metabolism and insulin resistance.

The two metabolic abnormalities most strongly associated with NASH are insulin resistance and an increased supply of FFAs from visceral adipocytes via the portal vein directly to the liver. There is evidence that NASH associated with obesity and type 2 diabetes is primarily due to peripheral insulin resistance and consequential hyperinsulinaemia.[9] Insulin blocks hepatic mitochondrial fatty acid oxidation, resulting in an increased concentration of intracellular fatty acids that may either be directly toxic or lead to oxidative stress. The link between central obesity and liver injury may be explained by the more rapid mobilisation of fatty acids from visceral (central) than from subcutaneous fat and because they drain directly to the liver via the portal vein (Fig 4).

Weight loss is generally associated with a reduction in the severity of the biochemical abnormalities and a regression of the steatosis. Nevertheless, sudden weight loss or 'weight cycling' (weight loss followed by weight regain) may predispose to NASH.

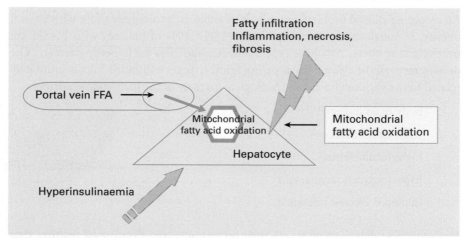

**Fig 4** A postulated mechanism for the development of nonalcoholic steatohepatitis (NASH). Increased release of free fatty acids (FFA) from visceral abdominal adipocytes into the portal vein has a detrimental action on hepatic cellular mitochondria. This results in fatty infiltration in the liver, inflammation, necrosis and, with time, fibrosis. The detrimental hepatic action is additionally compounded by hyperinsulinaemia.

## Haemostasis

The haemostatic system plays an important role in the pathogenesis of atherosclerotic plaques and associated complications. A prothrombotic environment and/or a situation in which thrombus is not cleared will predispose to the development of atherosclerosis and its clinical sequelae.

### Plasminogen activator inhibitor-1

The main inhibitor of fibrinolysis is PAI-1 which binds to and inactivates tissue plasminogen activator and urokinase-like plasminogen, the main activators of plasminogen. As PAI-1 levels increase, plasminogen activation is reduced and consequently fibrin accumulates. In this situation, the balance is in favour of thrombosis: high concentrations of PAI-1 are likely to favour the development of atherosclerosis and its acute complications. Furthermore, the prognostic value of PAI-1 appears to be related to its association with the metabolic syndrome.[10] Animal and human studies suggest that adipose tissue may be an important source of PAI-1 and responsible for elevated concentrations in obese subjects: as fat mass increases, so does PAI-1 production. There is evidence that elevated adipose tumour necrosis factor $\alpha$, as found in obesity, may increase PAI-1 mRNA expression in adipose tissue. Moreover, the production of PAI-1 from the liver appears to be regulated by insulin, in that chronic hyperinsulinaemia is associated with increased PAI-1 mRNA expression.[11]

PAI-1 levels are positively correlated with the degree of obesity, as judged by BMI and waist circumference. This correlation is confirmed by computed tomography measurements of visceral fat mass. PAI-1 concentration is also positively correlated with other variables that make up the metabolic syndrome: central obesity, hypertension, hypertriglyceridaemia and low HDL cholesterol concentration.

## □ IS LIFESTYLE CHANGE OF MEDICAL BENEFIT?

Physically inactive people are more likely to have impaired glucose tolerance, and type 2 diabetes is more common among people who are physically inactive. Prospective studies suggest that the more weekly exercise taken, the lower the risk of the development of diabetes.

Intervention studies demonstrate that a programme of lifestyle change focusing on improved diet and increased activity can delay, or possibly prevent, the development of type 2 diabetes in people at high risk because of impaired glucose tolerance. The North American Diabetes Prevention Program randomised 3,234 men and women with impaired glucose tolerance (mean age 50 years; mean BMI 34 $kg/m^2$) to placebo, metformin treatment or an intensive lifestyle intervention, with goals of at least 7% weight reduction and 150 minutes of physical activity each week. At three years, the individualised intensive lifestyle intervention group had achieved 58% reduction in the incidence of type 2 diabetes compared with 33% in the metformin group.[12] These highly significant results led to the cessation of the trial (Fig 5, overleaf). Identical results were found in a similar study in Finland.

Such findings strongly support the hypothesis for reversibility of the vicious cycle of events that follow increasing adiposity with increasing insulin resistance and systemic hyperinsulinaemia – provided that the lifestyle changes occur sufficiently early and prior to islet cell failure.

## □ CONCLUSIONS

The association between increasing body fatness, insulin resistance, impaired glucose tolerance and eventual type 2 diabetes is both predictable and avoidable. This chapter has described the biochemical and physiological changes and their links to alterations in lipid metabolism, hepatic function and haemostasis.

The important clinical message, based on compelling evidence, must be that such processes are avoidable provided that intervention strategies are implemented at an

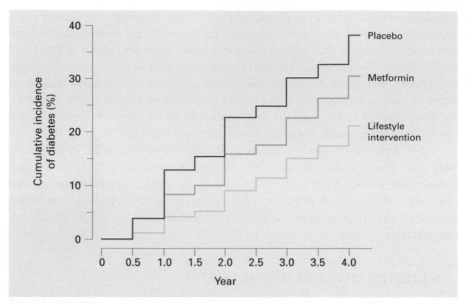

**Fig 5** The cumulative percentage incidence of diabetes in the three groups (placebo, metformin and lifestyle intervention) of the Diabetes Prevention Program (reproduced, by permission, from Ref 12).

early stage for those at particular risk. This requires a better understanding of the mechanisms involved in the metabolic syndrome by both clinician and patient alike.

## REFERENCES

1   Kopelman PG. Obesity as a medical problem. *Nature* 2000;**404**:635–43.

2   Lew EA. Mortality and weight: insured lives and the American Cancer Society studies. *Ann Intern Med* 1985;**103**:1024–9.

3   Reaven GM. Banting Lecture 1988. Role of insulin in human disease. Review. *Diabetes* 1988;**37**:1595–607.

4   Larsson B, Svardsudd K, Welin L, Wilhelmsen L *et al.* Abdominal adipose tissue distribution, obesity, and risk of cardiovascular disease and death: 13 year follow up of participants in the study of men born in 1913. *BMJ (Clin Res Ed)* 1984;**288**:1401–4.

5   Kolterman OG, Insel J, Saekow M, Olefsky M. Mechanisms of insulin resistance in human obesity. Evidence for receptor and postreceptor defects. *J Clin Invest* 1980;**65**:1272–84.

6   Frayn KN, Williams CM, Arner P. Are increased plasma non-esterified fatty acid concentrations a risk marker for coronary heart disease and other chronic diseases? Review. *Clin Sci (Lond)* 1996;**90**:243–53.

7   Bacon BR, Farahvash MJ, Janney CG, Neuschwander-Tetri BA. Nonalcoholic steatohepatitis: an expanded clinical entity. *Gastroenterology* 1994;**107**:1103–09.

8   James O, Day C. Non-alcoholic steatohepatitis: another disease of affluence. *Lancet* 1999;**353**:1634–6.

9   Wanless IR, Lentz JS. Fatty liver hepatitis (steatohepatitis) and obesity: an autopsy study with analysis of risk factors. *Hepatology* 1990;**12**:1106–10.

10  Eriksson P, Reynisdottir S, Lonnqvist F, Stemme V *et al.* Adipose tissue secretion of plasminogen activator inhibitor-1 in non-obese and obese individuals. *Diabetologia* 1998;**41**:65–71.

11  Shimomura I, Funahashi T, Takahashi M, Maeda K *et al.* Enhanced expression of PAI-1 in visceral fat: possible contributor to vascular disease in obesity. *Nat Med* 1996;7:800–3.

12  Knowler WC, Barett-Connor PH, Fowler SE, Hamman RF *et al.* Reduction in the incidence of type 2 diabetes mellitus by changes in lifestyle intervention or metformin. *N Engl J Med* 2002;346:393–403.

# Clinical nutrition in a district general hospital

W Rodney Burnham

## ☐ INTRODUCTION

Clinical nutrition is not a complex subject but it seems to be neglected by many able people both in university centres and in district hospitals. This chapter will address clinical nutrition with reference to this author's practice over the last 20 years, and review:

☐ the general organisation

☐ the role of the nutrition support team (NST) and, in particular,

☐ the role of the doctor as a member of that team and in the trust.

## ☐ DEFINITIONS

### What is a district general hospital?

A district general hospital (DGH) can be defined as one that provides a wide range of acute services mainly for the local community and is not part of a medical school site. It receives relatively few tertiary referrals and has less whole-time equivalent consultants per head of population than the teaching centres.[1]

### What is clinical nutrition?

Clinical nutrition encompasses both over- and undernutrition. In the context of this chapter, undernutrition will be mainly addressed. This is rare as a primary cause of admission to hospital in the Western world and is usually seen secondary to, or associated with, other pathology. Obesity is a relatively small part of my practice. Usually only one or two patients with morbid obesity are seen each week with either general medical problems or abnormal liver function secondary to a fatty liver.

## ☐ HOW THE SERVICE IS ORGANISED

The three district hospitals in which I work (Oldchurch, Harold Wood and St George's Hospital, Hornchurch) have about 1,000 acute and slow stream rehabilitation beds serving a population of over 450,000. Within a year of my appointment in 1981 a nutrition advisory group was established. This group, which still meets every two months, includes representatives from the catering department, dietitians, nursing staff (both specialist and ward nurses), medical and managerial staff. It provides a useful forum for discussing a wide range of issues relevant to food and nutrition; with regard to nutritional products, it serves a similar function to the drugs and therapeutics committee.

## □ THE NUTRITION SUPPORT TEAM

In 1987, a grant from the King's Fund enabled an NST to be set up. It was initially based at Oldchurch but, after obtaining additional funding from the health authority some years ago, it now goes to other hospitals and into the community. The NST receives an average of over 1,200 referrals a year. In addition, I am asked to consult on other patients with particular needs both in hospital and in the community (16–24 patients per week).

The nutrition team comprises specialist nurses, a nutrition support dietitian (two people doing a job share), medical staff (myself and a specialist registrar (SpR)), a pharmacist and other healthcare professionals including secretarial and administrative staff. There is close liaison with the biochemistry and speech and language departments.

### How to set up a nutrition support team

The first action in setting up a nutrition team is to identify strategic allies.

*Strategic allies*

*Dietitians and pharmacists.*   Because of their specialist knowledge, dietitians and pharmacists do not usually need persuading that a nutrition team is essential. They frequently see the consequences of the failure of medical and nursing staff to take seriously the problem of nutrition.

*Medical personnel.*   Medical colleagues can be somewhat more difficult to persuade. At the time of my appointment this large DGH did not have a dietitian, perhaps because it was not thought important. However, demonstrating to medical colleagues that an NST can provide safe nutritional support for their patients and avoid septic or metabolic complications usually persuades them of its value. It is important to start with an advice, rather than a 'take over', service.

*Managers and the director of nursing.*   For managers and the director of nursing, the emphasis is on efficiency and quality. In our case, the first step was taken relatively early when a research dietitian and a research nurse developed a computer programme that analysed the hospital diet. This showed that the recommended daily intake of a number of nutrients could not be achieved even if patients ate everything from the hospital menu. Another audit demonstrated, first, that 33% of patients on intravenous feeding had infected lines and, secondly, that a number of patients either had inappropriate nutrition support or developed metabolic complications. Research by the nurse showed how poor the provision of nutrition was on the wards.

*The community and primary care teams.*   If we were starting now, there would be much more emphasis on links with the community and primary care teams (PCTs). These links have developed over a period of time in our area as an increasing number of patients have gone home on nutritional support. The benefits need to be sold to PCTs, adapting the approach to local circumstances and needs.

### Promotion of the nutrition support team

Published data and reports can be used. This is easier now than when our NST was set up because there is much more in the literature, including the Royal College of Physicians (RCP) report, 'Nutrition and patients – a doctor's responsibility'.[2]

Once a team is established, it needs to be advertised and everyone encouraged to take an interest in the nutritional welfare of patients. We held a 'nutrition week', which included an exhibition attended by hospital and community staff, chaired by the chairman of the health authority, with well-known figures in nutrition as speakers.

Even when a team is established, frequent staff changes in the hospital mean that there is a constant need to educate. Guidelines and protocols are valuable only if someone (usually from the team) ensures implementation.

### The role of the nutrition support team

Nutrition support mainly provides support for the care of patients with various conditions. The Amsterdam definition of 'patients suffering from metabolic stress'[3] is probably too limited. In both hospital and community, patients needing nutrition support are mainly those with acute or chronic neurological diseases (stroke, Parkinson's disease or motor neurone disease (MND)), but also those with gastrointestinal diseases or who have had surgery. Malignant disease is another important area, particularly malignancies of the head and neck and pre- and postoperatively.

### ☐ THE DOCTOR'S RESPONSIBILITY

Consultants involved in clinical nutrition should provide leadership and encouragement both to the team and to the hospital as a whole. To do this, they require both medical and nutritional expertise; it is in the co-ordination of both aspects that the doctor is able to provide effective leadership. Communication with patients, relatives and colleagues, including managers, is vital to ensure that the activity of the nutrition team fits in with the management plan. Sometimes it is difficult to persuade surgical colleagues to share their management plan with the team, and occasionally necessary to be firm and say that the particular form of therapy requested is not appropriate for a patient. This can be done only by someone with medical training and extensive medical knowledge.

The British Artificial Nutrition Survey indicates that only 87 of 211 DGHs have an NST (R Stratton and M Elia; personal communication). The data on consultants are worse: only 14 respondents to the RCP census of over 7,000 consultants reported a timetabled commitment to nutrition.[1] No doubt others involve themselves in nutrition support but undertake it in the midst of many other demands on their time.

### How much time should a consultant spend on clinical nutrition?

Table 1 shows that I spend over three notional half days (NHD) per week on nutrition. My current timetabled commitment is only one NHD.

**Table 1** The average time per week spent on nutrition.

| Activity | Time (hours) |
|---|---|
| Team meeting | 1 |
| Team ward round | 2–3 |
| Other visits: | |
|    •  hospital | 2 |
|    •  outpatients | 1 |
|    •  community | 3 |
| Other meetings & administration | 2 |
| Total per week on nutrition | 11–12 (>3NHD) |

NHD = notional half days.

### What expertise does the consultant require?

Patients requiring intravenous nutrition are generally those with problems that prevent them taking nourishment by mouth or by tube. They may have problems with electrolyte balance, infection that complicates surgery or cardiorespiratory problems, or metabolic consequences of intravenous feeding such as hyperglycaemia. A danger for malnourished patients fed by any route is the refeeding syndrome, a potentially fatal complication of nutritional support that is rarely taught to undergraduates or postgraduates. It encompasses acute changes in plasma phosphate, potassium, magnesium and glucose metabolism as well as thiamine deficiency, and can lead to severe cardiovascular, neurological, renal and haematological impairment with potentially fatal consequences.[4]

The audit data on intravenous feeding in our hospitals over the past four years are shown in Table 2. Colleagues are given clear guidelines and there is not normally a large number of inappropriate referrals; it is usually possible to manage about 40% of the patients without intravenous feeding. Those who are fed intravenously are nourished via a peripheral or central cannula for over three weeks. During the past four years there have been no infected lines – a tribute to our nutrition sisters who care for these lines as well as training patients for home total parenteral nutrition.

**Table 2** Audit data for intravenous nutrition (IVN): average number of patients per year (1998–2002).

| | |
|---|---|
| Referrals (inpatients) | 35 |
| Accepted | 20 |
| Duration of feeding | 24 days |
| Lines inserted | 26 |
| | (52% PIC or PICC) |
| Infected lines | 0 |
| IVN averted | 15 |

PIC = peripherally inserted cannula; PICC = peripherally inserted central cannula.

## Ethical questions: what is the aim of treatment?

In both intravenous and enteral feeding, the doctor needs to consider ethical questions. The key question is 'what is the aim of treatment'? Feeding by these routes is equivalent to providing an antibiotic or putting someone on a ventilator. Treatment that will not help the patient is inappropriate. In cases of doubt, a time limited trial of therapy may be considered. Discussions involving the patient, relatives and the staff caring for them can be time-consuming but, in my experience, always rewarding.

## Specific problems

### Nasogastric tube displacement

A common problem is nasogastric tube displacement. This and other problems with nasogastric feeding may give rise to requests for gastrostomy feeding. It is our belief that frequent displacement of the nasogastric tube is not a reason to insert a gastrostomy because it can be secured using a nasal loop (Fig 1). Patients can be discharged with this in place if necessary and nasogastric feeding continued at home or in nursing home care.

### Gastrostomy

A gastrostomy may be considered appropriate in some patients. The doctor will be involved in discussions about this as well as local problems related to gastrostomies that have already been inserted such as leakage and infection. Another problem is the so-called 'buried bumper' (Fig 2). This occurs when there is inadequate supervision of energy balance after percutaneous endoscopic gastrostomy (PEG) insertion. The patient gains weight, thus increasing the distance from skin to gastric mucosa; the tube is unable to lengthen, so 'buries' the internal bumper within the stomach wall.

*Audit of percutaneous endoscopic gastrostomy insertions.*   All units performing gastrostomy should audit outcomes. Table 3 lists the results of a three-year audit at Old-church Hospital on 423 patients referred for PEG. The average age of the 206 patients who received a PEG, their various conditions and the 30-day mortality are shown.[5]

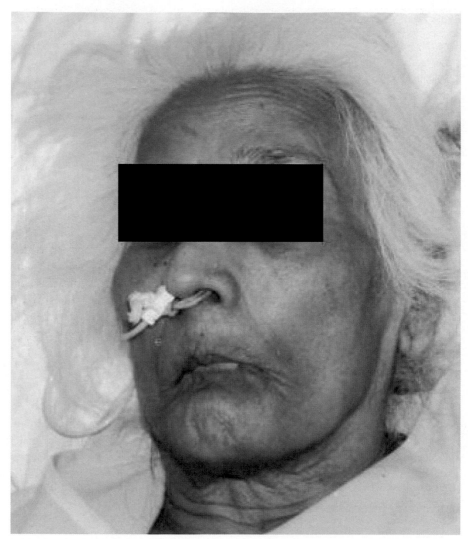

**Fig 1** Securing a nasogastric tube by means of a nasal loop.

The Nottingham group has recently published PEG results for two time periods 10 years apart (Table 3).[6] Fewer patients were involved than in our audit. Interestingly, the Nottingham 30-day mortality in 1988 was only 8% whereas in 1998 it was 19%. This increase was attributed to an older age group. This is probably not the real explanation as our patients were older too; it is likely that the answer lies in patient selection.

*Motor neurone disease*

A particularly difficult condition for patient selection is MND. Such patients are always able to discuss the condition and the risks and benefits of gastrostomy, even

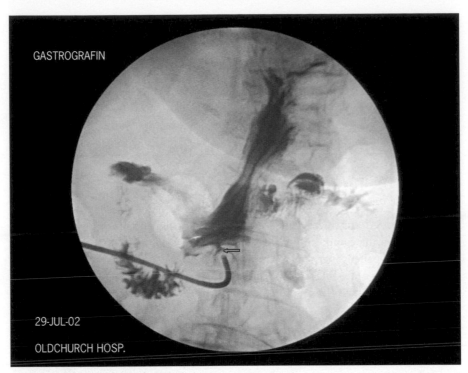

GASTROGRAFIN

29-JUL-02

OLDCHURCH HOSP.

**Fig 2** The so-called 'buried bumper'.

though communication may be difficult. Sometimes it is the first time they have discussed death, and conversations can be difficult. Our practice is to ask how they feel about resuscitation and ventilation (likely to be permanent) if they stop breathing. No patient has ever said that they want to be resuscitated or go on a ventilator. However, even with careful selection of patients, the 30-day mortality rate in MND was four times that of the overall audit for all PEGs (Table 4), but some patients survived for many months and they and their families appreciated this additional time.

**Table 3** Percutaneous endoscopic gastrostomy audits.

| | Oldchurch | Nottingham | |
|---|---|---|---|
| **Patient details** | **(1998–2001)** | **1998** | **1988** |
| Mean age (years) | 73 | 69 | 64 |
| 30-day mortality (%) | 7.3 | 19 | 8 |
| Patient types (%): | | | |
| • stroke | 60 | 42 | 33 |
| • head/neck cancer | 8 | 19 | 16 |
| • motor neurone disease | 6 | 4 | 27 |
| • other conditions | 26 | – | – |

**Table 4** Motor neurone disease (MND) and percutaneous endoscopic gastrostomy (PEG), Oldchurch (1998–2001).

---

- 25 patients referred over 3 years
- One patient found not to have MND
- 10 considered not fit for procedure
- 14 had PEG (4 (29%) died within 30 days)
- Average survival after insertion was 205 days, but some lived nearly twice as long
- Survival not related to age

---

*Home enteral tube feeding*

Patients on long-term enteral tube feeding should be fed either at home or in other care settings in the community if possible. Between 1998 and 2002, on average, we had nearly 140 patients per year on home enteral tube feeding, for each of whom the average duration of feeding was just under two years (530 days). During this period, 32% of all feeding days (hospital and community) were in the community.

### Teaching and training

A crucial role for the doctor in the NST is teaching and training. The aim should be to develop expertise among SpRs. It is encouraging that the new gastroenterology curriculum has reference to nutrition, albeit in a small way.[7] It is also important to share in the teaching of nurses and other healthcare professionals because nutrition requires a team approach.

## ☐ CONCLUSIONS

An NST requires medical expertise within it. Members of the team need to adapt to NHS changes. Every trust should have a consultant with training in nutrition who is allowed sufficient time in their timetable to be able to practise effectively. Clinical nutrition crosses the interface between primary and secondary care. Consultant expertise is valuable in preventing hospital admission and in ensuring that patients who are admitted do not stay in hospital any longer than is essential. It is important for SpRs to receive training within an NST so that they have a practical knowledge of the skills required (leadership, communication, medical and nutritional expertise). Courses are valuable but 'seeing is believing'.

## REFERENCES

1    Burnham WR . *Census of consultant physicians in the UK 2001*. London: Federation of Medical Royal Colleges, 2002.
2    *Nutrition and patients. A doctor's responsibility*. Report of a Working Party of the Royal College of Physicians of London. London: RCP, 2002.
3    Jonkers CF, Prins F, Van Kempen A, Tepaske R, Sauerwein HP. Towards implementation of optimum nutrition and better clinical nutrition support. *Clin Nutr* 2001;**20**:361–6.

4    Solomon SM, Kirby DF. The refeeding syndrome: a review. *J Parenter Enteral Nutr* 1990;14:90–7.

5    Chalmers-Watson TA, McKenzie CA, Burnham SP, Roberts G *et al.* An audit of the percutaneous endoscopic gastrostomy (PEG) service provided by a nutrition support team in a district general hospital over a three-year period. *Proc Nutr Soc* 2002;**61**:17A.

6    Skelly RH, Kupfer RM, Metcalfe ME, Allison SP *et al.* Percutaneous endoscopic gastrostomy (PEG): change in practice since 1988. *Clin Nutr* 2002;21:389–94.

7    *Higher Medical Training. Curriculum in gastroenterology.* London: Joint Committee for Higher Medical Training, January 2003.

# Nutrition in the intensive care unit

Simon Allison

## ☐ INTRODUCTION

It is difficult to prescribe a universal nutritional formula for use in the intensive care unit (ICU) in view of the heterogeneity of the patient population. Some high dependency units have a large proportion of patients, with or without prior malnutrition, recovering from major surgery or its complications. Other units have more patients with trauma, burns or sepsis, or suffering from catabolic illness and multiple organ failure (MOF). At the other extreme are patients with medical conditions such as status asthmaticus or diabetic ketoacidosis, who spend only two or three days in the unit before recovery and return to normal oral food intake.

There is little evidence that noncatabolic patients without prior malnutrition who spend less than five days in the unit benefit from aggressive nutritional support, or indeed suffer ill effects from a brief period of starvation. In contrast, those likely to spend more than five days in the unit should be started on artificial nutritional support without undue delay. There is growing evidence that the earlier this is begun, the better the outcome.[1]

Nutritional care must also be carefully integrated with other aspects of treatment with which it is interdependent, for example:[2]

☐ The administration of excessive amounts of glucose may increase oxygen consumption and carbon dioxide production, with corresponding embarrassment of lung function.

☐ Fluid and electrolyte overload may inhibit return of gastrointestinal (GI) function.

☐ Prolonged immobility may enhance muscle wasting, causing delays in recovery.

On the other hand, undernutrition impairs function in most organ systems resulting, for example, in muscle weakness (including respiratory weakness), impaired immunity and worse outcome.[1,3,4] Conversely, nutritional support produces striking improvements in function before regain of tissue mass, accompanied by better clinical outcome.[3,4] Impairment of function caused by malnutrition may embarrass organ systems.

A striking example of such integration is the enhanced recovery after surgery programmes developed by Scandinavian surgeons,[5] in which oral glucose given two hours before surgery reduces postoperative insulin resistance and negative nitrogen balance. This is combined with epidural analgesia, early mobilisation, oral intake on the first postoperative day and avoidance of excessive intravenous fluids. These measures have resulted in improved outcome and halving of hospital stay. Although these programmes have been developed in uncomplicated surgical patients, they have an important message for high dependency units devoted to recovery after major surgery.

## ☐ FACTORS AFFECTING NUTRITIONAL STATUS

### Prior malnutrition

Up to 40% of admissions to hospital have some degree of undernutrition, half of them sufficiently severe to affect clinical outcome.[2] Patients undergoing elective major surgery should therefore undergo nutritional screening before admission and, if found to be undernourished, receive some form of nutritional supplementation for 7–10 days prior to surgery.[6] Prior malnutrition is an important risk factor for mortality and morbidity in the ICU.[1] Malnutrition also tends to worsen during hospital stay due to inadequate nutritional care, with an average weight loss of 7–8%. This may continue following discharge unless appropriate measures are taken. At all stages, therefore, of the patient's journey through illness careful attention should be paid to adequate nutritional intake and monitoring. The main causes of disease-related malnutrition are anorexia and inability to take in, digest or absorb adequate amounts of food, although the catabolic response to injury is also an important factor.

### Response to injury[2]

In patients suffering severe trauma, major surgery or sepsis there is a neuro-endocrine and cytokine response to acute illness, causing an increase in metabolic rate and protein catabolism. This response has been divided into the initial shock or 'ebb' phase lasting a few hours, followed by the 'flow' phase, during which muscle protein is broken down to release amino acids for gluconeogenesis and the processes of healing and repair. This causes substrates such as glucose and amino acids to be diverted from the normal requirements for storage (eg glycogen) and muscle work. As protein and glycogen are broken down, potassium and phosphate are released from the cells and excreted, and there is an increased tendency to retain salt and water, or what Moore called the 'sodium retention' phase of injury.[7] These changes are mediated by the neuroendocrine response in which afferent signals reach the hypothalamus, stimulating high levels of catabolic hormones, catecholamines, cortisol and glucagon. During the ebb phase, insulin secretion is suppressed, but during the flow phase insulin and glucose levels are high, indicating insulin resistance.

Nutrition may ameliorate the wasting of lean mass in the critically ill but cannot abolish it. The metabolic tide does not turn until the convalescent or anabolic phase of injury is reached. Protein and glycogen synthesis are then restored, with cellular uptake of potassium and phosphate, causing a drop in the serum concentrations of these electrolytes. The capacity to excrete an excess salt and water load also returns: this is the sodium diuresis phase of injury.

The cytokine response,[8] with outpouring of interleukin-1 (IL-1), IL-6 and tumour necrosis factor, also stimulates the hypothalamus and an increase in metabolic rate with fever. It also has direct effects on tissues, enhancing catabolism. This phase is followed by secretion of counter-regulatory cytokines. These phases in the cytokine response have been termed the septic inflammatory response syndrome and compensatory anti-inflammatory response syndrome (CARS), although in practice there is considerable blurring of the two. The first phase is often associated with an initial septic episode, and the second with suppression of immune response and susceptibility to nosocomial infections and MOF.[1]

The extent of the cytokine response is genetically determined,[8] so patients who do not have an excessive response but who maintain adequate immune status are more likely to survive. Special substrates such as arginine, a precursor of nitric oxide (NO), may exaggerate the response, omega-3 fatty acids may suppress it, and both glutamine and arginine may enhance immunity in the second phase.

The whole subject of special substrates and immune-enhancing diets is bedevilled by the fact that different patients may respond differently to them, and because their response may be beneficial or adverse depending on the phase of the illness when such diets are introduced.

### Immobility[2,9]

Studies on immobilised normal subjects have shown muscle wasting, with corresponding negative nitrogen balance. This effect may be counteracted to some extent by physiotherapy using passive stretching exercises.[10]

### ☐ GOALS OF TREATMENT

Wolfe and colleagues summarised the goals of treatment as follows:

> The goal of nutritional management of critically ill patients is to promote wound healing and resistance to infection while preventing loss of muscle protein, since survival of critically-ill patients is inversely correlated with loss of lean mass.[11]

The limitations on achieving these goals have been described by Campbell:

> In the severely septic and injured patient, an improvement of nutritional status or increase of lean body mass by nutritional support alone is likely to be impossible. The most one can hope for is to slow the rate of decline. If lean body mass is to be maintained, it is likely that pharmacological methods will have to be found for doing so.[9]

### Minerals and micronutrients

To these aims should be added the correction or prevention of mineral and micronutrient deficiencies. Berger[12] has shown, for example, that burn patients lose excessive amounts of selenium, copper and zinc, and benefit from their supplementation. Many studies of nutritional support have had as their end-points reductions in mortality and complication rates, particularly infections. Lengths of stay in the ICU and in hospital have also been reduced.

### Complications of enteral and parenteral feeding

Another important goal is the avoidance of complications of feeding using enteral tubes or central venous lines. Expert nutrition teams can reduce the infection of central venous lines from around 30% to less than 1% using strict aseptic protocols when handling the catheters.[3] Mechanical complications may be similarly avoided by skilled operators. There is also a limit to the rate at which substrates may be administered without toxicity. The amount given enterally is limited by GI tolerance, but it is only too easy to give excess by the intravenous route.

Effects on outcome from nutritional or other interventions should be assessed not only for the period of ICU stay, but for the next 3–6 months since early interventions may have long-term benefits.

### ☐ TIMING OF FEEDS[11]

Although in many cases the priority over the first 24 hours after admission is cardiorespiratory resuscitation, there is increasing evidence that the earlier feeding is begun the more effective it is. This is certainly true for oral and enteral feeding after elective surgery, and there is evidence that this may also apply in other situations. It is reasonable to begin with half the patient's estimated requirements and build up to the full feed over 3–5 days. There are indications that failure to achieve 60% or more of requirements by this time diminishes the benefit of feeding.

### ☐ NUTRITIONAL REQUIREMENTS[2]

The former high metabolic rates of critically ill patients are now rarely seen due to improvement in other aspects of management, for example of wounds, infections, pain and fluid balance. The hyperalimentation regimens previously used in an attempt to bludgeon the response to injury into reverse have been abandoned in favour of a more conservative approach. Even burned patients rarely need an energy intake of more than 1.3 kcal/kg/day; although their resting energy expenditure may be increased above normal, this is partly offset by reduced energy consumption due to inactivity.

Resting energy expenditure may be estimated from the Harris-Benedict[13] or Schofield[14] equations, and total energy needs calculated, including carbohydrates (4 kcal/g), fat (9 kcal/g) and protein (4 kcal/g). In critically ill patients there may be considerable differences between estimated and measured energy expenditure, but the latter technique is available in only a few units and is demanding in expertise.

Intravenous glucose infusion at a higher rate than 5 mg/kg/min simply increases oxygen consumption and carbon dioxide production, with consequent respiratory embarrassment. Similarly, the administration of long-chain triglyceride fat emulsions above the recommended rate results in hyperlipidaemia and may cause respiratory, hepatic and immune problems, particularly in children. Studies of intravenous feeding have shown that when energy intake is adequate there is no advantage in increasing nitrogen intake above 0.25 g/kg/day, since excess nitrogen is simply converted to urea. The administration of fluid and electrolytes is also an important part of the calculation of nutritional requirements. Critically ill patients have difficulty in excreting an excess salt and water load and easily become oedematous, which may impair GI function, increase pulmonary complications and have other deleterious effects.

Patients who are re-fed after a period of starvation may also develop refeeding syndrome, with falls in serum potassium and phosphate concentrations as the cells take up these electrolytes. Biochemical monitoring, particularly in the early stages of feeding, is therefore important.

## ☐ ROUTES OF ADMINISTRATION[1]

### Enteral nutrition

Enteral feeding has advantages over parenteral feeding because of its specific effects on gut and immune function, so it is important to try to give at least some feed by the enteral route if this is tolerated. However, to achieve adequate nutritional intake in some cases, enteral feeding may need to be supplemented by parenteral feeding; this can be gradually withdrawn as GI tolerance improves.

Enteral feeding is not without its complications, particularly reflux and aspiration pneumonia. This complication is not diminished by nasojejunal, as opposed to nasogastric, feeding but is lessened by nursing the patient in the semi-recumbent position and giving the feed slowly.

Nasogastric feeding should begin at a rate of 20 ml/hour, aspirating the stomach four-hourly. If the residue does not exceed 300 ml, the feed rate may be cautiously increased. If there is prolonged impairment of gastric emptying, nasojejunal or jejunostomy feeding should be attempted. The needs of most patients are met using a standard polymeric feed with an energy content of 1 kcal/ml. Soluble fibre may improve intestinal function and diminish diarrhoea, although this complication is more often caused by concomitant antibiotics than by the feed *per se*. Bloating and abdominal distension may embarrass respiratory function, and necessitate reduction in the feed infusion rate. It should also be remembered that the micronutrient concentration of enteral feeds is such that the requirement for these nutrients can be met only if the full amount of feed is given per day. Micronutrient supplementation may be needed if this is not achieved.

### Parenteral nutrition

For the benefits of parenteral nutrition to outweigh the risks, it needs to be administered by a team experienced in its use in order to avoid the complications of central venous lines and the metabolic consequences of inappropriate feed formulae. It is doubtful if parenteral nutrition itself is harmful, provided that it is given properly. Indeed, studies comparing the combination of parenteral and enteral nutrition with enteral alone found a better outcome with the combination.

## □ SPECIAL SUBSTRATES[1]

So-called 'immune-enhancing diets' containing arginine (NO precursor and immune stimulant), omega-3 fatty acids (to decrease inflammatory response), nucleotides and, in some cases, glutamine have been studied extensively in critically ill patients. There is clear evidence of improved outcome, particularly in the reduction of infections, when the immune-enhancing cocktails are administered pre- and postoperatively to patients undergoing major GI surgery for cancer, and there is some evidence of benefit in major trauma. There is insufficient evidence, however, to warrant their general use in the ICU population.

In contrast, the data on glutamine are more convincing, particularly when given intravenously. Most enterally administered glutamine is metabolised by the upper GI tract, and little reaches the circulation to provide this important substrate for immune tissue and for the synthesis of glutathione, an important antioxidant.

Further studies are required using individual substrates in defined patient groups at particular phases of illness. For example, it may be deleterious to enhance NO production with arginine in a patient during the first few days of a huge inflammatory response. Conversely, the support of the immune system during the CARS phase could, on theoretical grounds, produce benefit.

## □ ADJUNCTIVE THERAPY[15]

Beneficial effects of insulin and growth hormone on protein metabolism in critically ill patients were shown many years ago. Unfortunately, studies of clinical outcome with growth hormone were negative, although recent studies of insulin administration to maintain normoglycaemia have shown striking improvements in outcome.[16] Hyperglycaemia is known to be associated with increased risk of infection, but it is still unclear whether the insulin effects described were caused solely by normalising the blood sugar or also by its other beneficial effects.

## □ PRE- AND PROBIOTICS[17]

The problem of infections in the ICU continues to outstrip current methods of management and the stock of antibiotics. Measures to increase resistance to invasive nosocomial infections are therefore of growing interest. One such measure is the manipulation of the intestinal flora using pre- and probiotics. The present position has recently been reviewed.[17]

## □ SUMMARY AND CONCLUSIONS

Nutritional care should be properly integrated into the overall management of critically ill patients, particularly those who spend more than five days in the ICU. Feeding should be started as early as possible and built up slowly to meet full requirements over 3–5 days, whether by the intravenous or enteral route. The latter is preferred for its effects on GI function and immunity, but may need to be supplemented or replaced by parenteral feeding where there is GI intolerance.

A skilled nutrition team reduces the complications of artificial nutrition and increases the benefits by giving appropriate formulae and avoiding excess of substrates, fluid and electrolytes which may produce toxicity. Care should be taken with adequate micronutrient administration, particularly in major trauma and sepsis.

The use of glutamine, particularly by the parenteral route, is well established, although immune-enhancing diet cocktails have proven their worth only when given perioperatively in major surgery and in some major trauma. Adjunctive therapy with insulin has benefits in terms of carbohydrate and protein metabolism, as well as improving outcome.

## REFERENCES

1   Griffiths RD. Nutrition support in critically ill septic patients. *Curr Opin Clin Nutr Metab Care* 2003;**6**:203–10.

2   Allison SP. Nutritional support. In: Healy TE, Knight PR (eds). *A practice of anesthesia*, 7th edn. London: Hodder Arnold, 2003:1063–77.

3   Allison SP. The uses and limitations of nutritional support. *Clin Nutr* 1992;**11**:319–30.

4   Stratton RJ, Elia M, Green CJ. *Disease related malnutrition: an evidence-based approach to treatment*. Oxford: CAB International, 2003.

5   Nygren J. Accelerated recovery from surgery. *Clin Nutr* 2002;**21**:171–3.

6   Allison SP. Perioperative nutrition in elective surgery. In: Pichard C, Kudsk KA (eds). *From nutrition support to pharmacologic nutrition in the ICU. Update in intensive care and emergency medicine*. Berlin: Springer Verlag, 2000.

7   Moore FD. *Metabolic care of the surgical patient*. Philadelphia: Saunders, 1959.

8   Grimble RF. Stress proteins in disease: metabolism on a knife edge. Review. *Clin Nutr* 2001;**20**:469–76.

9   Campbell IT. Limitations of nutrient intake. The effect of stressors: trauma, sepsis and multiple organ failure. Review. *Eur J Clin Nutr* 1999;**53**(Suppl 1):S143–7.

10   Griffiths RD. The 1995 John M Kinney International Award for Nutrition and Metabolism. Effect of passive stretching on the wasting of muscle in the critically ill: background. Review. *Nutrition* 1997;**13**:70–4.

11   Sakurai Y, Aarsland A, Herndon DN, Chinkes DL *et al.* Stimulation of muscle protein synthesis by long-term insulin infusion in severely burned patients. *Ann Surg* 1995;**222**:283–97.

12   Chiolero RL, Berger M. *Key vitamins and trace elements in the critically ill.* Nestlé Nutrition Workshop Series, Clinical and Performance Program, vol 8, Nutrition and Critical Care. Basel: Karger SA, 2003:99–118.

13   Harris JA, Benedict FG. *A biometric study of basal metabolism in man.* Publication no. 279. Washington, DC: Carnegie Institute, 1919.

14   Schofield WN. Predicting basal metabolic rate, new standards and review of previous work. *Hum Nutr Clin Nutr* 1985;**39C**(Suppl 1):5–41.

15   Martinez-Riquelme AE, Allison SP. Insulin revisited. *Clin Nutr* 2003;**22**:7–15.

16   Van den Berghe G, Wouters P, Weekers F, Verwaest C *et al.* Intensive insulin therapy in the critically ill patients. *N Engl J Med* 2001;**345**:1359–67.

17   Bengmark S. Gut microenvironment and immune function. Review. *Curr Opin Clin Nutr Metab Care* 1999;**2**:83–5.

☐ NUTRITION AND PATIENTS: A DOCTOR'S RESPONSIBILITY SELF
  ASSESSMENT QUESTIONS

### Why the metabolic syndrome?

1   The metabolic syndrome is characterised by:
    (a) Upper body obesity
    (b) Raised high-density lipoprotein (HDL) cholesterol
    (c) Type 2 diabetes
    (d) Hypothyroidism
    (e) Raised blood pressure

2   Factors contributing to insulin resistance:
    (a) Increased subcutaneous abdominal fat
    (b) Increased release of free fatty acids into the portal vein
    (c) Increased cytokines released from fat
    (d) Reduced hepatic gluconeogenesis
    (e) Increased glucose uptake by skeletal muscle

3   Non-alcoholic steatohepatitis (NASH):
    (a) Is characterised by fatty infiltration in the liver
    (b) May progress to cirrhosis in 50% of cases
    (c) Is always associated with overweight or obesity
    (d) The ratio of alanine transaminase to aspartate transaminase is greater than 1
    (e) Sudden weight loss reverses NASH

4   Plasminogen activator inhibitor-1:
    (a) Plasma levels correlate with degree of obesity
    (b) Plasma concentrations are correlated with degree of hypertriglyceridaemia
    (c) Plasma concentrations are important in determining the risk associated
        with the metabolic syndrome
    (d) Raised levels are associated with decreased thrombosis risk
    (e) Production in liver is regulated by insulin

### Clinical nutrition in a district general hospital

1   The role of a doctor in a nutrition team:
    (a) To liaise with medical colleagues about clinical and nutritional aspects of
        the care of patients
    (b) To educate doctors in training
    (c) To be a figurehead only
    (d) Does not require a timetabled commitment
    (e) Is important in considering issues involving medical ethics

2   Clinical nutrition is:
    (a) Not important in hospital
    (b) Relevant only to health education

    (c) Does not require medical input
    (d) Best delivered through a team approach
    (e) A complex subject and only for academics

3    A nutrition support team can:
    (a) Reduce infective complications in intravenous nutrition
    (b) Cure other medical problems by nutrition support alone
    (c) Help to reduce metabolic complications during artificial nutritional support
    (d) Deal only with metabolic problems in nutrition
    (e) Only help patients in hospital

4    Percutaneous endoscopic gastrostomy:
    (a) Is the only method of delivering long-term enteral tube feeding
    (b) Is a procedure without any risk to the patient
    (c) Requires no aftercare
    (d) Should always be given if patients remove their nasogastric tube
    (e) Is more risky in motor neurone disease

5    The refeeding syndrome is:
    (a) A minor problem
    (b) Associated with a high serum phosphate
    (c) Associated with a low serum potassium
    (d) Associated with a low serum albumin
    (e) Associated with a low serum magnesium

## Nutrition in the intensive care unit

1    The metabolic response to injury involves:
    (a) Decreased lipolysis
    (b) Increased metabolic rate
    (c) Impaired gluconeogenesis
    (d) Increased glucose production
    (e) Net protein catabolism

2    Energy intake in most patients during critical illness should:
    (a) Be double estimated resting metabolic rate (RMR)
    (b) Be 1.0–1.3 times estimated RMR
    (c) Be met by carbohydrate alone
    (d) Include carbohydrate less than 300 mg/kg/hour
    (e) Be calculated from combined intake of carbohydrate and protein

3    In most critically ill patients, nitrogen balance:
    (a) Is optimal when energy requirements are met
    (b) Is independent of energy requirements

   (c)  Is not improved above an intake of 0.15 g/kg/day

   (d)  Is not improved above an intake of 0.25 g/kg/day

   (e)  Is more negative because of immobility

4   There is good evidence of benefit from:

   (a)  Use of glutamine in critical illness

   (b)  Use of immune-enhancing diets in all critically ill patients

   (c)  Use of immune-enhancing diets prior to major upper abdominal surgery

   (d)  Maintenance of normoglycaemia in critical illness with high-dose insulin

   (e)  Giving saline despite an expanded extracellular fluid volume

# Imaging

# Interventional magnetic resonance imaging

Wladyslaw Gedroyc

## □ INTRODUCTION

The soft tissue contrast and discrimination capabilities of magnetic resonance (MR) are so much better than all other imaging modalities that its use for imaging in an interventional environment has been a long-term goal for many radiologists working in this field. If MR could be used for imaging during intervention, there should be great potential to carry out procedures with much greater accuracy and safety without the use of any form of ionising radiation. This would allow more to be done from less invasive approaches, thus decreasing patient morbidity and mortality and also substantially decreasing inpatient hospital stays.

Interventional MR (IMR) falls into the much larger grouping of image guidance of therapy. It uses many different forms of imaging modality, often integrated with computer assisted reconstructions producing 3D reformats and virtual reconstruction images which allow improved guidance of delivery of a wide range of therapies.

IMR has become a large field and the ability to discuss it comprehensively in one chapter is inevitably limited. Different practitioners focus on different specialist areas with this technique, so any single description is to some extent a personal review and interpretation of IMR.

## □ TECHNOLOGY

There are predominantly two types of environment in which IMR is carried out:

1    Procedures carried out at the side of an MR scanner, with some form of needle or instrument movement followed by pushing the patient into the scanner for imaging. After removing the patient from the scanner there is further instrument motion or biopsy in response to the images obtained. This type of procedure is usually carried out in a high field closed MR system which prevents the operator carrying out the procedure during the scan acquisition.

2    MR procedures in close to real-time, with instrument movement as in biopsies, are performed during MR acquisition with continuous updates produced. This type of procedure is almost inevitably carried out within some form of open scanner.

Open systems are becoming quite common and have two predominant configurations:

1    The so-called hamburger design where the patient lies between two of the magnet components placed horizontally above and below him. This configuration is usually at relatively low field strengths below 0.2 T.

2    A design in which there is a vertical split between two ring magnet components. These scanners are normally at 0.5 T field strength (Fig 1). The vertically separated midfield units allow both horizontal and vertical access to patients in the gap between the magnets which is the imaging field.

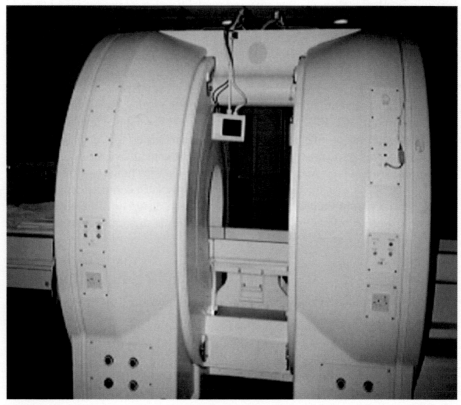

**Fig 1** 0.5 T open magnet (Signa SP10, GE medical systems, Milwaukee, USA). The vertical gap between the two vertical rings (the imaging volume) allows both horizontal and vertical access to the patient.

The more horizontal hamburger design limits access to horizontal approaches through the side of the patient in normal circumstances. The midfield units with vertically separated magnets allow a much greater range of procedures to be performed within the scanning environment because there is both horizontal and vertical access to the patient in the imaging volume. This is of particular benefit for open surgical procedures which are difficult in the lower field systems, requiring the patient to be intermittently removed from between the magnets if surgery is to be performed.

The disadvantage of both systems is that compromises have to be made in terms of imaging speed and gradient strength to achieve an open environment in which procedures can be performed. The quality of the images currently obtained is unequivocally inferior to that produced by conventional closed 1.5 T high-speed gradient machines.

Systems are available that attempt to utilise closed short-bore 1.5 T machines in an interventional environment. They are combined with a fluoroscopy unit located approximately 5–10 m from the magnet bore and connected to it by an MR compatible bed guide (rather like a short railway line) which can move the patient directly from the fluoroscopy area into the MR scanner. This hybrid system has advantages in that it is able to use better quality MR images from the 1.5 T scanner, but it does not allow real-time imaging of instrumentation in the MR scanner itself and introduces new difficulties into the procedure.

## □ APPLICATIONS

There are several applications of IMR imaging. This review will focus on the first three areas listed, rather than the other three areas of emerging application.

- □   Biopsies.

- □   MR guidance of open surgery.

- □   Thermal ablation procedures including focused ultrasound.

- □   Intravascular MR procedures.

- □   Endoscopic tracking.

- □   Erect biomechanical imaging.

## □ BIOPSIES

MR is selected for biopsies in several circumstances:

- □   When a complex multiplanar path is required to reach a particular target: for example, to puncture a liver lesion when only a small window can be found between low lying lung, high lying colon and gall bladder.

- □   When MR is the only modality that shows an individual area of pathology: for example, enhancing breast lesions not visualised on other modalities.

- □   Perhaps the most common indication overall is when there is a combination of these circumstances.

Many neurosurgical units now use MR guidance for frameless stereotactic biopsies of brain lesions.[1] This allows the biopsy needle to be guided in real-time to the lesion without the use of frames, and does not require information to be obtained from scans prior to carrying out a burr hole. There is frequent and significant motion of the brain after the skull is opened in these circumstances; this can result in scans prior to surgery providing misleading measurements for planning a regular stereotactic biopsy.

## ☐ MAGNETIC RESONANCE GUIDANCE OF OPEN SURGERY

Operative procedures to resect abnormalities from solid organs or solid tissues do not normally allow surgeons to visualise the entirety of the targeted area which is usually buried within the organ. Examples of this are resection of masses from brain or the breast. MR guidance can provide an extra dimension in this context, allowing an operator to assess the exact site of the target relative to adjacent structures. The extent of the resection as it proceeds and how it affects nearby vital structures can both be displayed.[2]

Surgery can be performed entirely within the magnet bore in some open magnets, particularly with vertical access to the patient which allows the procedure to be performed without having to move the patient in or out of the field. This has proved a popular approach for certain areas of neurosurgery, allowing rapid and easy targeting of lesions and assessment of the completeness of resection as an operation proceeds.

There are two obvious disadvantages of this approach:

1    The space is relatively limited within the bore of the magnet. This is unfamiliar to surgeons and may make the operation more difficult.

2    Conventional ferromagnetic instruments cannot be used easily within the high field system. Regular iron-based instruments have a significant magnetic moment in the scanner, and even non-magnetic steel instruments cause massive distortion of imaging if left in the field, although they may not experience a significant attraction to the magnet.

A substantial number of breast and perianal surgical procedures have been carried out at St Mary's Hospital.[2,3] Similar principles can be applied in many other areas where benign or malignant conditions are removed from solid tissues; MR can be used to control the site and extent of the surgical resection.

### Breast procedures

In the context of breast operations, the aim is to minimise repeat interventions by producing a more complete initial excision of the target mass using MR guidance.

### Perianal disease

In perianal disease, the surgeon is often faced with multiple fistulous tracks which may run through and around the anal sphincters in an unpredictable manner. MR imaging at intervals during surgery allows the ramifications of these tracks to be visualised and accessed. It also shows their relationship to the anal sphincters, enabling comprehensive treatment without damaging vital sphincter function.

## ☐ THERMAL ABLATION

Thermal ablation procedures are developing as effective local therapy for local disease in solid organs. Several methods are used to deliver energy to solid tissue including:

- ☐ laser fibres

- ☐ radio frequency ablation devices

- ☐ microwave electrodes, and

- ☐ cryotherapy probes.

All these devices except cryotherapy cause tissue heating and destroy cells by coagulating the cellular proteins without causing ischaemic syndromes. The great advantage of MRI in this field is that it can detect the heating or cooling effects of these probes within tissue as they occur. The operator is able to observe the amount of tissue being heated and the site of heating, and therefore to interact with the procedure to improve its accuracy, safety and reproducibility. No other modality can accurately provide such rapid feedback in this process. In effect, MRI can provide an *in vivo* thermal map of the whole heating process.[4]

Water cooled laser fibres are predominantly used as a heat source in MR guided procedures because they are entirely MR compatible. Current radio frequency probes cause significant distortion of the scanning process, preventing good imaging at the time of heat application. Modern interstitial laser fibres with water cooling are similar in overall tissue results to modern radio frequency systems.

Thermal ablation procedures have been carried out in a number of solid organs, but this section will focus on the main areas that we have treated with MR guided procedures:

- ☐ liver

- ☐ kidney, and

- ☐ uterine fibroids.

### Technique

A thermal map is produced using T1 magnitude subtraction images to give a colourised map of the heated area.[4] This works on the principle of comparing the signal loss with the initial template scan with that produced by heating within tissues during MR scanning. The amount of signal loss is displayed as a colourised scale which is then superimposed on the updated image to provide a sensitive colourised thermal map of the heated area which is refreshed every three seconds (Fig 2). In this situation, the colour scale is much more sensitive than the grey scale appearance of the raw data.[4]

One to three (or even four) water cooled laser fibres, each of which receives 25 W, are placed at the target site under MR guidance. MR guidance for puncturing the target lesion allows complex multiplanar oblique trajectories to be used, enabling lesions to

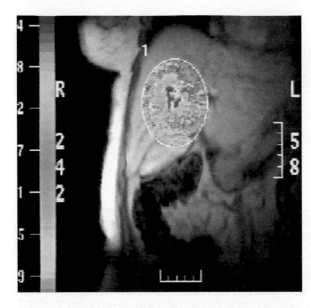

**Fig 2** Colourised thermal map of laser liver ablation procedure. The colour scale was calibrated by initial animal work: any colour beyond green is above 55°C (the temperature at which cellular proteins are coagulated). In this patient, who has a colorectal carcinoma liver secondary, the total size of ablated area was 5 cm using one water cooled fibre.

be accessed more safely in complex areas and in difficult patients, particularly where safe windows of passage into targets are strictly limited.[5] A typical example is a patient with chronic obstructive airways disease who has a lesion in the liver and in whom hyperinflated lungs cover large portions of the liver, thus making conventional punctures with ultrasound or computed tomography highly problematic.

Conventional iron and steel needles cannot be used for these punctures because of the artefact they would induce in the image. Modified needles made of titanium nickel alloys and similar substances provide adequate alternatives.

## Liver

This type of procedure has been used extensively in the liver. In local disease (fewer than five lesions, none >5 cm diameter) a mean survival of four years for all metastases treated is achievable in the best hands.[6] Five-year survival rates for hepatic colorectal carcinoma metastases of up to 30%, and slightly higher for patients with breast carcinoma hepatic metastases (34%), have been described.

Excellent results were obtained in a group of patients with predominantly hepatocellular carcinoma (Fig 3), with at least a doubling of normal survival. However, at present not nearly so many of these cases have been treated worldwide as for metastasis.[6]

## Kidney

A similar approach can be used in the treatment of renal cell carcinoma. Renal tumours can be punctured under MR guidance with needles and laser fibres, and heating used to destroy tissue (Fig 4). Our group has used this approach in a small number of patients[7] who:

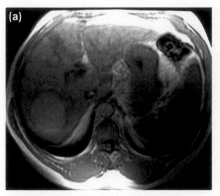
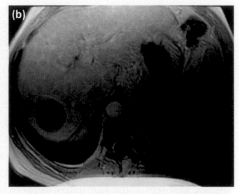

**Fig 3** A patient with a 4 cm diameter hepatocellular carcinoma on a background of cirrhotic change: **(a)** moderate enhancement post-contrast administration (gadolinium DTPA); **(b)** the same patient four weeks after an ablation procedure using the same post-contrast procedure as in (a). The same lesion no longer enhances following heat destruction, although it remains unchanged in size.

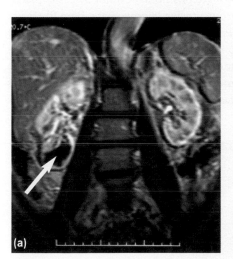
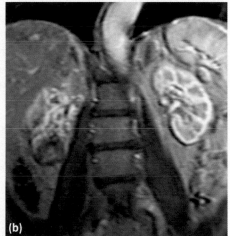

**Fig 4** A patient with a lower pole renal carcinoma: **(a)** after contrast (arrowed) in the right kidney, with peripheral enhancement; **(b)** the same patient 12 months after an ablation procedure. The same area in the lower pole now shows no significant enhancement, but is not greatly changed in size.

☐   had single kidneys

☐   would probably have needed dialysis following a significant surgical procedure

☐   were medically unfit for surgery

☐   refused surgery, or

☐   were unsuitable for surgery for some other reason.

Promising results have been obtained using this technique. Although half the small group of 12 patients treated in this way have died over the ensuing three years, none has died of the primary renal tumour.

## Uterine fibroids

Uterine fibroids are extremely common in women of childbearing age. They cause huge morbidity, and some estimates suggest that as much as $3 billion are spent annually on their treatment in the USA. Conventional therapy for uterine fibroids predominantly involves radical surgery such as hysterectomy or myomectomy. Increasing numbers of women now do not accept this type of treatment for a benign disease and seek some alternative approach.

The same principles as for liver and kidney have been used to treat uterine fibroids with a percutaneous heat ablation procedure. Laser fibres can be placed percutaneously under MR guidance in the centre of uterine fibroids (Fig 5) and heat applied. Water cooled fibres are not used because the plastic transparent thermostable tubes through which the fibres are positioned cannot be easily placed into the centre of extremely tough and fibrous uterine leiomyomata. Bare fibres are placed via metallic needles and heating performed at 5 W per fibre. MR guidance and thermal mapping are used as before to improve accuracy and safety. Our results in this field[8] indicate that the volume of the targeted fibroid may be reduced by 35% and symptoms by at least 70% over three months. This type of therapy usually gives sufficient symptomatic improvement in treated women for further surgical options to be rarely necessary.

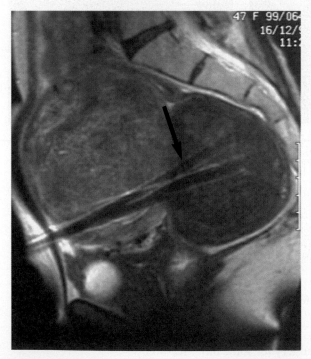

**Fig 5** Magnetic resonance (MR) compatible needles placed in a deep uterine fibroid mass (arrowed) deep in the pelvis. MR guidance was used prior to MR thermal ablation with laser fibres.

## High intensity focused ultrasound

The success of treating uterine fibroids with laser heating has led to the use of high intensity focused ultrasound in this field. This procedure uses a complex phased array ultrasound transducer with approximately 5–10,000 times the power of conventional diagnostic ultrasound. The transducer is carefully focused on an area in a uterine fibroid, causing rapid heating of this area leading to cell destruction. It is a completely non-invasive procedure, but is carried out in a conventional closed high-field MR scanner which allows careful targeting of the selected area of tissue (Fig 6). Thermal sensitive sequences are used to feed back the tissue response so that an accurate complete ablation can be obtained.

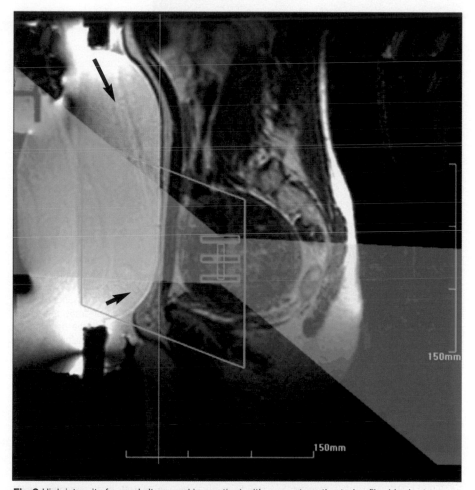

**Fig 6** High intensity focused ultrasound in a patient with a symptomatic uterine fibroid prior to onset of treatment. The green shaded area represents the potential path of the ultrasound beam for planning to assess whether any vital structures are in the path of the beam (eg bowel). Note large gel pad to assist in providing an acoustic window for treatment and to displace bowel from beam path (black arrows). Green rectangles projected over the fibroid represent three potential areas of sonication.

To date, 36 patients with uterine fibroids have been treated in this way as part of a multinational study. There are promising early results (Fig 7), which suggest that this modality may become an important way of treating abnormal tissue in solid organs. Focused ultrasound guided by MR provides a completely non-invasive method of tissue destruction which can be controlled by direct online tissue feedback, enabling the adjustment of factors to overcome the substantial variation in tissue response to this type of rapid tissue heating.

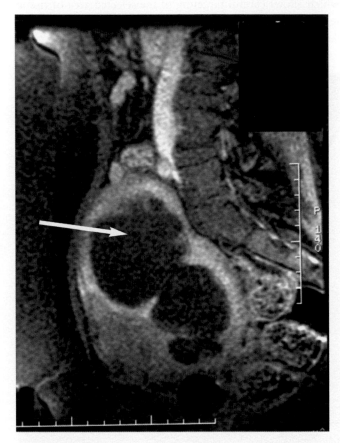

**Fig 7** Appearance of a fibroid uterus immediately after focused ultrasound treatment. The images were obtained after intravenous contrast and the whole uterus should be uniformly enhanced. The low signal areas represent areas of tissue destruction induced by multiple sonications in these positions (arrowed).

## REFERENCES

1   Kollias SS, Bernays R, Marugg RA, Romanowski B *et al.* Target definition and trajectory optimization for interactive MR-guided biopsies of brain tumors in an open configuration MRI system. *J Magn Reson Imaging* 1998;8:143–59.

2   Gould SW, Agarwal T, Benoist S, Patel B *et al.* Resection of soft tissue sarcomas with intra-operative magnetic resonance guidance. *J Magn Reson Imaging* 2002;15:114–9.

3   Gould SW, Lamb G, Lomax D, Gedroyc W, Darzi A. Interventional MR-guided excisional biopsy of breast lesions. *J Magn Reson Imaging* 1998;8:26–30.

4   Dick EA, Wragg P, Joarder R, De Jode M *et al.* Feasibility of abdomino-pelvic T1-weighted real-time thermal mapping of laser ablation. *J Magn Reson Imaging* 2003;17:197–205.

5    de Jode MG, Lamb GM, Thomas HC, Taylor-Robinson SD, Gedroyc WM. MRI guidance of infra-red laser liver tumour ablations, utilising an open MRI configuration system: technique and early progress. *J Hepatol* 1999;**31**:347–53.

6    Vogl TJ, Straub R, Eichler K, Woitaschek D, Mack MG. Malignant liver tumors treated with MR imaging-guided laser-induced thermotherapy: experience with complications in 899 patients (2,520 lesions). *Radiology* 2002;**225**:367–77.

7    Dick EA, Joarder R, De Jode MG, Wragg P *et al.* Magnetic resonance imaging-guided laser thermal ablation of renal tumours. *BJU Int* 2002;**90**:814–22.

8    Hindley JT, Law PA, Hickey M, Smith SC *et al.* Clinical outcomes following percutaneous magnetic resonance image guided laser ablation of symptomatic uterine fibroids. *Hum Reprod* 2002;**17**:2737–41.

# ☐ IMAGING SELF ASSESSMENT QUESTIONS

## Interventional magnetic resonance imaging

1   Magnetic resonance (MR) machines used in interventional MR:
    (a)  Are a minimum of 1.5 T field strength
    (b)  Are never greater than 0.5 T field strength
    (c)  Are problematic with ferromagnetic instruments
    (d)  Produce less rapid images at a lower field strength
    (e)  Are more adaptable to multiple procedures with a vertical gap

2   MR guidance of therapy can:
    (a)  Show tissue responses to heat
    (b)  Show tissue responses to cold
    (c)  Allow multiplanar oblique targeting of tissues
    (d)  Show tissue responses secondary to radio frequency application
    (e)  Demonstrate the path of a normal biopsy needle

3   MR guidance of surgery:
    (a)  Is commonly used in the brain
    (b)  Is rarely possible
    (c)  Indicates the extent of a tumour within solid tissue
    (d)  Limits the surgeon's appreciation of the surgical field
    (e)  Requires extensive MR compatible instrumentation

4   Laser thermal ablation of the liver:
    (a)  Can be guided by MR
    (b)  Can produce survival rates comparable with surgery
    (c)  Works best with power of over 100 W per fibre
    (d)  Can be used only for single liver lesions
    (e)  Works better with bare fibres than with water cooled fibres

5   High intensity focused ultrasound:
    (a)  Causes heating in a small focal spot in solid tissue
    (b)  Causes tissue damage by ischaemic necrosis
    (c)  Can be carried out only from within the body
    (d)  Requires five minutes per sonication
    (e)  Is well transmitted through bowel

# Infection:
# the Antiviral Revolution

# Treatment of HIV infection

Duncan Churchill

## □ INTRODUCTION

There were few precedents in twentieth century medicine for the rapid advances in the treatment of HIV infection that occurred in the late 1990s. Over a period of a few years, the outlook for someone with even advanced HIV disease was completely transformed: death rates fell dramatically and previously intractable opportunistic infections resolved.[1] For example, the number of deaths recorded in the clinic database at St Mary's Hospital, London, decreased from 172 in 1994 to only 23 in 1998, despite the clinic population increasing by around 30% during this period (Fig 1). These changes were mainly due to three innovations:

□   the introduction of new drugs, particularly protease inhibitors (PIs)

□   the routine use in clinical practice of measurements of plasma HIV viral load to guide decisions about starting therapy and to assess effectiveness of therapy, and

□   improved understanding of the dynamics of HIV replication, leading to more intelligent use of the available drugs.

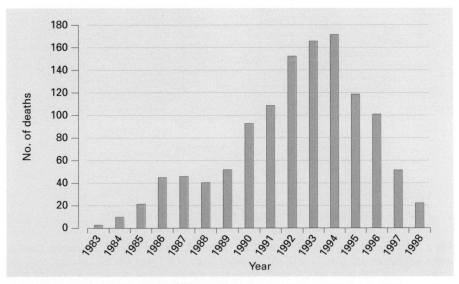

**Fig 1** The number of recorded deaths from all causes among patients attending HIV services at St Mary's Hospital, London, 1983–1998.

## ☐ ANTIRETROVIRAL THERAPY

The life cycle of HIV is illustrated in Fig 2. All except one of the currently available antiretroviral drugs (Table 1) are designed to inhibit the viral reverse transcriptase or protease enzymes. The exception is enfuvirtide, the most recently licensed antiretroviral agent, which inhibits fusion of the virus with the cell membrane. No drugs are available that inhibit HIV integrase, although several compounds are in development.

The first antiretroviral drug to be licensed was zidovudine, a nucleoside analogue reverse transcriptase inhibitor initially developed (before HIV was identified) as a cytotoxic agent. In contrast, the HIV PIs were synthesised after identification of HIV, specifically to inhibit HIV protease by acting as mimics of the cleavage sites in the viral polyprotein.

### Early studies

The initial licensing study of zidovudine[2] was a placebo-controlled, double-blind study in patients with advanced disease. It was terminated early following a planned

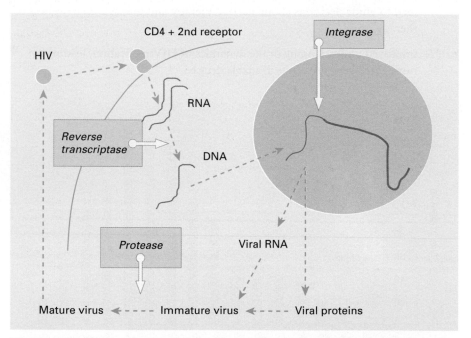

**Fig 2** HIV life cycle. Free virus is bound to CD4 on the surface of a CD4+ T lymphocyte, together with a second receptor (CXCR4 or CCR5). Following fusion of the virus with the cell membrane, two strands of viral RNA enter the cytoplasm where they are transcribed into proviral DNA under the control of the viral reverse transcriptase enzyme. Proviral DNA is then transported to the nucleus, where it is integrated into the cellular genome in a series of steps that are catalysed by the enzyme integrase. Proviral DNA then directs the synthesis of more viral RNA and viral proteins, which are packaged together to form immature virus. The action of a third viral enzyme, protease, cleaves viral proteins to form infectious virus, which is released from the cell to infect further cells.

**Table 1** Antiretroviral drugs licensed in Europe, June 2003.

| Fusion inhibitors | Reverse transcriptase inhibitors | | | Protease inhibitors |
|---|---|---|---|---|
| | Nucleoside analogues | Nucleotide analogues | Nonnucleosides | |
| Enfuvirtide | Zidovudine | Tenofovir | Nevirapine | Saquinavir |
| | Zalcitabine | | Efavirenz | Ritonavir |
| | Didanosine | | | Indinavir |
| | Lamivudine | | | Nelfinavir |
| | Stavudine | | | Amprenavir |
| | Abacavir | | | Lopinavir |

interim analysis because there had been 19 deaths in the placebo arm, and only one in the zidovudine arm. This led to widespread use of zidovudine monotherapy in advanced disease. Later studies suggested that earlier use of the drug was associated both with less toxicity and also with a reduction in the risk of some clinical indicators of immune suppression such as oral candidiasis. The limitations of monotherapy in early disease were not fully appreciated, however, until 1993 when the results of the Concorde study were first reported.[3] Concorde, a placebo-controlled study of early versus deferred treatment with zidovudine in 1,749 patients, found no benefit of early zidovudine versus later treatment on either disease progression or survival.

By this stage, it was clear that, although zidovudine delayed disease progression, the benefits were relatively short-lived (ca 6 months) and at the cost of considerable toxicity – relatively high doses were used, and side effects such as nausea and anaemia were common. The situation did not improve until September 1995 when the results of three studies comparing zidovudine monotherapy with dual therapy were first presented. The largest of these studies was the Delta study[4] in which 3,207 patients were randomised to receive zidovudine, zidovudine/didanosine or zidovudine/zalcitabine. The median follow-up was 30 months. The results showed that dual therapy was clearly superior to monotherapy, particularly in previously untreated patients – such patients in the zidovudine/didanosine arm had a 42% lower risk of death. Nevertheless, although these results indicated an important advance in antiretroviral therapy, there were still 699 deaths during the period of the study, and 936 of the 2,765 HIV infected patients without AIDS at entry developed an AIDS diagnosis during the study.

## ☐ HIV DYNAMICS

Earlier in 1995, groups in the USA led by David Ho, in New York,[5] and George Shaw, in Alabama,[6] reported a series of experiments in which plasma viral load was repeatedly measured in individual patients treated for brief periods with potent new antiretroviral agents, particularly the PI ritonavir. Plasma viral load varied substantially from one patient to another, but tended to be consistent in an individual at baseline. Large and rapid falls in viral load were seen with drug treatment in almost all patients. Data generated by these experiments showed that $10^9$–$10^{10}$ virions were produced each day in all infected individuals, regardless of the stage of disease.

There are a number of important implications of these data. First, given the high rate of viral production, potent regimens are needed in order to suppress viral replication more completely.

Secondly, because of the small size of the viral genome (around 10,000 bases), the high rate of (uncorrected) mutation (on average, about one mutation every time the genome of the virus is copied) and the high rate of viral replication, considerable genetic diversity of the viral swarm in an individual patient would be generated as time passed following infection. Given that a single specific mutation can confer high-level resistance to some drugs (such as the nonnucleoside reverse transcriptase inhibitors (NNRTIs)), and assuming that all possible single mutations occur with equal frequency, this implies that in any individual thousands of virus copies are produced every day that are inherently resistant to specific drugs. Before an individual patient has been treated with an antiretroviral agent, many copies of a virus that is resistant to any given drug are likely to be harboured. This suggests that monotherapy is likely to be ineffective in the long term as it will select out resistant virus, leading to drug failure.

This hypothesis has been borne out by experience: for example, the NNRTI nevirapine is extremely active as a single agent in the short term, typically producing 10–100 fold falls in plasma viral load over two weeks. However, by four weeks, plasma viral load returns to baseline and all the virus detected in plasma has a single mutation conferring resistance to nevirapine. Resistance to zidovudine is more complex, involving sequential acquisition of five or more mutations over a longer period of time, which explains why zidovudine monotherapy produces a short-lived clinical benefit.

For therapy to be effective over a longer period of time, more drugs taken in combination would be needed in order to suppress viral replication more powerfully and to delay the emergence of resistant virus. Although using two nucleoside analogue reverse transcriptase inhibitors together as in the Delta study led to a significant reduction in disease progression, it was clear that even more potent therapy would be needed.

## ☐ HIGHLY ACTIVE ANTIRETROVIRAL THERAPY

The first results from the Merck 035 study[7] were presented in January 1996. This was the first time a combination of three antiretroviral agents was studied, one of which was the PI indinavir. The study was much smaller than many previous studies such as Delta and Concorde, with only 97 patients randomised, and significantly shorter (the first results were presented after 24 weeks). Also, it did not have clinical end-points, such as disease progression or death, but the end-point was the proportion of patients in each arm of the study whose viral load was suppressed to below the cut-off of a commercial viral assay, initially 500 copies/ml plasma.

All patients had been previously treated with zidovudine, and were randomised to add lamivudine (like zidovudine, a nucleoside analogue reverse transcriptase inhibitor), indinavir or both drugs together. Despite their previous treatment with zidovudine alone (so that they harboured zidovudine-resistant virus), over 90% of patients who received the triple drug combination had achieved an undetectable plasma viral load after 24 weeks.

Follow-up of patients on the triple therapy arm has continued for over six years, and viral load remains suppressed in most patients. In the year following presentation of these results, treatment with three drugs, including a PI, became the standard of care (so-called highly active antiretroviral therapy (HAART)). This led to large and rapid reductions in the risk of disease progression and death. Later in 1996, results from the ACTG 320 study[8] confirmed that the improvement in plasma viral load response seen with HAART led to a corresponding improvement in disease progression and improved survival.

## ☐ CURRENT PROBLEMS IN THE TREATMENT OF HIV INFECTION

### Testing for HIV

The improvements in drug treatment of HIV infection have had profound effects on the epidemiology of HIV in the UK (Fig 3). Improved survival and ongoing transmission of infection have led to a steady increase in the prevalence of infection. The specialty of HIV medicine has changed focus from the care of acutely ill inpatients with major opportunistic infections to outpatient care of a much larger population of ambulant patients taking HAART. The availability of effective

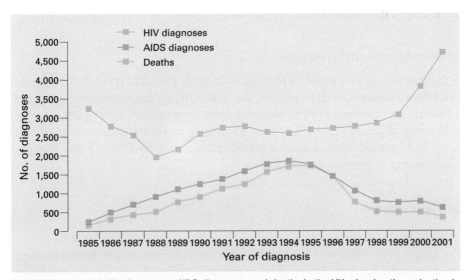

**Fig 3** Trends in new HIV diagnoses, AIDS diagnoses and deaths in the UK, showing the reduction in deaths following the introduction of effective antiretroviral therapy in the mid-1990s, despite increasing numbers of new HIV diagnoses. (*Source*: Communicable Diseases Surveillance Centre (UK), Scottish Centre for Infection and Environmental Health and Institute of Child Health (London).)

treatment means that there is now a strong argument for testing for HIV antibody in individuals who may have been at risk of HIV infection.

Despite this, there remains a major problem with late presentation of disease. Around one-third of patients in the UK do not have their HIV infection diagnosed until their CD4+ lymphocyte count has fallen below 200 cells/mm³, at which level they are at greater risk of death even if they start therapy. Many of them will already have developed a major opportunistic infection or tumour, sometimes with long-term ill effects. At the end of 2001, 31% of people with HIV infection in the UK were unaware of their status; in men with heterosexually-acquired HIV, this proportion was as high as 50%. More widespread availability of testing, enabling earlier recognition of HIV infection, is essential if such individuals are to benefit fully from antiretroviral therapy. This would also potentially help to reduce ongoing transmission of infection.

## Adherence

Some PI-based HAART regimens are highly demanding for patients to take regularly. For example, the once widely used regimen of zidovudine, lamivudine and indinavir requires patients to take a total of 10 pills a day at four precise times, ensuring that each of the three daily doses of indinavir are taken on an empty stomach. Despite the clear benefits of HAART, many patients find it hard to adhere to such complex regimens. Unfortunately, very high levels of adherence are necessary to have the best chance of treatment success. At least 95% of doses must be taken correctly; the chances of prolonged suppression of viral replication falls steeply with lower adherence.[9]

Simpler regimens based around NNRTIs such as efavirenz and nevirapine, which have much longer half-lives than the current PIs, are much less demanding, allow twice or even once-daily dosing and may be more effective than PI-based HAART.[10]

## Failure to control viral replication

If there is failure to control viral replication with HAART, typically because of suboptimal adherence, this leads to the selection of drug-resistant virus, and ultimately to treatment failure. Worrying data from the USA show that a large proportion of patients under follow-up harbour drug-resistant virus. A significant minority of patients with recently acquired infection (up to 25% in some cohorts) have evidence of primary drug resistance.

## Late drug toxicities

### *Lipodystrophy*

The longer-term efficacy of HAART has also been affected by the development of late drug toxicities. A syndrome of fat redistribution (lipodystrophy), in which loss of fat from subcutaneous tissues can occur together with central adiposity, was first recognised in 1997 and associated with the use of HAART.[11] The mechanisms by which lipodystrophy develops remain poorly understood, but recent data suggest that nucleoside analogues such as stavudine are strongly associated with loss of subcutaneous fat. This is a particularly distressing side effect of treatment, as the characteristic facial appearance of lipodystrophy adds to the stigma of HIV infection. Currently, there are limited management options for this complication of treatment. Switching drugs may be of some benefit, as may some plastic surgical procedures. Lipodystrophy is also associated with metabolic disturbances, including insulin resistance and hyperlipidaemia.

*Cardiovascular disease*

One large cohort study has suggested that the incidence of cardiovascular disease is increasing in patients treated with HAART.[12] Despite concerns about the risk of cardiovascular disease in the longer term, however, the risk to health associated with untreated HIV disease is much greater. Monitoring of plasma cholesterol and triglycerides is thus essential, and there is currently much interest in novel antiretrovirals, such as the PI atazanavir, which have minimal effect on plasma lipid concentrations.

## □ THE FUTURE

In countries where HAART is available, patients with HIV infection now have a good chance of living for many years, perhaps for decades, provided that they can adhere to treatment in the long term. Although HAART is highly cost-effective, it is an expensive treatment: the cheapest drug combination costs around £6,000 per patient per year in the UK. At the end of 2001, an estimated 40 million people worldwide were living with HIV infection, the majority of them in countries where HAART is unavailable for reasons of cost. This situation is changing, albeit slowly; differential pricing arrangements and local production of generic drugs mean that the annual cost of HAART can be as low as £200 per person.

Numerous small-scale projects in South Africa, Botswana, Haiti and Thailand have shown that delivery of HAART in resource-poor countries is possible and that the effects are as dramatic as in the West. The challenge now is to scale up the delivery of treatment in parallel with efforts to prevent infection. Failure to do this will consign 40 million people to a premature death, with devastating human and economic consequences for their countries.

## REFERENCES

1  Palella FJ Jr, Delaney KM, Moorman AC, Loveless MO *et al.* Declining morbidity and mortality among patients with advanced human immunodeficiency virus infection. HIV Outpatient Study Investigators. *N Engl J Med* 1998;338:853–60.

2  Fischl MA, Richman DD, Grieco MH, Gottlieb MS *et al.* The efficacy of azidothymidine (AZT) in the treatment of patients with AIDS and AIDS-related complex. A double-blind, placebo-controlled trial. *N Engl J Med* 1987;317:185–91.

3  Concorde: MRC/ANRS randomised double-blind controlled trial of immediate and deferred zidovudine in symptom-free HIV infection. Concorde Coordinating Committee. *Lancet* 1994; 343:871–81.

4   Delta: a randomised double-blind controlled trial comparing combinations of zidovudine plus didanosine or zalcitabine with zidovudine alone in HIV infected individuals. Delta Coordinating Committee. *Lancet* 1996;**348**:283–91. Erratum *Lancet* 1996;**348**:834.

5   Ho DD, Neumann AU, Perelson AS, Chen W *et al.* Rapid turnover of plasma virions and CD4 lymphocytes in HIV-1 infection. *Nature* 1995;**373**:123–6.

6   Wei X, Ghosh SK, Taylor ME, Johnson VA *et al.* Viral dynamics in human immunodeficiency virus type 1 infection. *Nature* 1995;**373**:117–22.

7   Gulick RM, Mellors JW, Havlir D, Eron JJ *et al.* Treatment with indinavir, zidovudine, and lamivudine in adults with human immunodeficiency virus infection and prior antiretroviral therapy. *N Engl J Med* 1997;**337**:734-_9.

8   Hammer SM, Squires KM, Hughes MD, Grimes JM *et al.* A controlled trial of two nucleoside analogues plus indinavir in persons with human immunodeficiency virus infection and CD4 cell counts of 200 per cubic millimeter or less. *N Engl J Med* 1997;**337**:725–33.

9   Paterson DL, Swindells S, Mohr J, Brester M *et al.* Adherence to protease inhibitor therapy and outcomes in patients with HIV infection. *Ann Intern Med* 2000;**133**:21-30. Erratum *Ann Intern Med* 2002;**136**:253.

10  Staszewski S, Morales-Ramirez J, Tashima KT, Rachlis A *et al.* Efavirenz plus zidovudine and lamivudine, efavirenz plus indinavir, and indinavir plus zidovudine and lamivudine in the treatment of HIV-1 infection in adults. Study 006 Team. *N Engl J Med* 1999;**341**:1865–73.

11  Carr A, Samaras K, Burton S, Law M *et al.* A syndrome of peripheral lipodystrophy, hyper-lipidaemia and insulin resistance in patients receiving HIV protease inhibitors. *AIDS* 1998;**12**:F51–8.

12  Friis-Møller N, Weber R, Reiss P, Thiebaut R *et al.* Cardiovascular disease risk fctors in HIV patients – association with antiretroviral therapy. Results from the DAD study. *AIDS* 2003;**17**:1179–93.

# Treatment of respiratory viruses

Patrick Mallia and Sebastian Johnston

## ☐ INTRODUCTION

The field of antiviral agents is expanding rapidly, with multiple new agents becoming available over recent years. Most of these have been for chronic viral infections such as HIV and viral hepatitis. The development of treatments for acute respiratory virus infections has lagged behind, probably because, except for influenza, they were considered as causing mild, self-limiting illnesses. However, it is now increasingly clear that respiratory viruses are a significant cause of mortality and morbidity, especially in those with pre-existing respiratory disease and at the extremes of life. This has led to increased interest in the development of antiviral agents for respiratory viruses, and several new drugs have recently become available or are in development.

## ☐ MORBIDITY ASSOCIATED WITH RESPIRATORY VIRUS INFECTIONS

### Influenza

Influenza is well recognised as a major cause of mortality during pandemics on four occasions over the last century. Outside these pandemics it is associated with even greater overall morbidity and mortality, causing an estimated 13,000 deaths per year in the UK. Surveillance data from a number of countries have shown a strong correlation between the incidence of reports of influenza-like illness and death rates. A UK study of mortality during 1975–1990 showed a strong correlation between influenza activity and mortality, even in years without a major influenza epidemic.[1] The majority of excess influenza winter deaths occur in the over-65s, with higher mortality in those with underlying medical conditions such as chronic obstructive pulmonary disease (COPD), congestive cardiac failure and diabetes.

### Respiratory syncytial virus

Respiratory syncytial virus (RSV) causes a wide spectrum of disease severity. Most people exposed to the virus develop upper respiratory tract infection only, but a small proportion of infants develop the lower respiratory tract syndrome bronchiolitis. RSV is the major cause of bronchiolitis in children, with 125,000 hospitalisations per year in the US, mostly in infants under the age of one year.[2] Immunity after RSV infection is incomplete and reinfection occurs.

There is now evidence that RSV is also a significant pathogen in adults and can result in a burden of disease similar in impact to influenza, mainly in the elderly and those with chronic cardiopulmonary disease. In these populations, RSV can cause severe lower respiratory tract syndromes, including pneumonia (5–15% of community acquired pneumonias in the winter months).[3]

## Respiratory viruses and asthma

Asthma affects an estimated eight million people in the UK (13% of the population). One in eight children receive treatment for asthma, making it the commonest chronic disease in childhood. Asthma is characterised by a varying level of chronic respiratory symptoms punctuated by intermittent exacerbations. Acute exacerbations are a major cause of emergency department visits, hospitalisations and excess medication use. They are caused by a number of factors, including allergen exposure, air pollution, stress and occupational exposures, but there is now convincing evidence that the major cause of asthma exacerbations in both children and adults is respiratory virus infection.

An association between colds and asthma exacerbations has been recognised for many years, but earlier studies of the association between viruses and asthma yielded low virus detection rates of around 30% in children and 10% in adults. Standard techniques of viral culture and serology have a low sensitivity for the detection of viruses, especially rhinoviruses and coronaviruses that account for over 50% of episodes of the common cold. The true association between viruses and asthma exacerbations was revealed only when polymerase chain reaction (PCR)-based methods for virus detection became available.

Studies using PCR have shown that respiratory viruses are responsible for a much higher proportion of asthma exacerbations than previously thought, with virus detected in 80–85% of exacerbations in children.[4] Rhinoviruses were detected most commonly (50% of exacerbations or 66% in which a virus was detected).

The contribution of individual respiratory viruses to wheezing in children varies according to age. Under the age of two years, RSV is the predominant virus detected whereas rhinoviruses are more common in children over two years old.[5] Coinfection with more than one virus is associated with more severe illness, more respiratory tract symptoms and greater falls in peak expiratory flow rate (PEFR) (unpublished data).

Viruses have also been detected in a high proportion of asthma exacerbations in adults. One study in adults detected virus in 44% of exacerbations in the community, with rhinoviruses again the most common (60% of episodes in which a virus was detected).[6] Cold symptoms preceded 70% of exacerbations in this study; virus shedding is of shorter duration in adults, so 44% may be an underestimate of the true association. Another study of adult asthmatics surveyed over 15 months detected a virus in 60% of exacerbations (67% rhinoviruses) (unpublished data).

Viruses are also associated with more severe asthma exacerbations that require hospitalisation. A virus was detected in 76% of adults presenting to the emergency department with an asthma exacerbation in an Australian study. Exacerbations in which a virus was detected were associated with a lower $FEV_1$, higher hospital admission rate and longer hospital stay, higher neutrophil count, neutrophil elastase and lactate dehydrogenase levels in induced sputum.[7]

Recent evidence has shown that respiratory viruses act synergistically with other factors such as allergic sensitisation and air pollution to exacerbate asthma. The risk of wheezing in children is increased by the concomitant presence of virus infection and allergy.[5] In adult asthmatics, admission to hospital with acute exacerbations is strongly associated with the combination of allergic sensitisation, exposure to high levels of an allergen and concurrent viral infection.[8]

The presence of high ambient levels of nitrogen dioxide prior to a viral infection in asthmatics is associated with more lower respiratory tract symptoms and greater falls in PEFR at exacerbation.[9]

### Respiratory viruses and chronic obstructive pulmonary disease

An estimated 600,000 people in the UK are affected by COPD, with 30,000 deaths per year. Acute exacerbations of COPD are a major cause of morbidity and mortality and the largest single cause of acute respiratory admissions in the UK. In 2000–2001 there were 135,000 hospital admissions for acute exacerbations of COPD, with a mean hospital stay of 10.3 days (almost one million bed-days).[10]

Exacerbations can be caused by a number of factors, with infection of the tracheo-bronchial tree the most common. Traditionally, COPD exacerbations have been considered as predominantly caused by bacteria – although the contribution of bacteria to exacerbations remains an area of controversy as they are also present in the airways in clinically stable COPD. There is now evidence that respiratory viruses can also cause exacerbations of COPD. Earlier studies suggested that they are responsible for only a minority of exacerbations but, as with asthma exacerbations, much higher viral detection rates have been achieved with PCR. In the COPD study in the East London area a virus was detected in 39% of exacerbations in a cohort of patients with moderate to severe COPD.[11] Again, as in asthma, the most commonly detected viruses were rhinoviruses (58% of viruses). Since 64% of the exacerbations were associated with symptoms of a cold, the true contribution of viruses may have been underestimated. There could be several reasons for this, including the following:

1   Samples were taken within 48 hours of the onset of lower respiratory tract symptoms. Upper respiratory tract infection may precede the exacerbation by several days and the virus may no longer be detectable by the time of the COPD exacerbation.

2   Nasal aspirate samples were taken from all patients, but sputum samples were tested for the presence of rhinovirus in only a subset of patients. In the latter, there were 40% more positive samples, indicating that if both upper and lower respiratory samples are tested the viral detection rate may be even higher.

A virus was detected in 56% of exacerbations in a study of hospitalised patients with COPD exacerbations, compared with a detection rate of 19% in a control group with stable COPD.[12] Picornaviruses were the most common viruses detected (36% of viruses). Some respiratory viruses (eg parainfluenza 1 and 2, and adenoviruses) were not tested for in this study, again suggesting that the actual contribution of viruses to acute exacerbations of COPD may be even higher.

These studies suggest that respiratory viruses are a significant cause of acute exacerbations of COPD, and that their importance was previously underestimated because low sensitivity methods of virus detection were used.

In the East London area COPD study, viral exacerbations were associated with:

☐   increased dyspnoea

☐   higher total symptom count at presentation

☐   longer median symptom recovery period, and

☐   slower rate of symptom return to baseline.

There was also a tendency to greater falls in PEFR, higher plasma fibrinogen and serum interleukin-6 (IL-6) levels in viral-associated exacerbations. Exacerbations caused by viruses are associated with more severe symptoms and an enhanced inflammatory response.

## ☐ SUSCEPTIBILITY TO VIRUS INFECTIONS

### Asthma

Respiratory virus infections lead to acute inflammatory changes in the airways, associated with a cellular inflammatory infiltrate due to activation of the innate and acquired immune systems, eventually leading to clearance of the virus and resolution of disease. Studies in naturally occurring infection have shown that respiratory virus infection in asthmatics is associated with more severe symptoms and changes in airway function.[13] Although much research interest has focused on the mechanisms of increased susceptibility to the effects of virus infection in asthmatics, they still remain obscure. One possible mechanism is the interaction between virus infection and type 2 inflammation in the asthmatic airway.

Asthma is characterised by a type 2 profile of inflammation, with CD4+ T cells that secrete IL-4, IL-5 and IL-13 and a relative defect in type 1 immunity. Asthmatics show impaired production of the type 1 cytokines interferon γ (IFNγ) and IL-12 in response to rhinovirus stimulation of peripheral blood mononuclear cells compared with nonasthmatics.[14] These cytokines are essential for effective viral clearance, so this defect in type 1 immune responses may underlie the pathogenesis of asthma exacerbation.

### Chronic obstructive pulmonary disease

Much less is known about the interaction between virus infection and COPD. COPD is also associated with increased severity of virus infections but not with type 2 inflammation. Impaired antiviral mechanisms may also be involved in COPD as it has been shown that COPD patients with lower serum IFNγ levels are more likely to have virus detected when clinically stable and have more frequent exacerbations.[15] A low IFNγ/IL-5 ratio is also associated with more severe exacerbations and longer time to recovery of PEFR to baseline.[15]

## ☐ TREATMENT

### Rhinoviruses

A number of different compounds with activity against rhinoviruses have been tested *in vitro*. Three targets in the viral life cycle have been targeted for pharmacological intervention:

- ☐ viral attachment
- ☐ viral uncoating, and
- ☐ the viral protease.

A capsid-binding inhibitor that blocks viral uncoating has shown most promise in clinical trials. By binding to the viral capsid, such compounds increase the stability of the virus and thereby prevent uncoating and replication of the viral RNA. In the major group of rhinoviruses whose cellular receptor is intercellular adhesion molecule-1 (ICAM-1), they also change the conformation of the receptor binding site and prevent attachment of the virus to ICAM-1.

Pleconaril, a capsid-binding inhibitor, is the first antipicornavirus agent developed for clinical use. Initial trials of pleconaril have shown that it reduces the duration and severity of picornavirus upper respiratory tract infections. In a Phase 2 double-blind, placebo-controlled trial, subjects over the age of 14 years presenting within 36 hours of onset of a cold were treated with pleconaril or placebo.[16] Subjects positive for picornavirus given pleconaril had a significant reduction (by 1.5 days) in the median time to complete resolution of symptoms, a significantly shorter time to 50% reduction of symptom severity score from baseline, and 16% reduction in disturbed nights.

### Respiratory syncytial virus

Only one agent, ribavirin, is currently licensed for the treatment of RSV infection. Ribavirin is a synthetic nucleoside that inhibits the synthesis of viral structural proteins and demonstrates antiviral activity against RSV *in vitro*. Despite being licensed for almost 20 years, controversy remains regarding its exact role in the treatment of RSV infection. Early clinical trials showed benefit in infants with underlying cardiopulmonary disease[17] and those with severe illness requiring mechanical ventilation,[18] but more recent studies[19] failed to confirm these results. Early enthusiasm for the use of ribavirin has waned; in 1996, the American Academy of Pediatrics changed their guidelines on the use of ribavirin from 'should be used' to 'may be considered' in high-risk children and those with severe illness.[20]

Palivizumab, a monoclonal antibody directed at the F surface glycoprotein of RSV, prevents fusion of the virus to host cells and is currently licensed for RSV prophylaxis in high-risk infants. Treatment of RSV-infected infants with palivizumab showed a reduction in viral load in the treated group, but no improvement in clinical parameters.[21]

New therapies are therefore required for RSV, and a number of new drugs are in development. An RSV fusion inhibitor VP14637 (Viropharma) has completed Phase I clinical trials and two other novel agents (R170591 (Janssen) and 433771 (Bristol Myers Squibb)) are in preclinical development.

## Influenza

### M2 inhibitors

M2, a membrane protein found in influenza A but not influenza B, is required for nucleocapsid release after viral fusion. Two M2 inhibitors are available (amantadine and rimantadine) that inhibit the function of the M2 protein and prevent viral uncoating following endocytosis. One drawback of treatment with M2 inhibitors is the rapid development of resistance after starting therapy. This does not usually lead to treatment failure in an immunocompetent host, but the resistant strains can spread and lead to failure of antiviral prophylaxis. A number of published clinical studies assessing the efficacy of the M2 inhibitors show that these agents reduce the duration of fever and symptoms in patients by about 24 hours. Their main limitation is the incidence of side effects in the elderly – the patient group at greatest risk of complications from influenza.

### Neuraminidase inhibitors

Neuraminidase, an enzyme expressed on the surface of influenza A and B, is essential for release of newly formed viruses from an infected cell. Two neuraminidase inhibitors, zanamivir and oseltamivir (not in Europe), are currently licensed for use and others are in development. Zanamivir has a low oral bioavailability and is delivered in inhaled form, whereas oseltamivir is available orally.

*Zanamivir.* In influenza, zanamivir reduces symptoms by 24 hours and also reduces the number of nights of disturbed sleep and use of over-the-counter medications. In a meta-analysis of zanamivir trials this agent resulted in a 40% reduction in lower respiratory tract complications and reduced antibiotic use. A retrospective analysis found that the benefit was even greater in high-risk patients (ie the elderly, those with chronic respiratory disease or cardiovascular disease).[22] In this group there was a 2.5 day reduction in the time to alleviation of symptoms, a three-day reduction in the time to return to usual activity, and a 43% reduction in complications requiring antibiotic use.

*Oseltamivir.* Oseltamivir has shown a similar efficacy to zanamivir in healthy adults and children, with reductions in illness severity and duration, viral shedding and lower respiratory tract complications. There are no published studies in high-risk groups so it is not known whether similar benefits are seen in such patients. However, oseltamivir has been used as a prophylactic agent in elderly nursing home residents without adverse effects.

## ☐ CONCLUSIONS

There have been exciting developments in antiviral agents for respiratory viruses in recent years and further new agents are expected to become available in the near future. However, their use will be tempered by issues of cost and patient selection.

Further research is required in high-risk groups such as the elderly and patients with chronic cardiopulmonary disease to assess whether these agents will lead to a reduction in the considerable morbidity and mortality associated with viral respiratory tract infections.

# REFERENCES

1   Nicholson KG. Impact of influenza and respiratory syncytial virus on mortality in England and Wales from January 1975 to December 1990. *Epidemiol Infect* 1996;**116**:51–63.

2   Schlesinger C, Koss MN. Bronchiolitis: update 2001. Review. *Curr Opin Pulm Med* 2002;**8**: 112–6.

3   Falsey AR, Walsh EE. Respiratory syncytial virus infection in adults. Review. *Clin Microbiol Rev* 2000;**13**:371–84.

4   Johnston SL, Pattemore PK, Sanderson G, Smith S *et al*. Community study of role of viral infections in exacerbations of asthma in 9-11 year old children. *BMJ* 1995;**310**:1225–9.

5   Rakes GP, Arruda E, Ingram JM, Hoover GE *et al*. Rhinovirus and respiratory syncytial virus in wheezing children requiring emergency care. IgE and eosinophil analyses. *Am J Respir Crit Care Med* 1999;**159**:785–90.

6   Nicholson KG, Kent J, Ireland DC. Respiratory viruses and exacerbations of asthma in adults. *BMJ* 1993;**307**:982–6.

7   Wark PA, Johnston SL, Moric I, Simpson JL *et al*. Neutrophil degranulation and cell lysis is associated with clinical severity in virus-induced asthma. *Eur Respir J* 2002;**19**:68–75.

8   Green RM, Custovic A, Sanderson G, Hunter J *et al*. Synergism between allergens and viruses and risk of hospital admission with asthma: case-control study. *BMJ* 2002;**324**:763. Erratum *BMJ* 2002;**324**:1131.

9   Chauhan AJ, Inskip HM, Linaker CH, Smith S *et al*. Personal exposure to nitrogen dioxide (NO(2)) and the severity of virus-induced asthma in children. *Lancet* 2003;**361**:1939–44.

10   www.doh.gov.uk/hes

11   Seemungal T, Harper-Owen R, Bhowmik A, Moric I *et al*. Respiratory viruses, symptoms, and inflammatory markers in acute exacerbations and stable chronic obstructive pulmonary disease. *Am J Respir Crit Care Med* 2001;**164**:1618–23.

12   Rohde G, Wiethege A, Borg I, Kauth M *et al*. Respiratory viruses in exacerbations of chronic obstructive pulmonary disease requiring hospitalisation: a case-control study. *Thorax* 2003; **58**:37–42.

13   Corne JM, Marshall C, Smith S, Schreiber J *et al*. Frequency, severity, and duration of rhinovirus infections in asthmatic and non-asthmatic individuals: a longitudinal cohort study. *Lancet* 2002;**359**:831–4.

14   Papadopoulos NG, Stanciu LA, Papi A, Holgate ST, Johnston SL. A defective type 1 response to rhinovirus in atopic asthma. *Thorax* 2002;**57**:328–32.

15   Seemungal T, Patel IS, Donaldson GC, Bhowmik A *et al*. Relationship between serum interferon-gamma levels and severity of stable COPD and COPD exacerbation. *Eur Respir J* 2003 (in press).

16   Hayden FG, Coats T, Kim K, Hassman HA *et al*. Oral pleconaril treatment of picornavirus-associated viral respiratory illness in adults: efficacy and tolerability in phase II clinical trials. *Antivir Ther* 2002;**7**:53–65.

17   Hall CB, McBride JT, Gala CL, Hildreth SW, Schnabel KC. Ribavirin treatment of respiratory syncytial viral infection in infants with underlying cardiopulmonary diseaase. *JAMA* 1985;**254**:3047–51.

18   Smith DW, Frankel LR, Mathers LH, Tang AT *et al*. A controlled trial of aerosolized ribavirin in infants receiving mechanical ventilation for severe respiratory syncytial virus infection. *N Engl J Med* 1991;**325**:24–9.

19  Law BJ, Wang EE, MacDonald N, McDonald J *et al.* Does ribavirin impact on the hospital course of children with respiratory syncytial virus (RSV) infection? An analysis using the pediatric investigators collaborative network on infections in Canada (PICNIC) RSV database. *Pediatrics* 1997;**99**:E7.

20  Reassessment of the indications for ribavirin therapy in respiratory syncytial virus infections. American Academy of Pediatrics Committee on Infectious Diseases. Review. *Pediatrics* 1996;**97**:137–40.

21  Malley R, DeVincenzo J, Ramilo O, Dennehy PH *et al.* Reduction of respiratory syncytial virus (RSV) in tracheal aspirates in intubated infants by use of humanized monoclonal antibody to RSV F protein. *J Infect Dis* 1998;**178**:1555–61.

22  Lalezari J, Campion K, Keene O, Silagy C. Zanamivir for the treatment of influenza A and B infection in high-risk patients: a pooled analysis of randomized controlled trials. *Arch Intern Med* 2001;**161**:212–7.

# Current issues in the treatment of genital herpes virus infections

Rajul Patel

## ☐ INTRODUCTION

The herpes virus group contains eight relatively large enveloped DNA viruses. There are three members of the alpha herpes virus subgroup: herpes simplex viruses type 1 and 2 (HSV-1, HSV-2) and varicella zoster virus. They are characterised by their ability to establish lifelong latency within the nervous system following initial infections of the skin. From within this immunologically privileged site they are able periodically to reactivate and reinfect the skin, causing usually mild, short-lived, recurrent cutaneous disease episodes.

## ☐ NATURAL HISTORY AND CLINICAL FEATURES

The natural history of genital herpes is summarised in Fig 1. First-infection genital HSV episodes may be due to HSV-1 or to HSV-2, they are symptomatic in up to 50% of individuals and vary widely in severity. Individuals with a non-clinical first episode will pass directly into the latent phase of infection.

There are variable systemic symptoms in clinical disease, with the local development of genital erythema and papules which rapidly evolve into superficial blisters that break easily to form clean, painful ulcers. Local lymphadenopathy is usual. Acquisition episodes tend to be more severe and prolonged than recurrent episodes which are usually unilateral. Disease, both at the time of acquisition and subsequently, tends to be milder in the presence of antibodies to the other HSV virus.

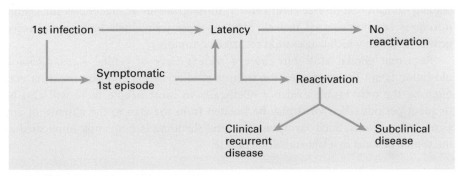

**Fig 1** Natural history of genital herpes infection.

Animal experiments suggest that a single episode of infection of HSV-1 or HSV-2 usually protects the ganglion from subsequent infection by a similar viral strain.

Following infection of the skin, an immunological response develops which clears the virus from local tissues. Both the cellular and humoral components are important in maintaining protection from subsequent reinfection.

HSV-1 and HSV-2 show different recurrence patterns depending on which neuronal ganglia are infected. HSV-2 recurs more frequently with lumbosacral involvement whereas HSV-1 recurs more often with cervical involvement. These differences are mediated by gene encoded factors and are not related to the relative frequency with which different anatomical sites may be infected with specific viral types. In the UK, HSV-1 is now the commonest cause of genital herpes infection and is frequently the cause of severe acquisition episode disease. Despite this, HSV-1 remains a rare cause of troublesome recurrent genital disease, with most of these cases (95%) being due to HSV-2.

There is considerable gene conservation between HSV-1 and HSV-2. Many codons are identical. The eleven envelope glycoproteins are mostly similar. Some significant variation is noted in gG, gC and gD. By looking for antibody responses to these type-specific antigens the humoral response following infection can be used to indicate specific exposure to HSV-1 or HSV-2.

## ☐ EPIDEMIOLOGY

Seroepidemiological surveys using type-specific tests show a number of trends in HSV infection. HSV-1 infection in childhood is becoming rare. Increased susceptibility to HSV-1 infection in latter life may explain the rising incidence of HSV-1 as the cause of first-episode genital disease in adult life. There is also an increasing prevalence of HSV-2 infection. Explanations for this include changes in sexual behaviour or increased susceptibility to adult HSV-2 in the population due to the decline in childhood HSV-1.

Studies in the adult UK population show that one in eight women and one in 25 men have antibodies to HSV-2. These rates are higher in people attending sexually transmitted disease clinics and in those generally at higher risk for genital infections (eg homosexual males). Most of these individuals have undiagnosed genital infection which causes mild recurrent symptoms.

Recurrent genital HSV can cause a wide variety of genital signs. Classical ulceration is not the most common feature; mild erythema and skin fissuring may often be the only visible evidence of disease. In most people there will also be frequent periods when virus may be isolated from the skin in the absence of any signs or symptoms. Such asymptomatic viral shedding is frequently implicated as the source of virus in a transmission episode.

## ☐ MEDICAL IMPORTANCE OF GENITAL HERPES SIMPLEX VIRUS

Studies using highly sensitive methods confirm HSV as the principal cause of genital ulceration in both the developed and developing world. Recurrent problems in patients with diagnosed genital herpes will often lead to significant psychosexual morbidity.

## Immunocompromised individuals

Although disseminated viral disease is a rare problem in the immunocompetent individual, there are several other serious complications in the immuno-compromised. Herpes lesions resistant to aciclovir (ACV) are increasingly being described in advanced HIV.

## Pregnancy

Herpes infections in pregnancy are associated with several possible severe outcomes. Dissemination is much more frequently seen in this group. New acquisitions in early pregnancy are associated with miscarriage, whilst infections in late pregnancy may lead to premature delivery and serious neonatal infection in up to 50% of babies. These risks can be modified by the prompt recognition of disease, avoidance of vaginal delivery and early treatment of infected babies. Recurrent disease carries much smaller risks to the baby, and advice regarding delivery cannot be so clear.

## Genital ulcerative disease

Genital ulcerative disease is an important cofactor in the transmission and acquisition of HIV infection. Modelling of the epidemic as well as HSV sero-prevalence studies show that herpes infections may be responsible for up to 30% of all new cases of HIV infection.

## □ TREATMENT OF GENITAL HERPES

Before the development of ACV in the 1970s life-threatening and serious HSV infections were treated with non-specific, highly toxic and poorly effective agents such as vidarabine and idoxuridine.

## Aciclovir

ACV is a structural analogue of guanosine. It passes easily across cell membranes, but is not active in uninfected cells since it requires phosphorylation for activity and is not a substrate for human cellular kinases. Within cells actively infected by HSV the drug is activated by viral thymidine kinase (TK) (a beta HSV gene product) to ACV monophosphate. This step occurs only if TK is being produced within infected cells. During latency there is no beta gene expression and drug activation will not occur. After activation, ACV monophosphate is further phosphorylated by human cellular kinases to the triphosphate and becomes a substrate for viral DNA polymerase. There is a high degree of specificity for viral DNA polymerase; ACV triphosphate is a poor substrate for human DNA polymerase. This agent has now been widely used and is extremely safe. The structure and mechanisms of action for ACV are shown in Fig 2.

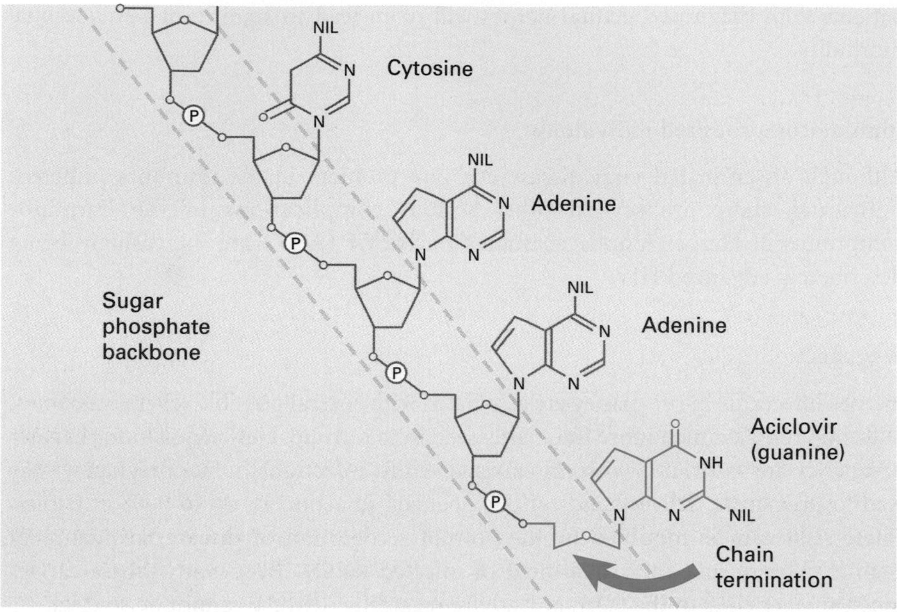

**Fig 2** Mode of action of aciclovir.

Amongst the herpes group, the simplex viruses have the highest sensitivity to ACV. Used episodically, ACV diminishes the severity and duration of first episode and recurrent disease and can be given continuously to prevent recurrent problems.[1] Used in this way the drug helps to reverse many of the psychosexual problems seen in these patients.[2]

Continuous therapy requires careful attention to dosing. ACV is poorly absorbed; given orally, it shows a saturation-type kinetic in its absorption profile. Increasing the dosage will not necessarily achieve higher levels of drug exposure, and maximum efficacy may be achieved by giving the daily dose in four or five divided doses. Such frequent daily dosing is often unacceptable to the patient; in many parts of the world once a day dosing with ACV prodrugs has become the standard of care in long-term management.

### Aciclovir prodrugs

Use of prodrugs bypasses the oral limitations to absorption of drugs such as ACV and penciclovir. Both valaciclovir and famciclovir can be given orally at doses that achieve exposures equivalent to intravenous therapy. The natural history of genital infection in man remains unchanged with these agents despite early high-dose antiviral treatment. Latency seems to be established early in the course of infection and is not amenable to standard drug treatment.

Prodrugs have not improved the efficacy of ACV treatment in genital herpes but have provided useful, simple drug therapy regimens. They have recently been shown to be effective as short courses of episodic therapy for recurrent disease.

## ☐ PREVENTION OF TRANSMISSION

Transmission of HSV is the major concern of most patients with diagnosed HSV.[3] Typically, it occurs early in relationships and is more frequent in relationships where HSV has not been discussed. Heterosexual transmission is more likely when the susceptible partner is female than male. Most transmissions occur in the context of asymptomatic shedding. The consistent use of condoms will diminish the risk of transmission but not necessarily prevent it indefinitely.[4]

### Use of prodrugs

The unpredictability of asymptomatic shedding and the failure of condoms have led to the investigation of other approaches to protect susceptible partners. Trials of antiviral therapy such as that shown in Fig 3 indicate that regular suppressive therapy controls most asymptomatic shedding.[5,6] However, sensitive polymerase chain reaction-based assays indicate that low levels of virus are present on some days. The clinical significance of this has recently been determined in a randomised, placebo-controlled study of once daily valaciclovir 500 mg to prevent genital herpes disease in serodiscordant monogamous couples.[7] Over an eight-month period 1,498 couples were regularly assessed clinically and serologically for genital herpes transmission. All suspected transmissions were confirmed by a laboratory test. The

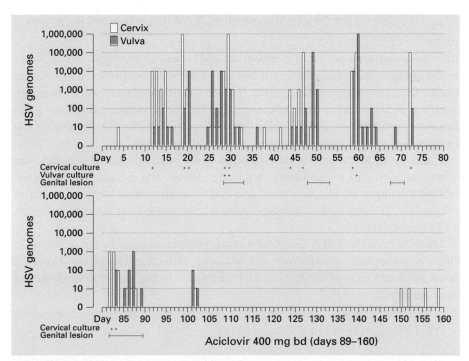

**Fig 3** Effect of aciclovir on asymptomatic herpes simplex virus (HSV) shedding.[6] Day 1–89: the subject is not taking any effective antiviral agent; day 89 onwards: whilst the patient is on suppressive aciclovir there is a marked reduction in symptomatic and asymptomatic shedding of herpes virus.

rate of disease transmission from patients on active suppressive therapy was 75% lower than in the placebo group. Transmission of infection was roughly halved.

This is the first demonstration of an antiviral medication interrupting the sexual transmission of an infection. The clinical place of this approach in genital herpes has yet to be clearly determined, particularly in other scenarios. However, suppressive therapy may well be seen as a useful adjunct to counselling, education and condom promotion, particularly in high risk situations.

## ☐ RESISTANT HERPES INFECTIONS

HSV-1 and HSV-2 will both generate mutations less susceptible to ACV under minimal genetic pressure, but the clinical significance of most of these mutations is usually minimal. Resistant strains are often of limited virulence and are cleared by normal immunological mechanisms.

Resistant strains are of much greater importance in the immunocompromised host and resistant disease should be suspected in any patient with possible immunodeficiency. Lesions will fail to clear on standard doses of ACV and become atypical (particularly large and deep ulceration). ACV resistance arises from three possible genetic mechanisms:

☐    TK variants that do not recognise ACV as a substrate

☐    TK deficient mutations, and

☐    DNA polymerase mutations in which ACV triphosphate is not recognised as a substrate.

If resistance is suspected, the patient should be placed on high-dose ACV (or prodrug) and cultures from the lesion taken for viral isolation and resistance testing (plaque reduction or dye uptake assays). If there is no improvement within five days, resistance is likely and a drug not requiring TK for activation should be given (foscarnet, cidofovir or trifluridine), the choice governed by the severity of the problem and whether topical treatment may be appropriate.

Clearance of the first resistant episode is usual but some resistant strains can achieve latency and subsequently reactivate. Unless the underlying immuno-deficiency is improved, relapse is usual and in time multiresistant herpes strains may well develop. Transmission of resistant strains is rare (due to their limited virulence), but has been reported.

Levels of prescribed ACV usage have steadily increased over the last 15 years. In addition, some ACV preparations are available without prescription. However, unlike resistance against antibiotics, ACV resistance is not expected to become a major problem.[8]

## ☐ THE FUTURE FOR HERPES VIRUS THERAPY

**Enzyme targets**

All current therapies exploit viral DNA polymerase as their target. Herpes viruses have other enzymes that can also be targeted and drugs are under development that target helicases and proteases. Candidate drugs will need to demonstrate exceptional safety similar to ACV if they are to be used in the general population.

## Immunotherapy

Topical immunotherapies are currently being developed for the treatment of early skin malignancies and are already licensed for genital wart virus infection. Trials of efficacy in genital herpes infections have generated mixed results.

## Vaccination

### Therapeutic vaccination

Therapeutic vaccination to boost host immune responses was efficacious in animal studies and a partial effect was demonstrated in one human study of a glycoprotein subunit vaccine. However, a number of agents showing promising results in the laboratory have failed to modify disease in clinical trials. At present, no therapeutic vaccine with proven efficacy is available for HSV infection.

### Prophylactic vaccines

In the laboratory, natural infection with herpes viruses is protective to a major extent against subsequent infection of the same area with a similar viral type. Some of this protection is mediated by the humoral and cellular components of the acquired immune response. Prophylactic vaccines have often demonstrated high levels of immunogenicity and protection in the laboratory but failed to protect subjects in human clinical trials.[9] A recent study of an HSV-2 glycoprotein D-alum-MPL vaccine has shown extremely promising results in two clinical studies.[10] This vaccine protected against disease in women, but interestingly not in men or in patients who had previously had HSV-1 infection. Infections occurred despite vaccination, but clinical disease during the period of follow-up was significantly diminished. This is the first vaccine with sex-specific efficacy. Large studies in HSV-1 and HSV-2 negative populations (ie no previous herpes simplex infections) are currently being planned in both Europe and North America. At present, this vaccine may not be appropriate for developing countries because of the high incidence of HSV-1 in childhood.

## ☐ CONCLUSIONS

Genital HSV (directly or indirectly) is a growing cause of morbidity. Safe, effective antiviral therapies are available which can manage the symptomatology and complications of acute and chronic genital herpes. In addition, continuous suppression has recently been shown to prevent transmission of genital herpes. Resistant disease is rare, but usually amenable to antiviral treatments and should always be suspected in immunocompromised patients.

## REFERENCES

1   National guideline for the management of genital herpes. Clinical Effectiveness Group (Association of Genitourinary Medicine and the Medical Society for the Study of Venereal Diseases). *Sex Transm Infect* 1999;75(Suppl 1):S24–8. (Updates available at www.mssvd.org)

2   Patel R, Tyring S, Strand A, Price MJ, Grant DM. Impact of suppressive antiviral therapy on the health related quality of life of patients with recurrent genital herpes infection. *Sex Transm Infect* 1999;75:398–402.

3   Patel R, Cowan F, Barton SE. Advising patients with genital herpes. *BMJ* 1997;314:85–6.

4   Casper C, Wald A. Condom use and the prevention of genital herpes acquisition. Review. *Herpes* 2002;9:10–14.

5   Wald A, Zeh J, Barnum G, Davis LG, Corey L. Suppression of subclinical shedding of herpes simplex virus type 2 with acyclovir. *Ann Intern Med* 1996;124(1 Pt1):8–15.

6   Wald A, Corey L, Cone R, Hobson A *et al*. Frequent genital herpes simplex virus 2 shedding in immunocompetent women. Effect of acyclovir treatment. *J Clin Invest* 1997;99:1092–7.

7   Patel R, Sacks S, Tyring S, Paavonen J *et al*. Once daily valaciclovir reduces transmission of genital herpes. Eurogin, Paris, 13–16 April 2003.

8   Blower SM, Porco TC, Darby G. Predicting and preventing the emergence of antiviral drug resistance in HSV-2. *Nat Med* 1998;4:673–8.

9   Stanberry LR. Control of STDs – the role of prophylactic vaccines against herpes simplex virus. Review. *Sex Transm Infect* 1998;74:391–4.

10  Stanberry LR, Spruance SL, Cunningham AL, Bernstein DI *et al*. Glycoprotein-D-adjuvant vaccine to prevent genital herpes. *N Engl J Med* 2002;347:1652–61.

# Immunotherapy for Epstein-Barr virus-associated lymphoma

Dorothy Crawford

## ☐ INTRODUCTION

Harnessing the immune response to treat cancer has long been the goal of tumour immunologists, but many became disillusioned when early workers failed to demonstrate specific immunity against tumour cells or to identify tumour-specific antigens. Recently, however, several tumour antigens have been identified and, with the ability now to generate designer antibodies and T cells with defined specificity, the concept of the 'magic bullet' has re-emerged. The past few years have seen many new and innovative immunological approaches to targeting and killing tumour cells that are now reaching the clinic.[1] T cell immunotherapy will never be simple to deliver because T cells function in an HLA restricted manner, which in practice means that T cells will recognise tumour cells only if they share common HLA antigens. For T cell immunotherapy to succeed, the T cells must be either derived from the patient themselves (autologous) or, if allogeneic, at least partially HLA matched to the recipient.

Up to 20% of human cancers have a viral aetiology, including common tumours such as hepatocellular cancer (hepatitis B virus) and cervical cancer (human papilloma virus).[2] The malignant cells in these tumours express viral antigens that are targets for immune attack, and therefore good models for developing tumour immunotherapy.

Epstein-Barr virus (EBV) has been used as a model in proof-of-principle trials of T cell immunotherapy. This review will concentrate on this work (for review of EBV and associated diseases, see Ref 3).

## ☐ BACKGROUND

EBV, a human herpes virus, was first discovered in 1964 in B cells grown from Burkitt's lymphoma tumour tissue. Since then, the virus has been shown to be the cause of infectious mononucleosis and associated with a wide variety of human malignancies, including common tumours such as Hodgkin's lymphoma (Table 1).

EBV readily infects B lymphocytes *in vitro*, transforming them into rapidly proliferating lymphoblasts which continue to grow indefinitely as lymphoblastoid cell lines (LCL). LCLs are latently infected, expressing few viral genes and producing no virus particles. These latent antigens include six nuclear antigens and three membrane proteins which act together to induce cell proliferation (Table 2).

**Table 1** Epstein-Barr virus (EBV)-associated tumours.

| Tumour | EBV association | % |
|---|---|---|
| B lymphoproliferative disease | PTLD | ca 90 |
| | HIV associated CNS lymphoma | <100 |
| | HIV associated peripheral lymphoma | ca 50 |
| Burkitt's lymphoma | African/endemic | 97–100 |
| | HIV associated | ca 25 |
| Hodgkin's disease | | ca 65 |
| T/NK cell lymphoma | | 10–100* |
| HIV-associated primary effusion lymphoma | | 70–80** |
| Nasopharyngeal carcinoma | Non-keratinised | 100 |
| | Keratinised | 30–100 |
| Gastric adenocarcinoma | Adenocarcinoma | 5–15 |

\* depending on histological type.
\*\* 100% contain human herpes virus 8.
CNS = central nervous system; NK = natural killer; PTLD = post-transplant lymphoproliferative disease.

**Table 2** Epstein-Barr virus (EBV) latent antigens.

| EBV antigen | Required for B cell transformation | Function (known/postulated) |
|---|---|---|
| EBNA 1 | + | Genome maintenance |
| EBNA 2 | + | Viral oncogene, transactivates cellular and other latent viral genes |
| EBNA 3A | + | Activates cellular genes |
| EBNA 3B | - | Activates cellular genes |
| EBNA 3C | + | Viral oncogene, increases LMP1 expression |
| EBNA LP | +/– | Coactivates EBNA 2-responsive genes |
| LMP 1 | + | Viral oncogene, induces B cell activation and adhesion, protects from apoptosis |
| LMP 2 | - | Repression of lytic cycle, enhances B cell survival |

EBNA = EBV nuclear antigen; LP = leader protein; LMP = latent membrane protein; +/- enhances efficiency of transformation.

Occasional cells in an LCL support a lytic infection with production of new viruses and cell death. This involves expression of about 70 viral genes, but the stimuli which induce the switch from latent to lytic infection are not fully understood.

EBV infects most people subclinically during childhood and thereafter persists in the body for life. If primary infection is delayed until adolescence or early adulthood, infectious mononucleosis may result. Following primary infection, the virus persists in the body by establishing a latent infection of B lymphocytes, while low level production of virus particles into saliva allows transmission between individuals. Primary and persistent EBV infections are mainly controlled by virus-specific T cells, classically HLA class I restricted CD8+ cytotoxic T cells (CTLs) which recognise viral peptides derived from both latent and lytic antigens displayed on EBV infected cells. In healthy individuals a lifelong balance is maintained between the persistent EBV infection of circulating B cells (viral load) and T cell immunosurveillance.

If T cell function is compromised by congenital, acquired or iatrogenic means, the EBV load increases; this accumulation of latently infected B cells can lead to B lymphoproliferative disease. This condition is mainly seen in AIDS and following solid organ or bone marrow transplantation (BMT) where the severe T cell immunodeficiency allows uncontrolled proliferation of EBV infected B cells. The lesions that arise in the context of transplantation are generally referred to as post-transplant lymphoproliferative disease (PTLD). This review will concentrate on T cell immunotherapy for PTLD (for general review of PTLD, see Ref 4).

## □ POST-TRANSPLANT LYMPHOPROLIFERATIVE DISEASE

PTLD occurs in up to 10% of transplant recipients, in over 50% of whom it is fatal despite treatment.

### Risk factors

Risk factors include high levels of immunosuppressive therapy. The dose of immunosuppression required to prevent graft rejection varies with the type of transplant, so the overall PTLD incidence rates vary accordingly (Table 3).[5] There is an increased risk of PTLD when high levels of immunosuppressive drugs, including additional agents such as OKT3, are given for rejection episodes, repeat transplants or mismatched transplants.

The second major risk factor for PTLD is primary EBV infection during immunosuppressive therapy. EBV may be acquired from the donor in the grafted organ. Thus, primary infection in a previously seronegative recipient often occurs early after transplant when immunosuppression is high and an effective immune

**Table 3** Incidence of post-transplant lymphoproliferative disease (PTLD) in different transplant types.

| Transplant type | PTLD incidence (%) |
| --- | --- |
| Kidney | 0.4–2.5 |
| Liver | 2.3–13.7 |
| Heart | 1.8–3.4 |
| Heart/Lung | 4.6–9.4 |
| Bone marrow | 0.2–1.6 |

response cannot be mounted. Children undergoing transplantation are more likely than adults to be seronegative and overall have a higher risk of developing PTLD.

### Tumour types

About 90% of PTLDs are EBV-associated B cell tumours. These show a wide spectrum of histological types, ranging from polyclonal proliferations to monoclonal lymphoma (most commonly of the large cell type). Progression from the former to the latter has been documented. Tumour cells generally express all the latent viral genes, although the rare post-transplant Burkitt-like and Hodgkin's lymphomas show a more restricted pattern. This indicates that the phenotype of most PTLDs is similar to *in vitro*-infected B cells in LCLs, suggesting that the tumour cells would be recognised and killed by CTLs specific for latent EBV antigens.

### Diagnosis

Clinically, PTLD often presents a diagnostic problem. Symptoms may be nonspecific and generalised (fever, weight loss, lymphadenopathy, anorexia), mimicking common post-transplant problems such as occult infection or graft rejection. This presentation is more common in – although not exclusive to – early PTLDs associated with primary EBV infection.

In contrast, PTLD in a seropositive recipient often appears late after transplant as localised tumour deposits, common sites being gut, brain and transplanted organ. EBV load in peripheral blood mononuclear cells (PMNC) is generally high in PTLD. This measurement has been used to predict those at risk of the disease, but levels as high as those in PTLD are also recorded in healthy transplant recipients so these results must be interpreted with caution. The negative predictive value of a low EBV load may be more reliable. Recently, a correlation between detection of EBV DNA in serum and PTLD development has been reported.

### Treatment

Standard first-line treatment for PTLD is reduction of immunosuppressive therapy. This approach frequently causes tumour regression, presumably by allowing regeneration of the CTL response. However, recovery is often incomplete, and recurrences commonly occur which are less sensitive to this conservative treatment. At this stage, classical lymphoma therapy is generally implemented but overall survival is poor.

### ☐ T CELL IMMUNOTHERAPY

PTLD is a severe and often fatal opportunistic tumour which develops in the immunocompromised setting because of a lack of T cell control of persistent EBV infection. Thus, PTLD is an ideal model for assessing T cell immunotherapy:

☐   The target antigens are expressed on tumour cells and not on normal cells.

☐ CTLs directed against viral latent antigens (with the exception of EBNA1) are present in the circulation of all healthy seropositive individuals and relatively easy to grow in culture.

☐ Tumours regress with reduction of immunosuppression when T cell activity is revived.

### Bone marrow transplants

T cell immunotherapy to prevent or treat PTLD was pioneered in BMT recipients because the BM donor is healthy and able to donate a blood sample from which the EBV-specific CTLs can be generated. In the initial study, donor-derived CTLs were infused into 10 recipients of mismatched or unrelated BMT recipients at a time (60–185 days) when the risk of PTLD was considered maximal. The CTLs remained functional in the recipients despite continued immunosuppressive therapy, and no PTLD developed in the infused recipients (compared with 30% in historical controls). These infused CTLs were gene marked and later shown to survive up to 18 months in the recipient's circulation. Additionally, donor CTLs successfully treated PTLD in BMT recipients.[6–8]

### Solid organ transplants

PTLD is more common in solid organ transplant recipients than following BMT, but here the donor is generally either not available to provide a blood sample or is not HLA compatible with the recipient. It may be possible to grow CTLs from the recipient at the time of PTLD diagnosis[9] but it is often difficult to grow them from patients taking iatrogenic immunosuppression. Furthermore, it takes about 12 weeks to generate enough T cells for infusion ($1–2 \times 10^6$/kg body weight); during this time patients often receive alternative forms of treatment while waiting for CTLs.

### Epstein-Barr virus-specific cytotoxic T cell bank

For these reasons we have generated a frozen bank of EBV-specific CTLs from healthy EBV seropositive blood donors. The bank includes around 100 CTLs, representing all the common UK HLA haplotypes which can now be used to treat PTLD on a best HLA match basis. The CTLs were generated in culture by stimulation of PMNCs with interleukin-2 and the irradiated autologous EBV transformed LCL (as antigen). They consist primarily of CD8+ T cells, although most contain a minority CD4+ population. After 8–12 weeks in culture the T cells show specific killing of the autologous LCL, with minimal non-specific killing of autologous EBV-negative cells, and are frozen in aliquots ready for infusion.

### *Pilot study*

To test the safety and efficacy of our banked CTLs, a pilot study was carried out in eight patients with progressive PTLD despite conventional treatment. In each case, the

CTLs were matched at least one HLA A and one HLA B locus, specific killing was high and non-specific cytotoxicity low. Three of the five patients who completed the course of treatment achieved complete remission and two showed no response.[10] No graft-versus-host disease was detected and graft function improved in the responders. Viral load fell to undetectable levels and no allospecific antibody response was observed. The longest disease-free survival is now over three years. Building on the success of this trial, a multicentre, randomised controlled trial is now underway.

## ☐ FUTURE PERSPECTIVES

The results of this and other trials demonstrate the feasibility of T cell immunotherapy for both infections and tumours, but many questions remain unanswered. It is now important to combine scientific knowledge with modern technology to ensure maximal killing of tumour cells. Thus, in the case of PTLD, it is essential to:

☐   understand the function of T cell subpopulations (CD4+, CD8+) in the CTLs and determine the most effective mix

☐   define the target viral epitopes which elicit the most effective killing, and

☐   identify cytokines and adhesion molecules which enhance T cell viability, activation and infiltration of tumour tissue.

When these questions are answered, it may be possible to produce designer T cell receptors and accessory molecules for transfection into patient T cells as required.

## REFERENCES

1   Smyth MJ, Godfrey DI, Trapani JA. A fresh look at tumor immunosurveillance and immunotherapy. Review. *Nat Immunol* 2001;2:293–9.

2   Talbot SJ, Crawford DH. Viruses and cancer. *Medicine* 2001;29:33–4.

3   Crawford DH. Biology and disease associations of Epstein-Barr virus. Review. *Phil Trans R Soc Lond B Biol Sci* 2001;356:461–73.

4   Hopwood P, Crawford DH. The role of EBV in post-transplant malignancies: a review. *J Clin Pathol* 2000;53:248–54.

5   Johannessen I, Crawford DH. *In vivo* models for Epstein-Barr virus (EBV)-associated B cell lymphoproliferative disease (BLPD). Review. *Rev Med Virol* 1999;9:263–77.

6   Rooney CM, Smith CA, Ng CY, Loftin S *et al.* Use of gene-modified virus-specific T lymphocytes to control Epstein-Barr-virus-related lymphoproliferation. *Lancet* 1996;345:9–13.

7   Heslop HE, Ng CY, Li C, Smith CA *et al.* Long-term restoration of immunity against Epstein-Barr virus infection by adoptive transfer of gene-modified virus-specific T lymphocytes. *Nat Med* 1996;2:551–5.

8   Rooney CM, Smith CA, Ng CY, Loftin SK *et al.* Infusion of cytotoxic T cells for the prevention and treatment of Epstein-Barr virus-induced lymphoma in allogeneic transplant recipients. *Blood* 1998;5:1549–55.

9   Khanna R, Bell S, Sherritt, M, Galbraith A *et al.* Activation and adoptive transfer of Epstein-Barr virus-specific cytotoxic T cells in solid organ transplant patients with posttransplant lymphoproliferative disease. *Proc Natl Acad Sci USA* 1999;96:10391–6.

10  Haque T, Wilkie GM, Taylor C, Amlot PL *et al.* Treatment of Epstein-Barr-virus-positive post-transplantation lymphoproliferative disease using partly HLA-matched allogeneic cytotoxic T cells. *Lancet* 2002;360:436–42.

## ☐ INFECTION: THE ANTIVIRAL REVOLUTION SELF ASSESSMENT QUESTIONS

### Treatment of HIV infection

1   Antiretroviral drugs:
   (a) All currently licensed drugs inhibit viral reverse transcriptase or protease enzymes
   (b) Zidovudine as a single agent is ineffective in delaying disease progression
   (c) Later use of zidovudine is associated with higher risk of toxicity
   (d) Common side effects of zidovudine are nausea and anaemia
   (e) Treatment with two nucleoside analogues offers few benefits compared with monotherapy with zidovudine

2   HIV dynamics:
   (a) Plasma viral load varies widely among untreated patients
   (b) Plasma viral load falls slowly after starting treatment with a protease inhibitor (PI)
   (c) Multiple mutations in the virus are required to produce resistance to antiretroviral drugs
   (d) Evidence of drug resistance in individuals with recently acquired HIV infection is common
   (e) $10^9$ virions are produced each day in an untreated individual with HIV infection

3   Current problems:
   (a) At least 95% of doses must be taken correctly to maximise the benefits of PI-based highly active antiretroviral therapy (HAART)
   (b) Non-nucleoside reverse transcriptase inhibitors such as efavirenz have short half-lives
   (c) There is an increase in cardiovascular disease in patients treated with HAART
   (d) Increased insulin sensitivity is seen in patients treated with HAART
   (e) Treatment with stavudine has been associated with loss of subcutaneous fat

### Treatment of respiratory viruses

1   Respiratory syncytial virus (RSV) infection:
   (a) Usually results in bronchiolitis
   (b) Causes long-lasting immunity
   (c) Is a significant pathogen in the elderly
   (d) Is the commonest virus in wheezing episodes in children under the age of two years
   (e) Accounts for less than 5% of cases of community acquired pneumonia in the winter

2    Rhinoviruses:
  (a) Are RNA viruses
  (b) Cause 80% of asthma exacerbations in children
  (c) Are the commonest viral cause of acute exacerbations of chronic obstructive pulmonary disease (COPD)
  (d) Have a higher detection rate in nasal samples than in sputum samples in COPD
  (e) Are readily detected by standard culture techniques

3    Respiratory viruses:
  (a) Are the commonest causes of asthma exacerbations
  (b) Act synergistically with allergens in causing asthma exacerbations
  (c) Are associated with more severe asthma exacerbations
  (d) Are cleared by type 2 immune responses
  (e) Increase interleukin-6 levels in acute exacerbations of COPD

4    Treatment of influenza:
  (a) M2 inhibitors are effective only against influenza B
  (b) M2 inhibitors often result in treatment failure due to the development of viral resistance
  (c) M2 inhibitors reduce the duration of symptoms by an average of three days
  (d) Zanamivir reduces lower respiratory tract complications only in high-risk patients
  (e) Oseltamivir exists in oral form

5    Pleconaril:
  (a) Is a viral protease inhibitor
  (b) Blocks viral uncoating
  (c) Has been shown to prevent virus-induced asthma exacerbations
  (d) Reduces the severity, but not the duration, of rhinovirus colds
  (e) Should be started within 36 hours of onset of a cold

**Current issues in the treatment of genital herpes virus infections**

1    Considering genital herpes transmission:
  (a) Transmission most often occurs early in relationships
  (b) Most transmission occurs during episodes of asymptomatic shedding
  (c) Risk of transmission is unaffected by regular condom use
  (d) Risk of transmission can be diminished with suppressive antiviral (prodrug) use
  (e) In heterosexual relationships the risk of acquisition is greater for women than for men

2    Considering resistant genital herpes infections:
  (a) Resistant herpes simplex viruses (HSV) cannot establish latency within the host neurone

(b)  They are more frequently seen in immunocompromised patients

(c)  Transmission of resistant herpes strains is a growing and significant problem

(d)  They should be suspected if a patient develops a recurrent episode whilst on suppressive aciclovir

(e)  They are most often due to mutations in the thymidine kinase gene

3    Aciclovir:

(a)  Is a substrate for viral thymidine kinase

(b)  Is an analogue of thymidine

(c)  Is phosphorylated only within cells actively infected with HSV

(d)  Requires human cellular kinases to become aciclovir triphosphate

(e)  Long-term use requires regular blood monitoring

## Immunotherapy for Epstein-Barr virus-associated lymphoma

1    Epstein-Barr virus (EBV):

(a)  Infects most of the human population

(b)  Causes disease in everyone infected

(c)  Is a tumorigenic virus

(d)  Is implicated in the aetiology of many cases of Hodgkin's disease

(e)  Causes glandular fever

2    Post-transplant lymphoproliferative disease:

(a)  Is usually a tumour of B lymphocytes

(b)  Is more common after bone marrow than solid organ transplantation

(c)  Is often associated with primary EBV infection

(d)  Always responds to immunosuppression dose reduction

(e)  Has a mortality of over 50%

3    Cytotoxic (CD8+) lymphocytes:

(a)  Are part of the innate immune system

(b)  Kill cells expressing 'foreign' antigens

(c)  Do not kill HLA mismatched target cells

(d)  Can be grown in tissue culture

(e)  Are an important control mechanism for persistent virus infections

# Rheumatology

# Glucocorticoids in rheumatoid arthritis

John Kirwan

## ☐ INTRODUCTION

Rheumatoid arthritis (RA) is a common disease affecting 1–2% of the population, usually starting in the 4th–6th decades, causing variable and increasing pain and loss of function due to joint inflammation and damage. Glucocorticoids were used therapeutically in RA when they were first discovered over 50 years ago, and some of the earliest randomised controlled trials (RCTs) in medicine tested gluco-corticoids in RA. Despite this, more continues to be discovered about their therapeutic benefits and risks, and much new information has emerged over the last decade. This chapter concentrates on new understanding about efficacy, mode of action and adverse effects of glucocorticoids.

## ☐ HOW GLUCOCORTICOIDS AFFECT CLINICAL SIGNS OF INFLAMMATION

Glucocorticoids in high doses rapidly and effectively suppress inflammation in many organs, including the joints, but severe adverse effects mean that long-term, high-dose therapy is contraindicated.[1] Low-dose oral glucocorticoids (eg 7.5 mg prednisolone daily) can also reduce the signs and symptoms of inflammation, but this effect is gradually lost.[2] Five long-term RCTs,[3-7] measuring clinical response and spread over half a century of investigation, can be summarised as shown in Fig 1. Some of these trials made no measurements until the third month, so the initial rate and size of increase in benefit are probably underestimated; nevertheless, the symptomatic benefits of glucocorticoids are lost by about six months of treatment. Although in most patients the benefits are lost completely, the persistence of a statistically nonsignificant benefit may represent a continuing true benefit in a small proportion of patients.

## ☐ HOW GLUCOCORTICOIDS AFFECT JOINT DESTRUCTION

The first clinical trial to show unequivocally that joint destruction can be stopped in RA was the Arthritis and Rheumatism Council (ARC) Low-Dose Glucocorticoids in Rheumatoid Arthritis study.[4,8] This was a double-blind RCT in 128 patients with active RA of less than two years' duration. Patients were randomised to prednisolone (7.5 mg) daily or identical placebo. Any other medication or physical treatments except oral glucocorticoids could be prescribed, and patients took the trial tablet each day in addition to their other medications. In practice, almost all

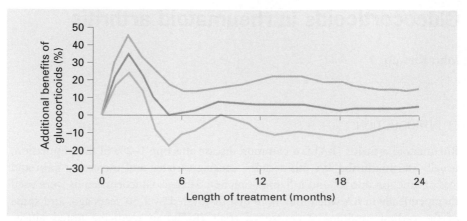

**Fig 1** Schematic illustration of symptomatic benefit from five trials of glucocorticoid therapy in early rheumatoid arthritis. All patients had disease duration of less than two years. The primary clinical outcome is used from each study. The additional benefit for the glucocorticoid treated group is calculated as a percentage of the comparator group (standard treatment) for each time point in the trial, with monthly values interpolated where necessary (only up to 12 months for one trial[5]). The unweighted mean value of the trials (centre line) and 95% confidence intervals (outer lines) were calculated for each month.[3-7]

patients were given first-line (nonsteroidal anti-inflammatory drug (NSAID)) and second-line (disease-modifying antirheumatic drug (DMARD)) therapy. After two years, trial tablets were reduced to alternate days for two weeks, then every third day for two weeks, then discontinued with follow-up for a further year.

The main results of this study are shown in Fig 2. The clinical response was similar to that summarised above (the additional benefits of glucocorticoids in reducing articular index were lost by six months) but the radiological response was markedly different. The progression of joint destruction, measured by the Larsen Score,[4] was almost completely halted by low-dose prednisolone. This effect continued throughout the period of treatment, but joint destruction resumed when prednisolone treatment was discontinued. Furthermore, the proportion of hands with erosions steadily increased in the placebo group (Table 1), but there was only a small increase in the prednisolone group while on treatment. The difference between the groups was greater after a third year even though the patients received no more glucocorticoids, raising the tantalising possibility that the treatment may have protected some patients from developing erosions in the future.

**Table 1** Percentage of hands with erosions in the Arthritis and Rheumatism Council Low-Dose Glucocorticoids in Rheumatoid Arthritis study.[4,8]

| Year | 0 | 1 | 2 | 3 |
|---|---|---|---|---|
| Placebo | 28.2 | 48.7 | 59.0 | 66.5 |
| Prednisolone | 27.8 | 29.2 | 34.7 | 39.2 |
| p (difference) | | 0.018 | 0.007 | 0.004 |

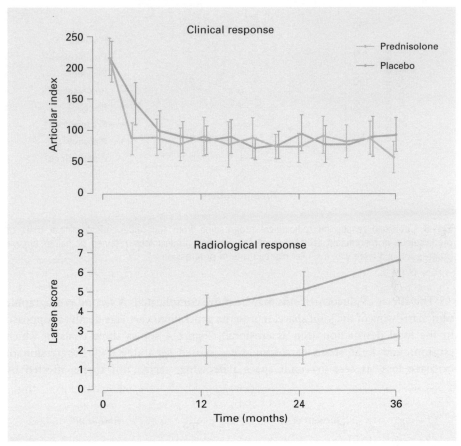

**Fig 2** Clinical and radiological response in the Arthritis and Rheumatism Research Council Low-Dose Glucocorticoids in Rheumatoid Arthritis study.[4,8] Treatment was for 24 months. Note the difference in effect on clinical and radiological responses.

Three further studies have now been undertaken[5-7] with low-dose prednisolone in patients with early disease (Fig 3, overleaf). Together with the ARC study they provide convincing evidence of the protective effect of glucocorticoids.

## ☐ IMPLICATIONS OF THE DISSOCIATION BETWEEN CLINICAL AND RADIOLOGICAL RESPONSE

The data reviewed above show that while low doses of glucocorticoids given in addition to conventional treatment suppress inflammation for only a few months, they substantially reduce the rate of radiographic progression for several years. One interpretation is that joint inflammation (as manifest by clinical symptoms) and joint destruction (as shown by the development and progression of radiographic erosions) occur through different pathological mechanisms. This is an observation of considerable interest and is supported by histological studies.[9]

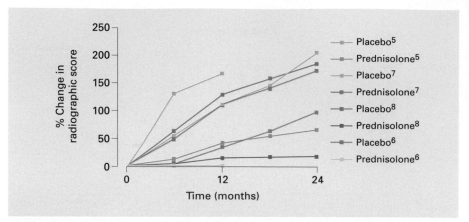

**Fig 3** Combined results on radiological progression from four independent clinical trials of prednisolone in rheumatoid arthritis. In all four studies prednisolone reduced or halted erosive progression and there was a similar placebo rate of progression.[5–8]

The effects of glucocorticoids may be more complicated. A second radiographic sign, narrowing of the joint space, represents generalised cartilage death (as opposed to the local destruction seen as erosions). Figure 4 shows three trials in which erosions and joint space narrowing were scored separately.[5,6,10] Progression of cartilage loss, as seen by joint space narrowing, seems not to be affected by

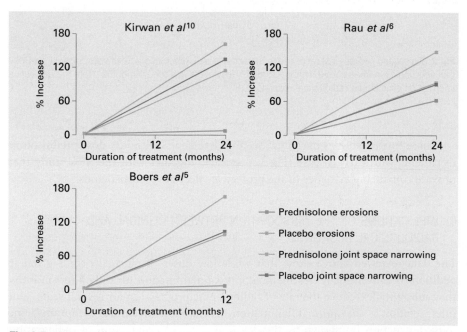

**Fig 4** Erosions and joint space narrowing in three studies of prednisolone in rheumatoid arthritis. The progression of erosions is reduced or halted, but there is no difference in the rate of increase in joint space narrowing.[5,6,10]

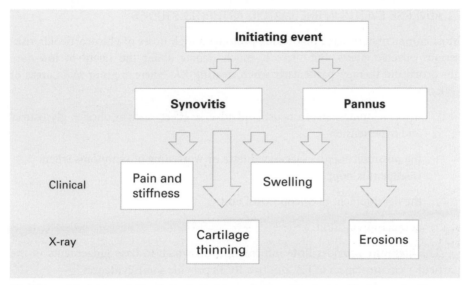

**Fig 5** A model of rheumatoid arthritis derived from studies of treatment with glucocorticoids.

glucocorticoid treatment. Thus, erosions and joint space narrowing may themselves have different aetiologies. Whereas in the past all the consequences of RA might have been considered to follow simply from inflammation, a more realistic model of the disease might now be sketched out as in Fig 5.

## ☐ GLUCOCORTICOIDS HAVE MORE THAN ONE ACTION

One possible reason that different pathologies might respond differently to glucocorticoids is because they have several modes of action. Current thinking proposes three mechanisms:

1   The traditional genomic mechanism by which glucocorticoid plus receptor move into the cell nucleus and control gene transcription. This takes 12–24 hours to have an effect, usually typified by the production of lipocortin-1.

2   Higher doses of glucocorticoid result in an increased number of receptor-glucocorticoid complexes in the cytoplasm which do not transfer to the nucleus but, through interactions with NF-κB and other control mechanisms, can more immediately change other cellular metabolic pathways.

3   When doses are extremely high (perhaps >200 mg prednisolone) there is sufficient glucocorticoid to occupy all receptors; free molecules dissolve in the cell membrane, immediately altering cell signalling and other functions.

These discoveries have led to a proposal to standardise glucocorticoid nomenclature in a way that reflects both clinical practice and mode of action.[11]

## □ ADVERSE EVENTS IN RHEUMATOID ARTHRITIS STUDIES

Most commentators agree that taking prolonged high doses of glucocorticoids risks serious adverse effects, but there is much debate about the safety of low-dose glucocorticoid therapy, particularly when treating RA. There are four main areas of concern:

- □    the development of glucocorticoid adverse effects such as obesity, glycosuria and hypertension

- □    the possibility of an exaggerated flare or worsening of symptoms when treatment is stopped

- □    the development of osteoporosis, and

- □    adrenal suppression.

The literature provides little information on which to base judgements in the particular circumstances of RA, but two RCTs provide some evidence:

1    The ARC Low-Dose Glucocorticoids in Rheumatoid Arthritis study.[4,8]

2    A study of budesonide in RA which included both prednisolone and placebo arms.[12] This was a double-blind RCT of 128 patients with active RA of less than two years' duration. Patients were randomised to budesonide (3 mg or 9 mg), prednisolone (7.5mg) or identical placebo. Concomitant first- (NSAID) and second-line (DMARD) therapy was given. Trial medication was stopped after 12 weeks with follow-up for a further four weeks. Particular attention was paid to glucocorticoid adverse events and to changes in the four weeks following discontinuation of therapy.

### Glucocorticoid adverse effects

Four patients in the ARC study had adverse events which might have been attributable to corticosteroid therapy. Two patients (hypertension, hypertension and weight gain) were on prednisolone, but the other two (diabetes, hypertension) were on placebo and there were no significant overall increases in weight or blood pressure in either group. In the budesonide study, every assessment included a checklist for adverse events (Table 2). Measurement of blood pressure and body weight and laboratory assessments, including blood glucose, were also performed at each visit. Potential glucocorticoid side effects were reported in many patients in all the groups and there were no clinically important differences between the groups (Table 3). In particular, there were again no changes in mean weight or blood pressure in any treatment group during the study.

### Change in symptoms on stopping treatment

Neither group in the ARC study showed any significant change in pain at 30, 33 or 36 months compared with 24 months or in the acute-phase response in the third

**Table 2** Check list for adverse events in the budesonide study.[12]

| | |
|---|---|
| • moon face | • hair loss |
| • buffalo hump | • swelling of ankles |
| • acne | • mood swings |
| • hirsutism | • depression |
| • purple skin striae | • insomnia |
| • bruising easily | |

**Table 3** Summary of adverse events (AE) in the prednisolone and placebo groups of the budesonide study.[12]

| | Prednisolone (7.5 mg) | Placebo |
|---|---|---|
| Evaluable patients | 39 | 31 |
| Exposure (days) | 3,255 | 2,312 |
| No. of AE | 88 | 70 |
| No. (%) of patients with AE | 33 (85) | 28 (90) |
| Reactions per 100 exposure days | 2.70 | 3.03 |

year either within or between groups. However, measurements were made only every three months, so it would have been possible to have had a short-term overshoot in disease symptoms not recorded in the study.

The budesonide study took particular care to analyse the response to termination of treatment, making assessments on diary cards over the following four weeks. There were deteriorations in all three treatment groups, but in no group were the results at four weeks after treatment termination different from placebo. Thus, in spite of the often reported difficulties of terminating treatment, patients are able to stop treatment satisfactorily when physicians are blind to the intervention.

## Osteoporosis

There is overwhelming evidence that glucocorticoids in high doses can cause osteoporosis, but almost no evidence of the effects of low-dose glucocorticoid treatment on bone mineral density (BMD) specifically in patients with active RA. BMD was measured in a subgroup of the patients (24) in the ARC Low-Dose Glucocorticoids in Rheumatoid Arthritis study. No difference was found between placebo and glucocorticoid treated patients in BMD loss at the proximal femur and the lumbar spine (Table 4). These data are insufficient to draw conclusions, but they point to the need to investigate this area further rather than to extrapolate from nondisease-specific data.

## Adrenal suppression

No evidence could be found about the effects of low-dose glucocorticoids on adrenal function in RA. It is reasonable to suppose that there may be an effect, but in the

**Table 4** Changes in bone mineral density in a subset of 24 patients from the Arthritis Research Council Low-Dose Glucocorticoids in Rheumatoid Arthritis study.[4,8]

| | Mean change (%) | | | |
| --- | --- | --- | --- | --- |
| | **1 year** | | **2 years** | |
| | **Lumbar** | **Femoral** | **Lumbar** | **Femoral** |
| Placebo | −1.4 | −2.3 | −4.8 | −6.3 |
| Prednisolone | −3.1 | −0.4 | −3.1 | −4 |

clinical trials which examined response to treatment withdrawal there appeared to be no clinical consequences. The budesonide study included an ACTH test the day after glucocorticoid withdrawal; these data will be of interest when they are published.

## ☐ CONCLUSIONS

Clinical trials have demonstrated that glucocorticoids can have several different effects on patients with RA, and current clinical practice has yet to catch up with recent findings. An evidence-based approach would use short-term treatment for the temporary relief of signs and symptoms of inflammation while other interventions to control the disease took effect. In patients with early, active disease, low-dose prednisolone will protect from erosive joint damage even after its effect on symptoms has declined.

Fears of adverse effects, based on a folk law derived from high-dose treatment in other diseases, is probably preventing many rheumatologists from adopting logical treatment strategies.

## REFERENCES

1   Saag KG, Kirwan JR. Glucocorticoid therapy in rheumatoid arthritis. In: Tsokos GC (ed). *Modern therapeutics in rheumatic diseases.* New Jersey, USA: Humana Press, 2002.

2   Kirwan JR. Systemic low-dose glucocorticoid treatment in rheumatoid arthritis. Review. *Rheum Dis Clin North Am* 2001;27:389–403.

3   Joint Committee of the Medical Research Council and Nuffield Foundation on Clinical Trials of cortisone, ACTH, and other therapeutic measures in chronic rheumatic diseases. A comparison of cortisone and aspirin in the treatment of early cases of rheumatoid arthritis. *BMJ* 1954;1:1223–7.

4   Kirwan JR, the Arthritis and Rheumatism Council Low-Dose Glucocorticoid Study Group. The effect of glucocorticoids on joint destruction in rheumatoid arthritis. *N Engl J Med* 1995;333:142–6.

5   Boers M, Verhoeven AC, Markusse HM, van de Laar MA *et al.* Randomised comparison of combined step-down prednisolone, methotrexate and sulphasalazine with sulphasalazine alone in early rheumatoid arthritis. *Lancet* 1997;350:309–18; erratum 351:220.

6   Rau R, Wassenberg S, Zeidler H and LDPT-Study Group. Low dose prednisolone therapy (LDPT) retards radiographically detectable destruction in early rheumatoid arthritis – preliminary results of a multicenter, randomized, parallel, double blind study. *Z Rheumatol* 2000;59(Suppl 2):II/90–6.

7   Van Everdingen AA, Jacobs JW, Siewertsz Van Reesema DR, Bijlsma JW. Low-dose prednisone therapy for patients with early active rheumatoid arthritis: clinical efficacy, disease-modifying properties, and side effects: a randomized, double-blind, placebo-controlled clinical trial. *Ann Intern Med* 2002;**136**:1–12.

8   Hickling P, Jacoby RK, Kirwan JR. Arthritis and Rheumatism Council Low-Dose Glucocorticoid Study Group. Joint destruction after glucocorticoids are withdrawn in early rheumatoid arthritis. *Br J Rheumatol* 1998;**37**:930–6.

9   Mulherin D, Fitzgerald O, Bresnihan B. Synovial tissue macrophage populations and articular damage in rheumatoid arthritis. *Arthritis Rheum* 1996;**39**:115–24.

10  Kirwan JR, Byron M, Watt I. The relationship between soft tissue swelling, joint space narrowing and erosive damage in hand X-rays of patients with rheumatoid arthritis. *Rheumatology (Oxford)* 2001;**40**:297–301.

11  Buttgereit F, da Silva JA, Boers M, Burmester GR *et al.* Standardised nomenclature for glucocorticoid dosages and glucocorticoid treatment regimens: current questions and tentative answers in rheumatology. *Ann Rheum Dis* 2002;**61**:718–22.

12  Kirwan JR, Hallgren R, Mielants H, Wolheim F *et al.* A randomised placebo-controlled trial of budesonide and prednisolone in rheumatoid arthritis. *Ann Rheum Dis* (in press).

# Primary systemic vasculitis

David Scott

## ☐ INTRODUCTION

Vasculitis simply means inflammation of blood vessels. The consequences of vasculitis depend on the size, number and site of blood vessels involved. When small or medium-sized arteries are involved there is frequently fibrinoid necrosis which usually leads to occlusion and infarction. If medium-sized arteries are involved and only part of the wall is inflamed, aneurysms can form due to the high pressure within the artery; aneurysmal rupture leading to severe haemorrhage is an important, serious complication of vasculitis. By contrast, small vessel vasculitis usually involves capillaries, venules and arterioles, is most commonly seen in the skin and is more rarely associated with serious consequences.

## ☐ CLASSIFICATION

A variety of classification systems has been devised, mainly over the last 50 years. Most are based on the size of blood vessel involved; the one we favour is shown in Table 1.[1] It is important to recognise that vasculitis can arrive *de novo* (primary

**Table 1** Classification of systemic vasculitis.

|  | Primary | Secondary |
|---|---|---|
| Large arteries | Giant cell arteritis<br>Takayasu arteritis | Aortitis (rheumatoid arthritis,<br>ankylosing spondylitis)<br>Infection (syphilis) |
| Medium arteries | Classic polyarteritis nodosa<br>Kawasaki disease | Infection (hepatitis B)<br>Malignancy (hairy cell leukaemia) |
| Small/medium vessels | Wegener's granulomatosis*<br>Microscopic polyangiitis*<br>Churg-Strauss syndrome* | Rheumatoid arthritis<br>Systemic lupus erythematosus<br>Sjögren's syndrome<br>Infection (HIV, hepatitis C)<br>Drugs |
| Small vessels | Henoch-Schönlein purpura<br>Essential cryoglobulinaemia<br>angiitis<br>Cutaneous leucocytoclastic<br>vasculitis | Rheumatoid arthritis<br>Systemic lupus erythematosus<br>Sjögren's syndrome<br>Infection<br>Drugs |

*diseases most commonly associated with antineutrophil cytoplasmic antibody (ANCA), with a significant risk of renal involvement and which are most responsive to immunosuppression with cyclophosphamide.

vasculitis) but also in association with many other conditions, including infections, connective tissue diseases, malignancy and some drugs (secondary vasculitis). Some classification systems include Wegener's granulomatosis (WG), microscopic polyangiitis (MPA), Churg-Strauss syndrome (CSS), Henoch-Schönlein purpura, cryoglobulinaemic angiitis and cutaneous leucocytoclastic vasculitis in one large group of small vessel vasculitides. Our preference is to separate WG, MPA and CSS because they are:

- [ ] strongly associated with the presence of antineutrophil cytoplasmic antibodies (ANCA) in contrast to the other small vessel vasculitides which are probably immune complex mediated

- [ ] the group of diseases most responsive to immunosuppressive treatment with drugs such as cyclophosphamide

- [ ] more prone to the development of severe glomerulonephritis, in contrast to renal infarction with frank haematuria which is more characteristic of classic polyarteritis nodosa (PAN), and

- [ ] associated with the poorest prognosis if untreated.

Table 2 summarises the usual treatments based on our classification:[1]

- [ ] Large vessel vasculitis (giant cell arteritis and Takayasu arteritis) is usually treated with high doses of prednisolone.

- [ ] Classic PAN, when associated with hepatitis B, can be successfully treated with plasma exchange and antiviral treatment.

- [ ] Kawasaki disease is treated with intravenous (iv) immunoglobulin.

- [ ] WG, MPA and CSS are usually responsive to cyclophosphamide combined with steroids.

- [ ] The pure small vessel vasculitides are treated either with relatively low doses of corticosteroids or perhaps with other drugs such as sulphones.

**Table 2** Relationship between vessel size and response to treatment.[1]

| Dominant vessels involved | Corticosteroids alone | Cyclophosphamide + corticosteroids | Others |
|---|---|---|---|
| Large arteries | + + + | − | + + |
| Medium arteries | + | + + | + +* |
| Small vessels and medium arteries | + | + + + | − |
| Small vessels | + | − | + + |

*includes plasmapheresis, antiviral therapy for hepatitis B associated vasculitis and intravenous immunoglobulin for Kawasaki disease.

## ☐ EPIDEMIOLOGY

The primary systemic vasculitides (WG, MPA and CSS) were originally thought to be rare but recent studies, especially from Europe, suggest an annual incidence of approximately 20 per million. They are slightly more common in men, and some studies suggest a slight increase in incidence with time (over the last 10–20 years), particularly since the introduction of ANCA. A comparative study in three centres in Europe (Tromsø, North Norway, Norwich and Lugo, North Spain)[2] used the same classification criteria applied by one researcher (Fig 1). It found that MPA is particularly common in Southern Europe, in contrast to WG which is commoner in North Europe, while CSS was commonest in Norwich. These diseases are also increasingly recognised in an older population (Fig 2, overleaf), with a peak onset in 65–75 year olds in the UK.

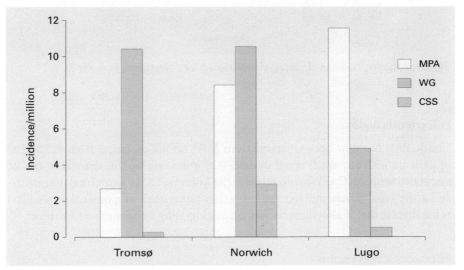

**Fig 1** Incidence of vasculitis in three regions of Europe (CSS = Churg-Strauss syndrome; MPA = microscopic polyangiitis; WG = Wegener's granulomatosis).[2]

## ☐ CLASSIFICATION CRITERIA

The introduction in 1990 of the American College of Rheumatology (ARC) classification criteria[4] allowed comparative studies in different parts of the world. Unfortunately, this did not include MPA, so the definitions used by a Chapel Hill Consensus Conference have been used as surrogate classification criteria. It is important to recognise that the Chapel Hill definitions were not introduced with this in mind but, in the absence of any other criteria, are all that are available. An adaptation of these was suggested by Sorensen and colleagues.[5] These criteria may be useful for separating one sort of vasculitis from another, but have not been found particularly useful when applied to an unselected group of patients with systemic disease. They are, however, important for differentiating the diseases.

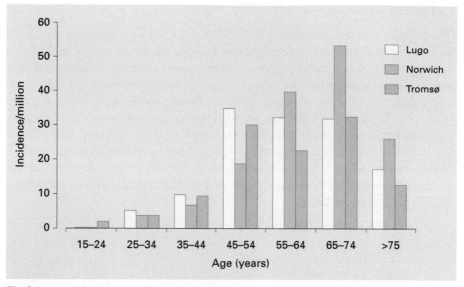

**Fig 2** Age-specific incidence of vasculitis[2] (reproduced, with permission, from Ref 3).

## Polyarteritis nodosa

Classic PAN has now been separated from MPA on the exclusion from classic PAN of patients with any small vessel disease. It is quite rare by this definition and not associated with ANCA. When it involves the kidneys, PAN causes frank haematuria and acute renal failure due to renal infarction rather than to glomerulonephritis. It is the disease that is also characterised on angiography by aneurysm formation.

## Microscopic polyangiitis

By contrast, MPA usually presents with renal involvement with a focal segmental glomerulonephritis without many immune deposits on immunofluorescence (pauci-immune). This disease is strongly associated with ANCA which has specificity against myeloperoxidase (MPO). It can overlap with classic PAN in that aneurysms are occasionally seen. Lung involvement is common, characterised by pulmonary haemorrhage.

## Wegener's granulomatosis

WG is characterised by the triad of:

☐    severe upper airways disease, leading to bone and cartilage destruction

☐    lower airway involvement with granuloma, sometimes leading to cavitation, and

☐    renal vasculitis identical to that seen in MPA.

The dominant feature of WG is the upper airway disease. The immunology is also different in that these patients frequently have ANCA with proteinase 3 specificity.

### Churg-Strauss syndrome

CSS usually presents with late-onset asthma, preceding a systemic vasculitis similar to the vasculitis in MPA and WG but with a higher incidence of peripheral neuropathy and cardiac involvement. These patients also frequently have ANCA, significant blood and tissue eosinophilia and usually MPO specificity.

## ☐ ENVIRONMENTAL/TRIGGER FACTORS

A number of factors have been described in controlled studies as associated with vasculitis (Table 3). For example, there was a doubling of the incidence of MPA after the Kobi earthquake compared with other regions of Japan. Two interesting studies highlight the importance of environmental factors:

1   The highest incidence (not confirmed in any subsequent study) of primary systemic vasculitis in the literature is from Kuwait in a study after the first Gulf War.

2   A large case-control study in Norwich[6] confirmed an association with silica, solvents and allergy (drug allergies). This study also identified for the first time an exposure to farming as a significant risk factor, particularly livestock rather than crops.

**Table 3** Environmental factors.

| |
| --- |
| • Silica |
| • Hydrocarbons |
| • Inhaled fumes and particulates |
| • Infections |
| • Drugs |
| • Allergy |
| • Vaccinations and desensitisation procedures |

### Drugs

The commonest drugs associated with vasculitis are propylthiouracil, hydralazine, allopurinol, minocycline and penicillamine. These drugs can act as a trigger for a systemic illness which can be as serious as the primary vasculitides. Propylthiouracil, hydralazine and allopurinol associated vasculitis can be associated with ANCA. Recent literature has also highlighted a relationship between leukotriene antagonists and CSS. Data from the Southampton Drug Surveillance Register suggest that these drugs probably unmask vasculitis by allowing steroid withdrawal, rather than acting as specific triggers for the disease.

## ☐ EXCLUSION OF DISEASES MIMICKING VASCULITIS

Before embarking on powerful immunosuppressive treatment it is essential both to classify systemic vasculitis and to exclude systemic diseases which can mimic vasculitis (Table 4). It is particularly important to recognise that cholesterol embolisation in patients who have severe atheromatous disease can cause skin infarction with an acute-phase response, eosinophilia, fever etc, as can subacute bacterial endocarditis and atrial myxoma. Calciphylaxis is rare and described almost always in patients with severe renal failure. Arterial and venous thrombosis, as characterised by the antiphospholipid antibody syndrome, is also an important mimic to exclude.

**Table 4** Important mimics of vasculitis.

- Subacute bacterial endocarditis
- Atrial myxoma
- Cholesterol embolism
- Antiphospholipid antibody syndrome
- Calciphylaxis

## ☐ OUTCOME

The introduction of cyclophosphamide changed diseases that were frequently fatal to diseases that could often be controlled and sometimes 'cured'. Early studies were from large tertiary referral centres and may have excluded patients dying of severe acute vasculitis. A summary of the current studies on outcome in vasculitis associated with ANCA suggests that:

☐  there is still a significant mortality (as high as 25% at two years)

☐  two-thirds of the patients continue to have low-grade disease

☐  up to 50% will relapse during follow-up

☐  up to 80% will have significant organ damage, despite apparently successful treatment, and

☐  up to 25% of patients with renal involvement have a significant risk of end-stage renal failure.

These diseases, therefore, are still serious, life-threatening and require long-term follow-up because of the risk of relapse and associated morbidity. In some ways, they now have many similarities with chronic rheumatic diseases such as rheumatoid arthritis, with a number of associated psychological problems.

## ☐ TREATMENT

### Cyclophosphamide

Treatment of choice is still cyclophosphamide, which has now been used for over 30 years. Early studies used continuous oral cyclophosphamide, but during follow-up this was found to be associated with serious long-term toxicity, particularly haemorrhagic cystitis and bladder cancer (>30-fold increased risk). The risk of infection is increased not only as a consequence of the cyclophosphamide but also because of the high doses of corticosteroids frequently used.

Because of the severe toxicity there has been a move over the last two decades to look at different ways of delivering cyclophosphamide and to use this drug for a shorter period of time. Pulsed iv cyclophosphamide has been particularly popular in the UK. In our experience, this is effective, with fewer side effects, although there may be a slightly higher risk of relapse. A meta-analysis of the published literature on pulse versus oral cyclophosphamide appears to confirm these findings (Table 5).[7] A study is currently underway, sponsored by the European Vasculitis Study (EUVAS) Group, to look at this more formally. EUVAS has also recently published the cycazarem study[8] which shows that converting patients from continuous oral cyclophosphamide to oral azathioprine within 3–6 months is as effective as continuous cyclophosphamide. Whatever dose or route of cyclophosphamide is used, there is now a general acceptance that treatment should be as short as possible, perhaps 3–6 months.

**Table 5** Pulse versus continuous cyclophosphamide in systemic vasculitis (143 evaluable patients).[6]

Pulse cyclophosphamide:
- less toxic than oral
- equally potent at inducing remission
- slightly higher risk of relapse

| Outcome | Pulse vs continuous | |
| --- | --- | --- |
| | Odds ratio | Confidence interval |
| No remission | 0.29 | 0.12–0.73 |
| Infection | 0.45 | 0.12–0.89 |
| Leucopenia | 0.36 | 0.17–0.78 |
| Relapse | 1.79 | 0.85–3.75 |

### Severe relapsing disease

A variety of other treatments has been considered in patients with severe relapsing disease, including:

- the new biological agents (eg antitumour necrosis factor α)

- other immunosuppressive drugs

- plasma exchange, and

- high doses of cyclophosphamide (Hi-Cy 3).

In an unpublished study comparing iv methylprednisolone with plasma exchange in severe cases with marked renal impairment, the EUVAS group found that plasma exchange was the most effective treatment. Current studies include a Hi-Cy 3 regimen aimed to reduce the damage which exists in early disease.

## □ SUMMARY

Current thoughts on management are summarised in Table 6. It is important to remember that the primary vasculitides still have a significant effect on morbidity and mortality and must be considered in the differential diagnosis of systemic illness in the elderly. Treatment has significantly improved outcome, so it is important to make an early accurate diagnosis and to use appropriate immunosuppression when the diagnosis is confirmed. Clearly, the treatment of vasculitis depends on its classification. Cyclophosphamide is still the gold standard for the severe primary vasculitides. It is probably safer given iv, although this route is possibly associated with a slightly increased risk of relapse. Cyclophosphamide should be given for as short a time as possible, by whatever route. Azathioprine can be used effectively after remission, and plasma exchange may be helpful for severe refractory disease.

Although these diseases are more common than previously recognised, they still occur in relatively small numbers in most units. Thus, collaborative, long-term prospective studies are essential, and long-term monitoring is important because of the risk of relapse.

**Table 6** Current management of systemic vasculitis.

| |
|---|
| • Still severe life-threatening diseases, often affecting elderly |
| • Treatment usually includes significant immunosuppression, so accurate diagnosis essential |
| • Different treatments for different types of vasculitis |
| • Cyclophosphamide the 'gold standard' for severe disease |
|     – intravenous pulse safer |
|     – continuous oral fewer relapses |
|     – give for only 3–6 months if possible |
| • Switch to azathioprine (?or methotrexate) after 3—6 months |
| • Plasma exchange helpful for refractory disease |
| • Collaborative multicentre studies (eg EUVAS) essential |
| • Long-term monitoring essential |

EUVAS = European Vasculitis Study group.

## REFERENCES

1    Scott DG, Watts RA. Classification and epidemiology of systemic vasculitis. *Br J Rheumatol* 1994;33:897–9.

2    Watts RA, Koldingsnes W, Nossent H, Gonzalez-Gay MA *et al.* Annual incidence of primary systemic vasculitis in three regions of Europe (letter). *Ann Rheum Dis* 2001;60:1156–7.

3    Hochberg MC, Silman AJ, Smolen JS, Weinblatt M, Weisman MH (eds). *Rheumatology*, 3rd edn. Edinburgh, Toronto: Mosby, 2003.

4    Leavitt RY, Fauci AS, Bloch DA, Michel BA *et al.* The American College of Rheumatology 1990 criteria for the classification of Wegener's granulomatosis. *Arthritis Rheum* 1990;**33**:1101–7.

5    Sorensen SF, Slot O, Tvede N, Petersen J. A prospective study of vasculitis patients collected in a five year period: evaluation of the Chapel Hill nomenclature. *Ann Rheum Dis* 2000;**59**:478–82.

6    Lane SE, Watts RA, Bentham G, Innes NJ, Scott DG. Are environmental factors important in primary systemic vasculitis? A case-control study. *Arthritis Rheum* 2003;**48**:814–23.

7    de Groot K, Adu D, Savage CO; EUVAS (European Vasculitis Study Group). The value of pulse cyclophosphamide in ANCA-associated vasculitis: meta-analysis and critical review. *Nephrol Dial Transplant* 2001;**16**:2018–27.

8    Jayne D, Rasmussen N, Andrassy K, Bacon P *et al.* A randomized trial of maintenance therapy for vasculitis associated with antineutrophil cytoplasmic antibodies. *N Engl J Med* 2003;**349**:36–44.

## FURTHER READING

1    Watts RA, Scott DG. Epidemiology of vasculitis. In: Ball GV, Bridges SL Jr (eds). *Vasculitis.* Oxford: Oxford University Press, 2002:211–26.

2    Jennette JC, Falk RJ, Andrassy K, Bacon PA *et al.* Nomenclature of systemic vasculitides. Proposal of an international consensus conference. Review. *Arthritis Rheum* 1994;**37**:187–92.

3    Wechsler M, Finn D, Gunawardena D, Westlake R *et al.* Churg-Strauss syndrome in patients receiving montelukast as treatment for asthma. *Chest* 2000;**117**:708–13.

4    Fauci AS, Haynes BF, Katz P, Wolff SM. Wegener's granulomatosis: prospective clinical and therapeutic experience with 85 patients for 21 years. Review. *Ann Intern Med* 1983;**98**:76–85.

5    Guillevin L, Lhote F, Gayraud M, Cohen P *et al.* Prognostic factors in polyarteritis nodosa and Churg-Strauss syndrome. A prospective study in 342 patients. *Medicine (Baltimore)* 1996;**75**:17–28.

6    Watts RA, Scott DG. Primary systemic vasculitis. *Rheum Dis Topical Rev* 2003;No. 11:1–8.

# Joint replacement in rheumatoid arthritis

Robert Marston

## □ INTRODUCTION

Rheumatoid arthritis (RA) is a chronic inflammatory condition affecting about 1–2% of the British population. Three times as many women as men are affected and the commonest age of onset is in the 4th–6th decades.

Joint replacement is a highly successful treatment for patients experiencing pain and disability as a result of articular cartilage destruction. However, it is only one of a number of surgical procedures which benefit RA sufferers:

1   Surgical synovectomy.

2   Excision arthroplasty (eg in the forefoot or distal ulna).

3   Arthrodesis.

4   Interpositional arthroplasty.

5   Total joint replacement.

## □ SPECIAL CONSIDERATIONS

Unlike patients with osteoarthritis, those with RA have several systemic factors which make both the surgery and rehabilitation much more complex and prone to complications.

### Multiple joint involvement

The presence of upper limb involvement hampers postoperative care and essentially precludes the use of any procedure which requires partial weight bearing as part of the rehabilitation. Instead of elbow crutches, gutter crutches are required in order to protect deformed wrist and finger joints from further damage.

### Medical treatment

*Steroids*

Immunity is reduced by steroids, so there is a higher rate of postoperative infection. They also inhibit wound healing. Both the disease process and the prolonged use of steroids cause osteopenia. The risk of periprosthetic fracture in the perioperative period increases as well as the risk of aseptic loosening due to poor cement bone interface. The stress of surgery also means that steroid doses must be increased at the time of surgery. Immunity is similarly reduced by tumour necrosis factor.

### Methotrexate

Until recently, methotrexate, another disease-modifying agent, was stopped prior to surgery; this is now considered unnecessary because the increased morbidity of surgery in these patients is a reflection of the severity of their disease and not of the methotrexate.

## Anaesthetic problems

Atlanto-axial or subaxial subluxation is present in 30–40% of rheumatoid patients which can make intubation perilous. All patients should have lateral flexion and extension views of the cervical spine to look for instability (Fig 1). Severe cases may warrant cervical magnetic resonance imaging to assess the amount of peri-odontoid pannus and how much space is available for the cord. An anaesthetist with nasoendoscopic intubation expertise must be available.

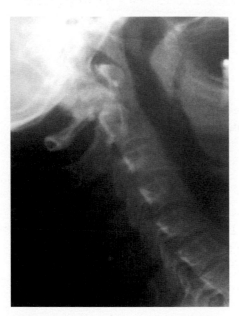

**Fig 1** A lateral cervical spine view in flexion clearly demonstrates atlanto-axial subluxation.

## Systemic disease

Patients may be anaemic or neutropenic, which may again increase the rate of postoperative complications. Lung involvement is more common in male patients, but may be manifest by interstitial lung disease, pleural effusions, haemorrhage and bronchiectasis. Pericarditis and arrhythmias due to myocardial nodules affecting the conduction system can be seen in up to 40% of patients.

## □ EPIDEMIOLOGY

A study of 103 patients over a 25-year period found that 22 (19 female) had undergone a total of 41 large joint replacements:[1]

- □   17 total hip replacements (mean of 14 years from disease onset)

- □   four total knee replacements (mean of 17 years from onset)

- □   three total shoulder replacements after 18 years, and

- □   seven total elbow replacements after 21 years.

The recommendation for the greater use of disease-modifying drugs, and at an earlier stage, should delay the time to replacement and reduce the overall number requiring surgery. In the UK it remains to be seen whether the National Institute for Clinical Excellence will be forward thinking or humane enough to license these drugs or whether financial imperatives will intervene.

A 30-year study in Minnesota found that at 14–18 years following diagnosis 35% of patients had undergone one or more procedures; by 30 years, this figure had risen to 53%. Overall survival was equal to that of rheumatoid patients not requiring surgery.[2] The study revealed that surgery was more likely in the following groups:

- □   those with positive rheumatoid factor

- □   those with rheumatoid nodules

- □   young patients

- □   female patients.

## □ REPLACEMENT SURGERY

### Hip replacement

About 40% of patients with RA have hip involvement. The cost/benefit ratio of replacement is low, but the peri- and postoperative complication rate is higher than for osteoarthritic patients.

Standard cemented components on the femoral and acetabular side are the components of choice (Fig 2). Cement allows excellent primary fixation of the hip into poor bone and immediately allows full weight bearing. Fracture is more common due to osteopenia, and great care must be taken to avoid femoral fracture when dislocating the damaged hip or relocating it after replacement (Fig 3). Protrusio acetabuli is also common (Fig 4), and it is important that the floor of the acetabulum is grafted so that the centre of rotation of the acetabular component does not lie too medially. Malposition will lead to premature failure, usually due to failure of the floor of the acetabulum, and successful reconstruction can be a significant challenge.

Intracapsular fracture of the neck of the femur in rheumatoid patients is associated with a high rate of nonunion, if treated with internal fixation, due to poor bone. With displaced intracapsular fractures, total hip replacement is the procedure

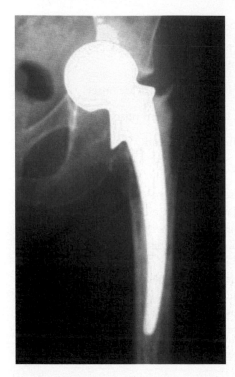

**Fig 2** Hip replacement using a standard cemented prosthesis, with excellent results.

**(a)**    **(b)**

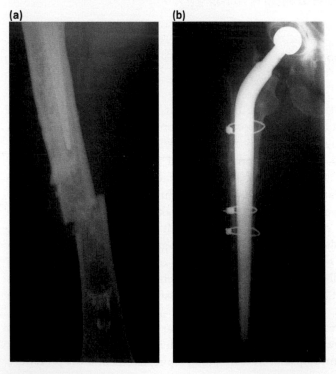

**Fig 3 (a)** A periprosthetic fracture of the femoral shaft below the prosthetic stem; **(b)** revision of a similar fracture to a long stem prosthesis using cerclage wires.

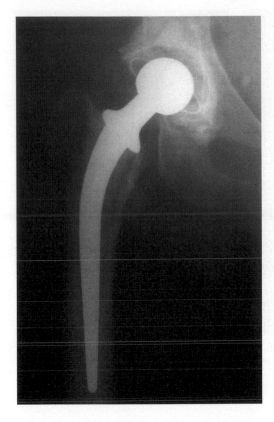

**Fig 4** The loose acetabular component shows substantial protrusio and an acetabular fracture.

of choice since hemiarthroplasties migrate medially through the acetabular floor becoming protrusio (Fig 5). The revision required is complex with a high complication rate.

### Knee replacement

Up to 90% of rheumatoid patients have knee involvement, bilateral in 75% (Fig 6). The cost/benefit ratio of replacement is favourable. The components are cemented and the patella must be resurfaced. Most patients will have retained a much better range of flexion than their osteoarthritic counterparts, and this seems to continue to be retained postoperatively. It is probably due to a less severe degree of soft tissue scarring in ligaments, tendons and the joint capsule, possibly as a result of long-term anti-inflammatory treatment. If the patient has a stiff hip on the same side, this must be replaced before the knee.

A small subgroup of patients develop 'windswept' knees – a significant valgus deformity in one knee and a varus deformity in the other. A stabilised knee replacement is required because of collateral ligament damage. The articulating components are partially constrained so they compensate for the damaged ligaments.

Good or excellent results are obtained in only 83% of RA patients compared with 95% in osteoarthritis, and the percentage of poor results is higher.[3]

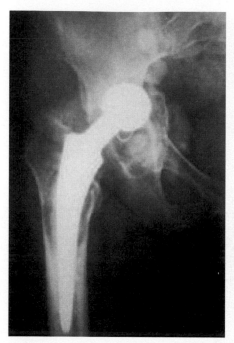

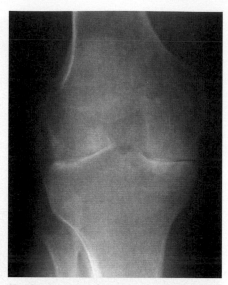

**Fig 6** Anteroposterior view of the knee shows changes characteristic of rheumatoid, with concentric joint space loss and little sclerosis or subchondral cyst formation.

**Fig 5** Following treatment for an intracapsular fracture, the hemiarthroplasty is eroding into the pelvis.

### Ankle replacement

Although ankle replacement is much less common than hip or knee prostheses, the rheumatoid patient is a much better candidate for this than the osteoarthritic patient. This has been attributed to the lower activity levels of the rheumatoid patient due to multiple joint involvement, thus reducing stresses on the prosthetic bone interface.

The results are improving, but many patients need conversion to arthrodesis which remains the treatment of choice. In a series reported from the Hospital for Joint Diseases in Wrightington, two-thirds of the Thompson-Parkridge-Richards replacements were loose at two years, half of which required fusion.[4]

### Shoulder replacement

Shoulder replacement gives good results. Of 105 patients from Wrightington with good long-term follow-up, 92% of total shoulder replacements were still in situ at nine years.[5] The results were much better if the rotator cuff muscle tendon unit was intact (Fig 7). This prevents superior and medial migration of the joint which is associated with a poor outcome. The results of hemiarthroplasty of the shoulder, where the glenoid fossa is not replaced or resurfaced, are as good as total shoulder replacement.

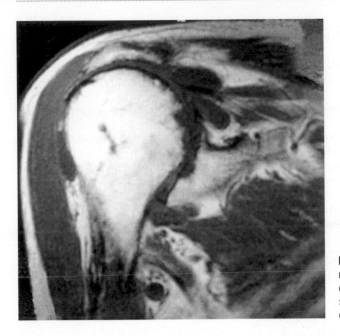

**Fig 7** A T1-weighted coronal magnetic resonance image demonstrates widespread shoulder erosions and a tear of the rotator cuff.

## Elbow replacement

The success of elbow replacement in the rheumatoid patient is related to previous surgery. Patients who have had resection arthroplasties are particularly prone to complications. In a series of 59 patients undergoing total elbow replacement, 44% had RA.[6] This group had a 20% complication rate. Revision elbow replacement is challenging, even when possible.

## Wrist replacement

In a study of 76 wrist replacements at a mean follow-up of 52 months, 74% had good to excellent results.[7] More than half the patients who had a contralateral arthrodesis would have preferred an arthroplasty on that side. Five patients required a revision or fusion, and nine had radiological loosening, of which three were symptomatic. Implant survival was 83% at eight years.

## ☐ CONCLUSIONS

Joint replacement in RA patients is a beneficial procedure. Total hip and knee replacements are the most well evaluated, but shoulder, elbow and wrist are increasing in reliability.

## REFERENCES

1   Palm TM, Kaarela K, Hakala MS, Kautianen HJ *et al.* Need and sequence of large joint replacements in rheumatoid arthritis. A 25-year follow-up study. *Clin Exp Rheumatol* 2002;20:392–4.

2    Massardo L, Gabriel SE, Crowson CS, O'Fallon WM, Matteson EL. A population based assessment of the use of orthopedic surgery in patients with rheumatoid arthritis. *J Rheumatol* 2002;29:52–6.

3    Wright J, Ewald FC, Walker PS, Thomas WH *et al.* Total knee arthroplasty with the kinematic prosthesis. Results after five to nine years: a follow-up note. *J Bone Joint Surg Am* 1990;72: 1003–9.

4    Wood PL, Clough TM, Jari S. Clinical comparison of two total ankle replacements. *Foot Ankle Int* 2000;21:546–50.

5    Trail IA, Nuttall D. The results of shoulder arthroplasty in patients with rheumatoid arthritis. *J Bone Joint Surg Br* 2002;84:1121–5.

6    Fink B, Krey D, Schmielau G, Tillmann K, Ruther W. Results of elbow endoprosthesis in patients with rheumatoid arthritis in correlation with previous operations. *J Shoulder Elbow Surg* 2002;11:360–7.

7    Takwale VJ, Nuttall D, Trail IA, Stanley JK. Biaxial total wrist replacement in patients with rheumatoid arthritis. *J Bone Joint Surg Br* 2002;84:692–9.

## ☐ RHEUMATOLOGY SELF ASSESSMENT QUESTIONS

### Glucocorticoids in rheumatoid arthritis

1   Rheumatoid arthritis (RA):
   (a) Occurs in about 1–2% of people
   (b) Starts usually in people over the age of 60
   (c) Progresses relentlessly
   (d) May be a mixture of intra-articular pathologies
   (e) Causes joint inflammation and joint destruction

2   In RA:
   (a) Joint destruction can be slowed by treatment
   (b) Low-dose glucocorticoids usually suppress inflammation for many years
   (c) Joint destruction has at least two components
   (d) Erosions can be prevented by low-dose glucocorticoids for some years
   (e) Cartilage thinning correlates with joint inflammation

3   Glucocorticoids:
   (a) In low doses affect cell metabolism by dissolving in the cell membrane
   (b) Probably work by different mechanisms at different doses
   (c) Can prevent the progression of joint erosions in RA
   (d) Affect inflammation and joint destruction differently
   (e) Are too expensive to use in many patients

4   Adverse effects of low-dose glucocorticoids in RA:
   (a) Are obvious in most patients
   (b) Are well recorded in the literature
   (c) Include weight gain and hypertension
   (d) May be associated with inappropriate dose increases
   (e) Include a 'rebound flare' after treatment withdrawal which makes patients worse off than before

5   The evidence in the literature related to RA points to:
   (a) A difference in the effects of glucocorticoids on inflammation and joint damage
   (b) A potential therapeutic benefit from treating patients with glucocorticoids early in the disease
   (c) The need for long-term glucocorticoid treatment to control symptoms
   (d) Clear-cut information about the balance of risks and benefits of low-dose glucocorticoid treatment in patients with long-standing disease
   (e) Histological support for the notion of different intra-articular pathologies

**Primary systemic vasculitis**

1  Antineutrophil cytoplasmic antibodies with specificity against proteinase 3 are commonly found in:
   (a) Polyarteritis nodosa (PAN)
   (b) Vasculitis associated with rheumatoid arthritis (RA)
   (c) Wegener's granulomatosis (WG)
   (d) Henoch-Schönlein purpura (HSP)
   (e) Kawasaki disease

2  Focal segmental necrotising glomerulonephritis in the absence of significant immune deposits (immunoglobulin G (IgG), IgA, IgM, complement component 3) is a characteristic of:
   (a) Systemic lupus erythematosus
   (b) WG
   (c) HSP
   (d) Microscopic polyangiitis
   (e) Churg-Strauss syndrome

3  Aneurysms detected on angiography may be seen in patients with:
   (a) PAN
   (b) HSP
   (c) WG
   (d) Vasculitis complicating RA
   (e) Cutaneous leucocytoclastic vasculitis

4  The following are statements about the treatment of vasculitis:
   (a) Cyclophosphamide is the drug of choice in patients with Takayasu arteritis
   (b) Oral cyclophosphamide should be continued until patients have been in remission for at least one year
   (c) Azathioprine and methotrexate are appropriate alternatives to cyclophosphamide in primary systemic vasculitis when patients have achieved remission
   (d) Pulsed intravenous cyclophosphamide is as effective as continuous oral cyclophosphamide
   (e) Bladder toxicity is a serious complication of daily oral cyclophosphamide

**Joint replacement in rheumatoid arthritis**

1  In rheumatoid arthritis (RA):
   (a) The disease process can be modified by metronidazole
   (b) Atlanto-axial subluxation can cause anaesthetic complications in 35%
   (c) A pericardial rub may be heard
   (d) 5% of the population is affected
   (e) Lung disease is more common in women

2    Concerning hip replacement in RA:
   (a) The complication rate is similar to that seen in osteoarthritis
   (b) Cemented components are used
   (c) 70% of patients have hip involvement
   (d) Undisplaced intracapsular fractures can be treated conservatively
   (e) Protrusio acetabuli is common

3    Concerning knee replacement in RA:
   (a) 90% of patients have knee involvement
   (b) Windswept knees have bilateral patellar subluxations
   (c) Postoperative flexion is better than in osteoarthritis patients
   (d) Results of surgery are better than in osteoarthritis patients
   (e) The knee must be replaced before the hip

# Respiratory Medicine

# Chronic obstructive pulmonary disease

Peter Calverley

## ☐ INTRODUCTION

Chronic obstructive pulmonary disease (COPD) remains a major cause of morbidity and mortality in the UK and worldwide. Despite substantial falls in the prevalence of its principal cause, cigarette smoking, over the last 40 years, the number of patients presenting with COPD to family doctors, and especially to the hospital services, continues to rise. Hospitalisations due to COPD increased by 50% between 1991 and 2000. The most recent estimate for the UK suggests there were 308,355 admissions for COPD in 1999, with an average stay in hospital of 7.9 days.

This has led to an interest in the underlying pathophysiology of the disorder and a concern to try to standardise patient management in order to lessen the substantial burden this disease poses for those affected and to the healthcare system. This chapter will briefly review some of the more important current insights into the pathophysiology that underlies this condition and summarise current management approaches (as of 2002).

## ☐ DEFINITION

Defining COPD continues to cause significant problems for both patients and doctors. The term now includes individuals with either chronic bronchitis or a pathological diagnosis of emphysema, who have persistent airflow obstruction operationally described as an $FEV_1/FVC$ below 0.7. Ideally, this measurement should be performed post-bronchodilator, with the ratio expressed as a percentage predicted for age, although in clinical practice this is frequently not done.

The emphasis on airflow obstruction reflects the known natural history of the condition and the association of airflow obstruction, but not regular cough and sputum production, with mortality. This issue has been revisited as the recently published Global Initiative in Obstructive Lung Disease (GOLD) classification suggested a group at risk of COPD.[1] These patients do not have airflow obstruction but have suggestive symptoms such as the presence of cough or sputum production. The value of defining people in this way remains controversial, particularly as those who have these symptoms but no airflow obstruction do not appear to be more likely to develop COPD than the general population.[2]

The presence of persistent airflow obstruction requires spirometry to ensure its correct diagnosis, but several other aspects have been emphasised by GOLD. Airflow obstruction:

- [ ]   should not be fully reversible – although what constitutes reversibility is not stated

- [ ]   is normally progressive and, by inference, persistent, and

- [ ]   is associated with an abnormal inflammatory response within the lungs – again, what is abnormal is not specified.

This inflammation is the result of the inhalation of noxious particles or gases, principal amongst which is tobacco smoke. However, in many parts of the world other non-tobacco based organic dust and smoke inhalation can produce significant airflow obstruction among non-smokers. Thus, the pathogenesis of COPD is slightly more complex than the traditional western view of 'tobacco-induced obstructive lung disease', although this remains by far the most important factor in the UK.

## ☐ PATHOLOGICAL BASIS

COPD takes time to develop, reflecting the chronic exposure to a low dose of an inhaled irritant. It is difficult in any individual to quantify the total exposure of the respiratory tract to inhaled particles and gases as patients adopt different patterns of tobacco smoking for different periods of the day and, when inhaled, the particulate and gaseous phases impact rather differently upon the respiratory tract. It is no surprise that some individuals show changes which predominate in the large airways. However, most people who develop airflow obstruction show an increase in peripheral airways resistance, reflecting damage to airways narrower than 2 mm in diameter and also to the alveoli.

Chronic bronchitis is characterised by enlargement of the mucus glands in the large airways which then become infiltrated with inflammatory cells. Cilia are frequently lost or damaged in the central airways, impairing mucociliary clearance and contributing to the cough and sputum production, cough being the principal clearance mechanism for the airways. More dramatic changes are normally seen in the respiratory bronchioles, with increased cellular inflammation beneath the epithelium around the airways smooth muscle and in the adventia together with peribronchial fibrosis.[3] Macroscopic emphysema predominates in the upper lobe, but can be more widespread in some patients.

Lymphocyte numbers are increased in the airways, with relative equivalence of helper and suppressor cells, a rather different pattern from bronchial asthma. Recent quantitative pathological studies found that almost all major inflammatory cells increase as COPD progresses, including macrophages, lymphocytes and neutrophils.[4]

## ☐ PATHOGENIC MECHANISMS

There is currently no generally agreed scheme that explains the pathogenesis of COPD; proponents of individual mechanisms continue to collect data in support of their favoured theory. There are several suggested mechanisms.

## Protease-antiprotease imbalance

The concept of protease-antiprotease imbalance is of significant historical interest. This mechanism is strongly supported by the naturally occurring form of emphysema due to alpha1-antitrypsin deficiency.[5] Classically, emphysema is basal in distribution and may be ameliorated by intravenous antitrypsin replacement treatment. Proteases released from neutrophils can digest elastin within the interstitium of the lung, which would explain the occurrence of emphysema. Their role in the potentially more important bronchiolar disease remains more speculative.

## Oxidant-antioxidant defence imbalance

Another important candidate mechanism is an imbalance between oxidant and antioxidant defences. Cigarette smoke is a potent source of oxidant molecules that not only damage lipid membranes but also induce inflammation and inactivate antitrypsins. Elegant studies in mice exposed to cigarette smoke suggest that macrophage-produced proteases may be particularly important in this model. Coupled with studies in other animal models with genetically engineered overexpression of specific cytokines (eg interleukin-13 and interferon gamma), these new approaches offer potentially important insights into how the different mechanisms interact to produce disease.[6]

## Amplifying and predisposing factors

There is increased interest in the role of amplifying or predisposing factors in the genesis of COPD. One group has proposed that latent viral infections may make some individuals particularly susceptible. The search for genetic correlates, in particular polymorphisms of specific genes in ordinary human COPD, is now beginning and a number of candidate genes have already been identified. This is likely to be an area of rapid growth in the coming years.

## ☐ PHYSIOLOGICAL ADVANCES

### Bronchodilator reversibility

There is now increasing evidence that testing for bronchodilator reversibility, whether with an inhaled bronchodilator or a course of corticosteroids, is of limited value at least in established COPD. The small changes in lung function produced by these drugs can easily be overinterpreted when arbitrary reversibility criteria are applied, and their reproducibility on repeated testing is poor. Long-term mortality is unrelated to the magnitude of the bronchodilator response.

### Expiratory airflow limitation

New methods have been developed to identify expiratory airflow limitation non-invasively during tidal breathing, the most widely accepted being the application of a negative expiratory pressure at the beginning of expiration.[7] This test easily distinguishes patients whose expiratory flow increases when the negative pressure is applied from those in whom this does not occur. The latter group represents individuals who can increase their expiratory flow only by changing their end-expiratory lung volume. Many studies show that this occurs during exercise in severe COPD patients,[8] that it correlates with breathlessness and can be reduced by bronchodilator treatment.

Not all patients have tidal flow limitation at rest, and other factors determine their exercise performance. So far these have been less well studied, although it is likely that problems with oxygen delivery to the peripheral muscles and associated cardiovascular factors are relevant in at least some individuals.

## □ SYSTEMIC EFFECTS

COPD is defined in terms of airflow obstruction, but there is renewed interest in the impact of this disorder on the whole body. Good data indicate that COPD is associated with both an increased loss of bone mass as the disease progresses and an unexpectedly high incidence of osteoporosis. Nutrition in general is often poor in COPD and a reduced body mass index is an independent prognostic factor. Exercise capacity is related to this loss of muscle mass and a specific 'COPD myopathy' may occur in patients with severe disease. Quality of life (now called 'health status') is impaired in COPD; it is a predictor of mortality, as is the level of breathlessness reported on the Medical Research Council dyspnoea scale.[9]

## □ MANAGEMENT

A series of clear, evidence-based steps towards COPD management has been agreed following the publication of the GOLD guidelines, and forms the basis of many subsequent guideline documents. The GOLD approach emphasises the need to make a firm diagnosis based on:

- □   an appropriate clinical history

- □   relevant exposure to a noxious agent, and

- □   confirmation by spirometry.

Having obtained a firm diagnosis, the main focus of management in the stable condition is twofold:

1   Preventing disease progression.

2   Pharmacological management.

### Preventing disease progression

Removal from an identified environmental exposure can halt disease progression. By far the most important is stopping smoking tobacco – a task that remains difficult, but attainable, even in COPD patients. Appropriate counselling, nicotine replacement or pharmacological support during withdrawal can help patients quit successfully.

## Pharmacological management

### Long-acting inhaled bronchodilators

First-line therapy with long-acting inhaled bronchodilators in patients who have persistent symptoms due to COPD is now supported by good data. Long-acting inhaled beta-agonists (eg salmeterol, formoterol) and anticholinergics (eg tiotropium) not only produce sustained improvements in lung function but also reduce the number of exacerbations and improve health status. Adding in an inhaled corticosteroid helps patients with an $FEV_1$ below 50% predicted who have a history of previous exacerbations.[10]

## Pulmonary rehabilitation

All stages of COPD are helped by pulmonary rehabilitation; it produces quantitatively larger improvements in exercise performance and health status than any drug treatment. Unfortunately, maintaining this has proved difficult, although substantial clinical benefit persists for 12–18 months after a course of rehabilitation. The optimum way of trying to lengthen this period has not been defined. Most patients can undergo outpatient rehabilitation courses and benefit from this relatively cost-effective therapy.

## Domiciliary oxygen therapy

Continuous domiciliary oxygen therapy is of benefit only to patients with an arterial $PO_2$ below 7.3 kPa when clinically stable. It can improve exercise tolerance when given while exercising, but the value of short-burst treatment is less certain.

## Lung volume reduction surgery

Lung volume reduction surgery is not appropriate for those with an $FEV_1$ and/or carbon monoxide diffusion in the lungs below 20% predicted and in patients with generalised emphysema. However, reported randomised control trials suggest that others may benefit.

## Managing exacerbations

Short courses of oral corticosteroids as an adjunct to bronchodilator therapy improve lung function recovery and shorten hospital stay during COPD exacerbations.[11] Nasal positive pressure ventilation is effective in controlling respiratory acidosis, even when used in the district general hospital setting,[12] and represents a major step forward in improving hospital care of the acutely ill COPD patient.

## □ CONCLUSIONS

Real progress has been made in understanding the factors that produce COPD and in developing rational approaches to its management. Applying available technologies, particularly spirometry, to confirm the diagnosis, represents an important step forward in management. There is now a real chance that insights derived from clinical and laboratory studies will enable the construction of a rational scheme of treatment to prevent progression of this major source of ill health in our society.

## REFERENCES

1   Pauwels RA, Buist AS, Calverley PM, Jenkins CR, Hurd SS. Global strategy for the diagnosis, management, and prevention of chronic obstructive pulmonary disease. NHLBL/WHO Global Initiative for Chronic Obstructive Lung Disease (GOLD) Workshop summary. Review. *Am J Respir Crit Care Med* 2001;**163**:1256–76.

2   Vestbo J, Lange P. Can GOLD Stage 0 provide information of prognostic value in chronic obstructive pulmonary disease? *Am J Respir Crit Care Med* 2002;**166**:329–32.

3   Turato G, Zuin R, Miniati M, Baraldo S *et al.* Airway inflammation in severe chronic obstructive pulmonary disease: relationship with lung function and radiologic emphysema. *Am J Respir Crit Care Med* 2002;**166**:105–10.

4   Hogg JC, Senior RM. Chronic obstructive pulmonary disease – part 2: pathology and biochemistry of emphysema. Review. *Thorax* 2002;**57**:830–4.

5   Stockley RA. Alpha-1-antitrypsin deficiency: what next? Review. *Thorax* 2000;**55**:614–8.

6   Shapiro SD. Evolving concepts in the pathogenesis of chronic obstructive pulmonary disease. Review. *Clin Chest Med* 2000;**21**:621–32.

7   Koulouris NG, Valta P, Lavoie A, Corbeil C *et al.* A simple method to detect expiratory flow limitation during spontaneous breathing. *Eur Respir J* 1995;**8**:306–13.

8   O'Donnell DE, Revill SM, Webb KA. Dynamic hyperinflation and exercise intolerance in chronic obstructive pulmonary disease. *Am J Respir Crit Care Med* 2001;**164**:770–7.

9   Domingo-Salvany A, Lamarca R, Ferrer M, Garcia-Aymerich J *et al.* Health-related quality of life and mortality in male patients with chronic obstructive pulmonary disease. *Am J Respir Crit Care Med* 2002;**166**:680–5.

10  Calverley P, Pauwels R, Vestbo J, Jones P *et al.* Combined salmeterol and fluticasone in the treatment of chronic obstructive pulmonary disease: a randomised controlled trial. *Lancet* 2003;**361**:449–56.

11  Davies L, Angus RM, Calverley PM. Oral corticosteroids in patients admitted to hospital with exacerbations of chronic obstructive pulmonary disease: a prospective randomised controlled trial. *Lancet* 1999;**354**:456–60.

12  Plant PK, Owen JL, Elliott MW. Early use of non-invasive ventilation for acute exacerbations of chronic obstructive pulmonary disease on general respiratory wards: a multicentre randomised controlled trial. *Lancet* 2000;**355**:1931–5.

# Sleep apnoea

John Stradling

## ☐ INTRODUCTION

Obstructive sleep apnoea (OSA) is now firmly part of mainstream medicine. An appreciation of its pathophysiology, relevance and the effectiveness of treatment has moved it from a medical curiosity to a disease that most doctors will encounter. Recent particularly relevant developments relate to:

- ☐ the increased incidence of road traffic accidents (RTAs) in these patients

- ☐ a realisation that OSA is an independent risk factor for essential hypertension, and

- ☐ an acceptance that simplified methods of diagnosis and treatment are appropriate.

This chapter will concentrate on these three areas which are influencing practice.

## ☐ PATHOPHYSIOLOGY

The upper airway needs dilator muscles to hold it open. Failure of this function during unconsciousness or anaesthesia is familiar to all doctors; the recovery position was introduced partly to overcome pharyngeal obstruction (as indeed does the forward jaw thrust). Sleep produces the same failure of pharyngeal dilator function in some people.[1] The initial result is snoring, then significant narrowing engendering increasing inspiratory effort, and finally complete collapse with frustrated inspiratory efforts. This represents a spectrum of increasing pharyngeal failure, along which snoring and apnoea are two easily recognisable points. The body's main defence against this problem is transient arousal which restores the dilator tone so that ventilation can return. These arousals are provoked mainly by the increased effort to breath in, rather than the attendant hypoxia (which usually occurs during each event). Heavy snoring on its own, without easily detectable hypoxia, can also provoke these recurrent arousals (so-called upper resistance syndrome).

Imaging studies show that the dominant area of obstruction is retroglossal, even if the collapse begins higher up in the vicinity of the soft palate. Significant upper airway narrowing during sleep can be caused by any condition or situation that encourages this process and amplifies the normal, irrelevant narrowing due to the reduced pharyngeal dilator tone coincident with sleep onset.

## Risk factors

### Obesity

The most prevalent risk factor is obesity, in particular neck obesity. Not only does neck obesity produce a smaller pharyngeal airway, but it also 'loads' the airway and overcomes the reduced dilator activity during sleep. Most of the neck fat is subcutaneous, but there is some evidence that enlarged peripharyngeal fat pads crowd the airway directly and fatty infiltration of the relevant dilator muscles may reduce their effectiveness. Thus, neck circumference is the best predictor of the presence of OSA, with the likelihood rising rapidly if it is above 17 inches.

### Retro- or micrognathic lower face

In addition to obesity, a retro- or micrognathic lower face will also crowd the upper airway. Most studies have shown a degree of retropositioning of both the mandible and maxilla. This is not usually obvious from the outside, but inspection inside the mouth may show crowded teeth, no room for third molars and/or molars displaced backwards off the horizontal into the angled part of the mandible, as well as a small retroglossal space antero-posteriorly. Large tonsils, mainly seen in children, also crowd the airway, provoking obstruction when the pharyngeal dilators relax with sleep onset.

### Other causes

Other causes of OSA are listed in Table 1. Neuromuscular failure is a rare cause – indeed, there is evidence that the pharyngeal dilators usually work harder than normal to defend the airway, even when awake. However, if a neuromuscular disease does weaken pharyngeal dilators, OSA can result, for example following stroke and in motor neurone disease, muscular dystrophies etc.

**Table 1** Causes of obstructive sleep apnoea and snoring.

| | |
|---|---|
| • Obesity, particularly upper body | • Alcohol taken in the evening |
| • Lower facial shape | • Smoking |
| • Hypothyroidism | • Nasal congestion |
| • Enlarged tonsils | • Menopause |
| • Acromegaly | • Neuromuscular diseases/stroke |
| • Mucopolysaccharidoses | |

## □ EPIDEMIOLOGY

OSA is common: epidemiological surveys show that up to 25% of middle-aged men have a certain number of obstructive apnoeas at night. However, there is a problem of definition. As with hypertension, the exact prevalence heavily depends on the threshold chosen to define the disease. In hypertension it is judged according to the longer-term outcomes, but in OSA such data are only in their infancy. In addition, current measures of OSA may not accurately define the disease, just as one-off clinic blood pressure measurement may not define an individual's true risk from hypertension. None the less, in the spectrum from light snoring to severe OSA, a stage is reached when morbidity rises to unacceptable levels. Most studies have found a prevalence of severe symptomatic OSA in middle-aged men of about 1–2%, and about half or less than that in women.[2] The figure will also depend on prevailing levels of obesity and is likely to be higher in the US, with the UK rapidly catching up. There also appear to be racial differences; even after correction for differences in obesity, there is a higher prevalence in black Americans and Orientals. Because of the high prevalence in the UK, OSA is now one of the top three reasons for referral in some respiratory units, and a general practice of 10,000 patients is likely to have 5–10 such patients.

## ☐ SYMPTOMS

### Daytime sleepiness

The dominant and most obvious symptom of OSA is excessive daytime sleepiness, which is unfortunate for several reasons, including the following:

1   Sleepy patients are often poorly motivated and irritable, a combination that may retard their presentation.

2   Sleepiness is also often viewed as a minor symptom (by doctors), and further trivialised when associated with the symptom of snoring, itself usually the butt of jokes.

3   Sleepiness produces poor performance at work and at home.

4   There is an increased rate of RTAs.

Sleepiness is different to tiredness, and patients need to be asked whether they fall asleep during the day, and this tendency assessed. The Epworth Sleepiness Score is the most validated way of doing this (Fig 1). The vast majority of patients with OSA are sleepy and not tired, although some, particularly women, may choose the word 'tiredness' to describe the result of their sleep fragmentation.

### Road traffic accidents

Of greater concern is the increased RTA rate in these individuals. Particularly in severe OSA, the accident rate may be 8–10 times higher than normal. In driving simulator studies, the control of the car is worse than in normal subjects and, on average, as bad as subjects over the legal blood alcohol level. It is not clear if this is the result only of sleepiness and microsleeps, or whether eye-hand co-ordination is also affected by sleep deprivation.

The good news is that the increased RTA rate falls with treatment of OSA,[3] and that effective treatment seems to reverse the simulator abnormality.[4] Thus, driving is regarded as safe in patients with OSA once successful treatment has removed the

## EPWORTH SLEEPINESS SCALE

Name: ................................................................. Hospital number ..............................

Date:...................... Your age (Yrs) ............... Your sex (Male = M / Female = F) .............

- How likely are you to doze off or fall asleep in the situations described in the box below, in contrast to feeling just tired?
- This refers to your usual way of life in recent times.
- Even if you haven't done some of these things recently try to work out how they would have affected you.
- Use the following scale to choose the <u>most appropriate number</u> for each situation:–

      0 = would <u>never</u> doze           2 = <u>Moderate</u> chance of dozing

      1 = <u>Slight chance of dozing</u>      3 = High<u> chance of dozing</u>

| Situation | Chance of dozing |
|---|---|
| Sitting and reading | |
| Watching TV | |
| Sitting, inactive in a public place (eg a theatre or a meeting) | |
| As a passenger in a car for an hour without a break | |
| Lying down to rest in the afternoon when circumstances permit | |
| Sitting and talking to someone | |
| Sitting quietly after a lunch without alcohol | |
| In a car, while stopped for a few minutes in the traffic | |

**Thank you for your cooperation**

**Fig 1** Epworth Sleepiness Score. A validated way to assess the impact of sleepiness on daily activities. The overall score (the addition of each individual item, scored 0–3) can vary between 0 (no sleepiness) and 24 (maximum sleepiness). Normal subjects average 5.9 (standard deviation (SD) 2.2) with 9 the upper limit of normal. Patients with sleep apnoea average 16.0 (SD 4.4).

excessive daytime sleepiness. In professional class 2 drivers, verification of satisfactory treatment and response by a specialist clinic is required.

### Other symptoms

In addition to sleepiness, there are a variety of other symptoms, some more obvious than others (Table 2). The nocturia represents a true increase in urine production, with a reversal of the usual day/night pattern.

Despite this plethora of symptoms, it is the sleepiness that most often drives treatment from the patient's point of view.

**Table 2** Symptoms of obstructive sleep apnoea.

| Common | • Loud snoring |
|---|---|
| | • Excessive daytime sleepiness |
| | • Choking or shortness of breath sensations during sleep |
| | • Restless sleep |
| | • Unrefreshing sleep |
| | • Changes in personality |
| | • Nocturia |
| Less common | • Morning headaches |
| | • Reduced libido |
| | • Nocturnal sweating |
| | • Spouse worried by apnoeic episodes |
| Rarely | • Enuresis |
| | • Symptomatic oesophageal reflux |
| | • Recurrent arousals/insomnia |
| | • Nocturnal cough |

## ☐ CARDIOVASCULAR CONSEQUENCES

Early in the history of OSA it was realised that dramatic cardiovascular changes occur with every apnoeic event (Fig 2): there are large blood pressure (BP) surges with every arousal, and dips with every frustrated inspiratory effort during the apnoea (pulsus paradoxus). It has been difficult to prove whether OSA is an independent risk factor for hypertension and cardiovascular disease, basically because most of these patients are men in a high-risk group anyway, overweight (with an upper body distribution) and middle-aged. However, recent careful studies

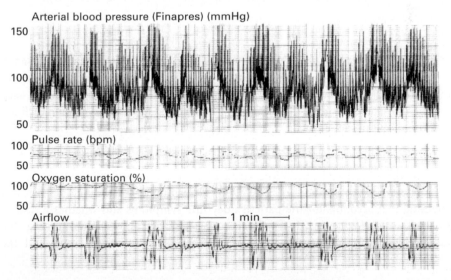

**Fig 2** Five-minute recording of continuous blood pressure (arterial), pulse rate, oxygen saturation in arterial blood (%) and airflow from a patient with obstructive sleep apnoea. In the blood pressure line, note the large rises due to the arousal at the end of each episode of apnoea (resumption of airflow) and the transient dips (pulsus paradoxus) with each frustrated inspiratory effort during the apnoea.

have shown an independent effect of OSA on diurnal hypertension. Both matched-pair and randomised controlled trials (RCT) with placebo versus real nasal continuous positive airway pressure (CPAP) suggest that OSA produces an average BP rise of about 5 mmHg.[5] However, in subsets with severe disease, who use their CPAP for over five hours a night and are already on antihypertensives, the fall on treatment is over 10 mmHg. Such a fall would be expected to produce a substantial reduction in adverse cardiovascular events.

It is not clear whether OSA produces an increase in stroke and myocardial infarction, either through hypertension or other mechanisms. However, the evidence is mounting, although definitive RCTs are unlikely to be possible.

☐ INVESTIGATION

Sleep apnoea management in the UK has been severely held back by the prevailing US view that the diagnosis of this condition needs expensive investigative techniques based on polysomnography (involving electro-encephalography, electro-oculography, electromyography, thoracic and abdominal movements, airflow at the nose and mouth, oximetry, and sometimes even more physiological signals).[1] This view has been shown to be indefensible, with clear evidence that simpler techniques are at least as good at identifying patients likely to respond to CPAP treatment.[6] It is now incorrect to insist on more expensive polysomnographic studies when the same financial resources could be better used to investigate and treat more patients.

Figure 3 shows the output from a simple sleep study system, based on oximetry and computer-processed video signals. The use of such simplified systems has enabled many units in the UK to set up services which would not otherwise have been possible. Even in North America, a more pragmatic approach is beginning to be taken.[7]

Diagnosis

The diagnosis of symptomatic OSA is not based solely on the sleep study. OSA used to be defined according to arbitrary thresholds found on a sleep study (eg >15 apnoeas or hypopnoeas per hour). However, because of the poor correlation between sleep studies and symptoms, the definition is now much more clinically useful and includes no numerical thresholds:

> *Sleep apnoea syndrome* is defined as 'sleep induced upper airway obstruction, leading to symptomatic sleep disturbance'.

The sleep study is thus interpreted by determining whether it has revealed anything that accounts for the patient's daytime symptoms and whether a trial of treatment would be justified. Clearly, the decision involves balancing the inconvenience of treatment against the history, the sleep study result and the patient's own assessment of their symptoms.

☐ TREATMENT

Treatment of OSA has to be tailored to the patient's symptoms (Table 3).

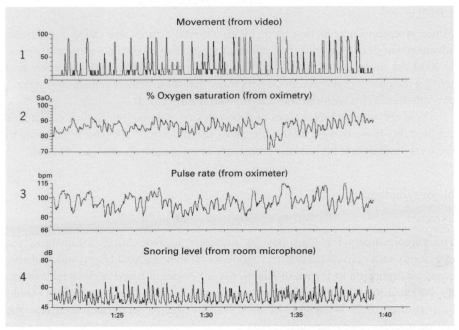

**Fig 3** Twenty-minute tracing (left to right) from a patient with obstructive sleep apnoea. Channel 1: body movement derived from computer processing the video signal; channel 2: % oxygen saturation in arterial blood ($SaO_2$) (finger oximetry); channel 3: pulse rate (bpm) (from the oximeter); channel 4: sound level (snoring) (dB) from an overhead microphone. Note the frequent dips in $SaO_2$ accompanied by recurrent arousal (seen on both the movement and pulse rate channels) and the snore/silence/snore pattern of obstructive sleep apnoea (Visilab, Stowood Scientific Instruments, Oxford).

**Table 3** Treatments for obstructive sleep apnoea and snoring.

- Treat any underlying disorder (eg acromegaly, hypothyroidism)
- Stop evening alcohol and sedatives
- Stop smoking
- Lose weight (very difficult)
- Posture training (avoiding supine position)
- Dental devices/mandibular advancement devices
- Nasal continuous positive airway pressure
- Obesity surgery

## Minor symptoms

### Lifestyle changes

Trivial symptoms may require only changes in lifestyle, whereas major symptoms will require nasal CPAP. However, a recent evidence-based guideline found no evidence that lifestyle alterations are likely to work for OSA and that sustained weight loss is extremely difficult to achieve.[8]

## Dental devices

Minor symptoms may be best treated with a dental device (also called mandibular advancement device) or concerted efforts at weight loss. Dental devices are designed to hold the lower jaw forward during sleep, enlarging the retroglossal space and tensing the pharyngeal walls. Good data show that these devices reduce snoring and partially treat OSA, with significant symptom improvement.

There are many different types of dental device and no clear favourite. The best are probably those that are adjustable, allow jaw movement laterally, attach only to the teeth (and do not occlude the gums), are of minimal bulk and easy to clean.

## Major symptoms

### Surgery

*Pharyngeal surgery* for OSA has an unhappy history. Initial enthusiasm for operations such as uvulopalatopharyngoplasty (with or without lasers) was probably based on regression to the mean effects. Recent evidence-based reviews have found no real evidence of benefit; it is therefore recommended that such operations should be performed only as second- or third-line treatments, preferably in a research setting in order to provide further data.[9]

Prior *palatal surgery* makes it harder subsequently to tolerate nasal CPAP, due to loss of the sealing effect of the palate blowing down on to the back of the tongue.

In children, *tonsillectomy* is effective even when the tonsils are not very big. In adults, it is probably worth doing a tonsillectomy only if the tonsils are clearly enlarged, but the benefit seems to be less in the more obese. *Mandibular,* or *mandible and maxilla, advancement surgery* in selected cases has a better research base, and is a reasonable – if rather heroic – approach in individual patients.

*Obesity surgery.* The best, and perhaps most beneficial, operation for overweight patients with OSA is obesity surgery. This has recently been assessed by the National Institute for Clinical Excellence, which concluded that in the right setting it is good practice and economically sensible.

When effective appetite suppressants are available in a few years' time, the management of many patients with OSA (and many other diseases) will be revolutionised.

## Nasal continuous positive airway pressure

Nasal CPAP involves wearing a small mask over the nose (Fig 4) connected to an air blower, maintaining an airway pressure of about 10 cm $H_2O$. This pressure splints open the pharynx and allows regular breathing with no obstruction and therefore no arousals. An added bonus is that the snoring also disappears. The pressure required varies between individuals, most needing 5–15 cm $H_2O$.

There is no doubt that nasal CPAP is the treatment of choice for moderate to severe OSA. The research evidence is impeccable, with several RCTs available,[10] some

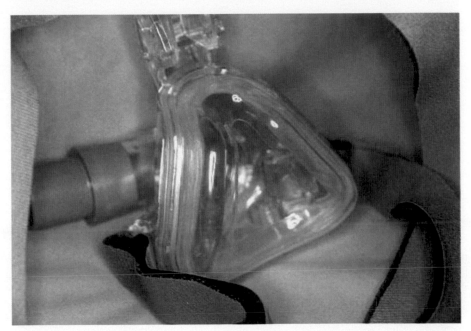

**Fig 4** Recent nasal mask for delivering continuous positive airway pressure. There is a soft inner membrane that blows down on the skin, providing a seal with minimum tightening of the head straps. This increases comfort and reduces the incidence of nasal bridge ulceration (Ultra mirage from Resmed).

even using sham CPAP as the control arm. The improvements in sleepiness (objective and subjective) and measures of self-reported quality of life (health status) are enormous compared with other therapies for other disorders. The controlled trials have also shown improvements in driving simulator performance[4] and 24-hour BP profiles.[5]

### Delivery

Nasal CPAP is cumbersome and unattractive in appearance, although virtually without significant side effects. The delivery of a CPAP service therefore needs to concentrate on making the experience as reasonable as possible, involving a sensitive multidisciplinary approach from referral to follow-up on CPAP. It has proved a good area to enlist the help of specialist nurses, who now run most of the clinical service in Oxford. Other disciplines can also be usefully involved, with lung function staff taking on the role of CPAP provision in some units.

### Training patients

Setting up patients on nasal CPAP used to require a training session, an overnight stay in hospital for manual titration of the pressure requirement, assessment the next morning and close initial follow-up. The increase in patient referrals (Fig 5), without

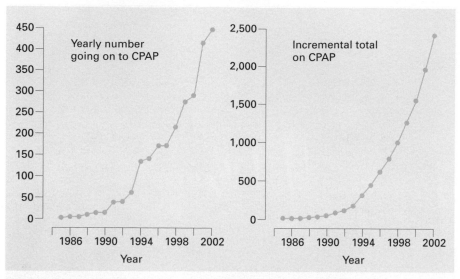

**Fig 5** The number of patients requiring nasal continuous positive airway pressure (CPAP) in the Oxford clinic between 1984 and 2002, showing the considerable increase.

commensurate funding, has meant the continuing introduction of alternative strategies. Patients are now educated in groups of four or five during an afternoon clinic session. Their CPAP pressure is set according to an algorithm (based on CPAP severity and neck circumference) and they spend their first night at home. Telephone help is available on weekdays (9 am to 5 pm).

Audit of this change of practice shows identical outcomes to the original service, with considerable savings. Our belief is that such a programme works only because of the input of expertise and dedication mainly from the specialist nurses and other support staff. Depending on the symptomatic thresholds chosen to initiate treatment, about 80% of patients offered treatment stay on it long term, with a compliance of 5–6 hours a night. This compares extremely favourably with acceptance and compliance rates for other symptom-driven treatments.

## ☐ CONCLUSIONS

The take-home message for doctors who may see these patients (which will be the majority) is that OSA is a common condition with much morbidity and probably some mortality. Newer simplified and cheaper approaches make this condition easy to diagnose and treat, as long as the expertise is there to understand the limitations of these simplified systems. Diagnostic services should be available in all district general hospitals, even if CPAP services remain tertiary for some time. The evidence base is there to justify this effort, and it is this author's experience that these patients are most grateful and enthusiastic about their treatment, despite its peculiarity.

# REFERENCES

1  Malhotra A, White DP. Obstructive sleep apnoea. Review. *Lancet* 2002;**360**:237–45.

2  Davies RJ, Stradling JR. The epidemiology of sleep apnoea. Review. *Thorax* 1996;**51**(Suppl 2): S65–70.

3  George CF. Reduction in motor vehicle collisions following treatment of sleep apnoea with nasal CPAP. *Thorax* 2001;**56**:508–12.

4  Hack M, Davies RJ, Mullins R, Choi SJ *et al*. Randomised prospective parallel trial of therapeutic versus subtherapeutic nasal continuous positive airway pressure on simulated steering performance in patients with obstructive sleep apnoea. *Thorax* 2000;**55**:224–31.

5  Pepperell JC, Ramdassingh-Dow S, Crosthwaite N, Mullins R *et al*. Ambulatory blood pressure after therapeutic and subtherapeutic nasal continuous positive airway pressure for obstructive sleep apnoea: a randomised parallel trial. *Lancet* 2002;**359**:204–10.

6  Bennett LS, Langford BA, Stradling JR, Davies RJ. Sleep fragmentation indices as predictors of daytime sleepiness and nCPAP response in obstructive sleep apnea. *Am J Respir Crit Care Med* 1998;**158**:778–86.

7  Kryger M. What data do we need to diagnose and treat obstructive sleep apnoea syndrome? *Sleep Med Rev* 2002;**6**:3–6.

8  Shneerson J, Wright J. Lifestyle modification for obstructive sleep apnoea (Cochrane Review). In: *The Cochrane Library*, Issue 1, 2003. Oxford: Update Software Ltd.

9  Bridgman SA, Dunn KM, Ducharme F. Surgery for obstructive sleep apnoea (Cochrane Review). In: *The Cochrane Library*, Issue 1, 2003. Oxford: Update Software Ltd.

10  White J, Cates C, Wright J. Continuous positive airways pressure for obstructive sleep apnoea (Cochrane Review). In: *The Cochrane Library*, Issue 1, 2003. Oxford: Update Software Ltd.

## □ RESPIRATORY MEDICINE SELF ASSESSMENT QUESTIONS

### Chronic obstructive pulmonary disease

1   In chronic obstructive pulmonary disease (COPD):
   (a)  Airflow obstruction is mainly due to large airway disease
   (b)  A low body mass index is a poor prognostic finding
   (c)  Bronchodilator reversibility testing is needed to make the diagnosis
   (d)  A history of tobacco exposure is needed to make the diagnosis
   (e)  Osteoporosis is a common finding in men

2   Exercise capacity in COPD:
   (a)  Is limited by increases in end-expiratory lung volume
   (b)  Can be predicted by the presence of inspiratory flow limitation
   (c)  Is a major determinant of health status
   (d)  Can be limited by skeletal muscle weakness
   (e)  Improves more with bronchodilator treatment than after rehabilitation

3   Management of stable disease involves:
   (a)  Regular use of oral corticosteroids in severe cases
   (b)  Prescription of inhaled corticosteroids to patients with an $FEV_1$ above 50% predicted
   (c)  Routine use of long-acting inhaled bronchodilators in symptomatic patients
   (d)  Prescription of domiciliary oxygen if the $PaO_2$ is below 7.3 kPa
   (e)  Referral for lung volume reduction surgery in patients with diffuse emphysema

### Sleep apnoea

1   Adult sleep apnoea is often due to:
   (a)  Upper body obesity
   (b)  Weak pharyngeal dilator muscles
   (c)  Certain lower face anatomical characteristics
   (d)  Brainstem abnormalities
   (e)  Enlarged uvula

2   Obstructive sleep apnoea (OSA) can result in:
   (a)  Greater probability of having a road traffic accident
   (b)  Increased blood pressure (BP) during sleep
   (c)  Increased BP awake
   (d)  Subjective and objective increases in daytime sleepiness
   (e)  Reduced physical activity and a greater tendency to weight gain

3   Nasal continuous positive airway pressure:
   (a)  Works by stimulating pharyngeal dilators
   (b)  Produces objective improvements in sleepiness compared with placebo

(c) Reduces daytime blood pressure compared with placebo

(d) Is continued long term in only about 50% of patients who try it

(e) Is harder to tolerate following palatal surgery

4 The following are useful treatments for OSA:

(a) Mandibular advancement devices or dental devices

(b) Surgical resection of the palate

(c) Tonsillectomy in children

(d) Laser surgery to the palate

(e) Surgical advancement of the mandible and maxilla in selected cases

5 Treatment of OSA:

(a) Should be given whenever the sleep study indices of activity reach a certain threshold, regardless of symptoms

(b) Is most likely to be accepted by the more sleepy patient

(c) May produce falls in diurnal BP

(d) May reduce nocturia

(e) Would not be expected to improve snoring

# Gastroenterology

# Helicobacter pylori

Mark Thursz

## ☐ INTRODUCTION

*Helicobacter pylori*, a Gram-negative spiral bacterium, was identified in 1983 by Warren and Marshall.[1] It is a ubiquitous organism which infects over half the population worldwide for most of their lives. Fortunately, only a minority of individuals with this infection suffer any significant sequelae, of which duodenal and gastric ulcers are the most common. However, in some parts of the developing world gastric cancer remains the most important consequence.

*H. pylori* establishes infection of the gastric mucosa below and within the mucous bicarbonate barrier which protects epithelial cells from the hostile lumenal environment. It is invariably associated with an active, chronic gastritis characterised by infiltration of the gastric epithelium by neutrophils and lymphocytes. *H. pylori* infection interferes with the epithelial defences and control of acid secretion, leading to the adverse consequences of peptic ulcer, gastric cancer and lymphoma.

The prevalence of *H. pylori* in many developed countries is decreasing so rapidly that the infection and associated diseases may disappear from the indigenous populations by 2010.

## ☐ EPIDEMIOLOGY

*H. pylori* infection is associated with low socio-economic status and residence in developing countries. In developed countries, infection is associated with bed sharing during childhood and use of an outside lavatory. Infection appears to be acquired during early childhood. Although the precise mode of transmission is unknown, it is likely to be by oral-oral spread – that is, by transfer of regurgitated stomach contents from one infant to another. Evidence for faeco-oral spread or transmission from zoonotic reservoirs is not convincing. Age-specific prevalence rates reflect the rapidly changing socio-economic situation in many countries, in that they are high in older cohorts of the population. This does not reflect a cumulative infection process as the incidence of new infection is low in young adults.

Once established, *H. pylori* infection appears to persist for the life of the individual unless treated. Loss of infection may occur when atrophy of the gastric mucosa destroys the unique ecological niche preferred by the organism. In children, recurrent self-limiting infections have been documented prior to chronic infection becoming established. When the infection has been eradicated, re-infection is a rare event in adults.

## ☐ DUODENAL ULCER

Duodenal ulcers are associated with *H. pylori* infection in 95% of cases. Marshall established the link between *H. pylori* infection and duodenal ulcer disease by demonstrating that recurrence of duodenal ulcer did not occur in patients after eradication of the organism, whereas persistent infection was associated with 80% relapse within one year.[2]

Considerable research over the last few years has revealed the mechanism underlying the association of *H. pylori* with duodenal ulcer disease. *H. pylori* infection and gastritis are predominantly confined to the gastric antrum in duodenal ulcer patients where the inflammation is thought to interfere with somatostatin secretion by neuroendocrine D cells (Fig 1).[3] Low levels of somatostatin fail to

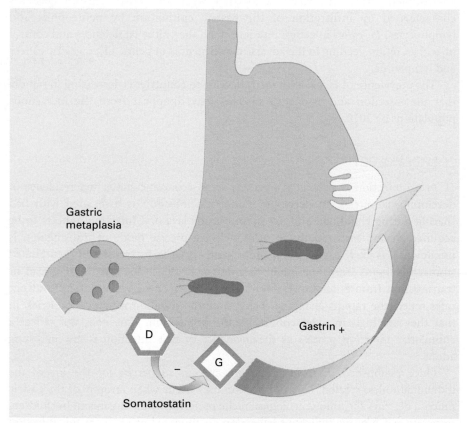

**Fig 1** In duodenal ulcer disease antral inflammation induced by *Helicobacter pylori* interferes with somatostatin secretion by D cells, leading to excess gastrin secretion by G cells and increased acid production. Excess acid induces gastric metaplasia in the duodenum which may be infected with *H. pylori*, leading to duodenitis.

control gastrin release from G cells, leading to higher levels of acid production from the parietal cells in the stomach body. Excess acid induces gastric metaplasia in the duodenal mucosa, providing a niche for *H. pylori* infiltration.[4] The resultant duodenitis is responsible for duodenal ulceration and the associated complications. Duodenal ulcer disease may therefore be managed with a combination of acid suppression and *H. pylori* eradication.

### Outcome of infection

Duodenal ulcer disease arises in only a minority of individuals with *H. pylori* infection. Several factors may influence the outcome of infection. Bacterial virulence factors have been widely studied. Some strains of *H. pylori* carry an additional genetic segment, the cag pathogenicity island (PAI) which encodes 25 genes, one of which, the *cagA* gene, is often used as a marker for the presence of this genetic segment.[5] *H. pylori* strains with the cag PAI are associated with more intensive inflammation in the gastric mucosa and higher levels of induction of pro-inflammatory cytokines such as interleukin (IL)-8.[6] Within the cag PAI is the *VacA* gene which encodes a vacuolating toxin. Polymorphism in the *VacA* gene has been associated with increased risk of duodenal ulcer disease.[7]

Individuals carrying the most virulent strains of *H. pylori* can develop the full range of clinical outcomes from their infection. This can include suffering no clinical consequences, suggesting that other factors must also influence the outcome of infection. Duodenal ulcer disease often clusters in families and has been linked to blood group status. Host genetic background is therefore probably another important influence on the outcome of infection.

## ☐ GASTRIC CANCER

Epidemiological studies associate 70% of gastric cancer cases with *H. pylori*. The use of serology to identify past as well as current *H. pylori* infection reveals that the organism increases the risk of gastric cancer eightfold. The link between *H. pylori* and gastric cancer has been strengthened by the development of gastric cancer in Mongolian gerbils infected by the organism.[8]

### Mechanism of development

The mechanism linking *H. pylori* infection to the development of gastric cancer is not fully understood. One hypothesis is that *H. pylori* infection promotes gastric cancer through a stepwise progression. There is first chronic gastritis which leads to gastric atrophy and intestinal metaplasia, and eventually to dysplasia and invasive malignancy.[9] *H. pylori* probably plays a role in the early phases of this carcinogenic sequence, but once atrophy is established environmental factors such as diet and smoking play an important role. Furthermore, in the achlorhydric stomach overgrowth of other organisms promotes the production of carcinogenic nitrosamine compounds.

*Gastric atrophy and hypochlorhydria*

Gastric atrophy and hypochlorhydria are important phases in the development of cancer. The inflammation associated with *H. pylori* infection induces secretion of the cytokine IL-1, a powerful inhibitor of acid secretion. It is plausible that either the chronic inflammation or the constant suppression of parietal cells leads to loss of gastric glands over prolonged periods of infection in susceptible individuals.

*Genetic predisposition*

Only a minority of individuals infected with *H. pylori* develop gastric cancer, raising the question of what are the predisposing factors. A genetic predisposition has been postulated for some time. El-Omar and colleagues recently demonstrated an important role for polymorphisms in the IL-1 receptor antagonist and the IL-1 receptor beta.[10]

## ☐ GASTRIC LYMPHOMA

Gastric lymphoma is a rare complication of *H. pylori* infection. It is usually a low-grade B cell lymphoma arising from the mucosa-associated lymphoid tissue (MALT). Lymphoid tissue is not normally found in the stomach mucosa, unlike the small and large intestine. *H. pylori* infection induces lymphoid aggregates. In some individuals it is thought that the T cell response to the antigens drives a nonspecific polyclonal B cell response which eventually becomes oligoclonal and then a monoclonal malignancy. Interestingly, intervention with *H. pylori* eradication at the oligoclonal stage when the tumour is low grade may be sufficient to cure the lymphoma.[11]

## ☐ DIAGNOSIS OF HELICOBACTER PYLORI INFECTION

Several diagnostic techniques are available for detection of *H. pylori* infection. Many of these are noninvasive (Table 1), whereas others are designed to be used in conjunction with endoscopic assessment (Table 2). Both the sensitivity and specificity of each test must be carefully monitored, as well as its applicability to post-eradication monitoring.

**Noninvasive tests**

- ☐ Serological tests have become popular in recent years due to their convenience but are not particularly sensitive or specific and cannot be used to monitor effectiveness of treatment.

- ☐ $^{13}$C-urea breath tests and faecal antigen tests are recommended for noninvasive assessment.

- ☐ Urease-based tests are cheap and convenient to use in association with endoscopy.

**Table 1** Noninvasive diagnostics.

| Test | Sensitivity (%) | Specificity (%) | Cost (£) | Post-eradication |
|---|---|---|---|---|
| Lab serum | 88–94 | 74–95 | 15 | No |
| Salivary Ab | 65–89 | 72–90 | N/A | No |
| ¹³C-UBT | 90–96 | 88–98 | 25–30 | Yes |
| Faecal Ag | 88–95 | 82–99 | ? | Yes |

Ab = antibody; Ag = antigen; UBT = urea breath test.

**Table 2** Invasive diagnostics.

| Test | Sensitivity (%) | Specificity (%) | Cost (£) | Post-eradication |
|---|---|---|---|---|
| Urease | 88–95 | 95–100 | 1.50 | Yes |
| Histology | 93–96 | 98–99 | 45–50 | Yes |
| Culture | 80–90 | 100 | 20 | Yes |

**Invasive tests**

☐ Histological assessment by expert histopathologists may provide useful guidance when patients have recently taken proton-pump inhibitors (PPIs) or antibiotics.

☐ Biopsy and culture are helpful when antibiotic resistance is suspected as a cause of eradication failure.

## ☐ WHO TO TREAT?

A number of national and international guidelines make recommendations about which patients should be treated for *H. pylori* infection. Unfortunately, only a minority of the guidance is supported by strong experimental evidence, some of which may be regarded as controversial.

### Peptic ulcer disease

Treatment of patients with duodenal ulcer disease or gastric ulcers who are not taking nonsteroidal anti-inflammatory drugs (NSAIDs) is not controversial. *H. pylori* should probably be eradicated in patients with duodenal ulcers who are taking NSAIDs. However, in patients taking NSAIDs who have gastric ulceration there is evidence that leaving *in situ* the *H. pylori* may assist with ulcer healing.[12] If NSAIDs are still required after ulcer healing, prophylaxis with PPIs is recommended.

## Low-grade MALT lymphoma

*H. pylori* should be eradicated in patients with low-grade MALT lymphomas, but regular and intensive endoscopic follow-up is also required.

## Intestinal metaplasia/gastric atrophy

It might be advisable to eradicate *H. pylori* in patients with histologically confirmed intestinal metaplasia or gastric atrophy. It is not yet clear whether reversal of these histological lesions occurs after *H. pylori* eradication, and it would be impractical to demonstrate whether this policy would prevent gastric cancer.

## Relatives of gastric cancer patients

There is a good rationale for treating first-degree relatives of gastric cancer patients, but no evidence to support this practice.

## Nonulcer dyspepsia

The most controversial group of patients considered for *H. pylori* eradication are those with nonulcer dyspepsia. In the several trials in this group of patients, a roughly equal number demonstrated benefit or no benefit for *H. pylori* eradication. Most trials found that a proportion of patients in the noneradicated groups developed ulcer disease during follow-up, indicating that the original disease classification, based on a single endoscopic examination, was incorrect.

Although the data do not support widespread use of *H. pylori* eradication for all patients with nonulcer dyspepsia, it is interesting to note that in one study relief of symptoms was associated only with complete resolution of the gastritis including the lymphocytic infiltrate. This usually occurs more that three years after successful eradication, suggesting that a longer period of follow-up may be required to determine the efficacy of *H. pylori* eradication in this group of patients.[13]

## Gastro-oesophageal reflux disease

Labenz published a retrospective study in 1997[14] suggesting that eradication of *H. pylori* in duodenal ulcer disease patients exacerbates or induces gastro-oesophageal reflux disease (GORD). This study was criticised on a number of counts, but corroborating evidence suggested that these findings are true, for example:

☐   the declining prevalence of *H. pylori* mirrors the increasing prevalence of GORD, and

☐   in many individuals *H. pylori* infection suppresses gastric acid secretion and eradication leads to hyperacidity.

The Labenz study has recently been refuted by well designed prospective studies in which many patients with a diagnosis of duodenal ulcer disease at endoscopy have symptoms of GORD – indicating that the two conditions frequently coexist.

In patients with GORD but without duodenal ulcer disease, *H. pylori* status is not relevant. If *H. pylori* is present, there is an argument for leaving the bacterium alone as PPIs are more effective in infected patients.

### Dyspepsia algorithms

*H. pylori* infection impacts on algorithms of dyspepsia management. Dyspeptic patients presenting over the age of 50 or with symptoms of concern (Table 3) are appropriately assessed by endoscopy. However, most patients do not fall into these categories and it is impractical and unnecessary to subject all of them to this invasive investigation. Noninvasive testing for *H. pylori* and treating those patients found to be positive has become an increasingly popular protocol. It inevitably means that some patients with dyspepsia unrelated to *H. pylori* infection will be treated, but several studies have demonstrated the efficacy of this regimen.

**Table 3** Symptoms of concern in patients over the age of 50 with dyspepsia.

Dyspepsia with:
- age >50, onset within 1 year
- weight loss
- anorexia/early satiety
- anaemia
- haematemesis
- family history of >2 first-degree relatives with carcinoma of the stomach
- pernicious anaemia
- Barret's oesophagus

### ☐ ERADICATION

A large number of regimens are used to eradicate *H. pylori* infection, mainly based on a PPI and two antibiotics (metronidazole and clarithromycin) (Table 4). *In vitro*, *H. pylori* is susceptible to a wide range of antibiotics but resistance is rapidly increasing:

☐ *Metronidazole* is a common component of eradication regimens but resistance is widespread worldwide, particularly in developing countries. However, metronidazole resistance is not an absolute predictor of eradication failure.

**Table 4** *Helicobacter pylori* eradication regimens.

|  | **Eradication regimen** |
| --- | --- |
| **First-line** | • PPI + clarithromycin 500 mg + amoxycillin 1 g bd one week<br>• PPI + clarithromycin 500 mg + metronidazole 1 g bd one week |
| **Second-line** | • Bismuth subcitrate 120 mg qds + PPI bd + clarithromycin 500 mg bd + amoxycillin 1 g bd *or* metronidazole 500 mg *or* tetracycline 500 mg qds tds two weeks |

PPI = proton-pump inhibitor.

☐    *Clarithromycin* resistance is associated with very low eradication rates; it is not common in the UK although the prevalence is increasing. In France, where this antibiotic has been widely used for a long time, the prevalence of clarithromycin resistance approaches 15%.

## ☐ PROSPECTS FOR VACCINATION

Eradicating all *H. pylori* infection using PPIs and antibiotics has been questioned on a number of grounds including cost, complications and possible benefit of *H. pylori* infection in some individuals. An alternative means of controlling the infection on a population scale would be vaccination, either prophylactic or therapeutic. Several candidate vaccines have been tested in mouse models of *H. pylori* infection, including vaccines based on recombinant proteins as well as some based on inactivated organisms. These show promise in the models and a number of the vaccines are now in clinical phase human trials.

## ☐ POPULATION SCREENING

Infection with *H. pylori* clearly has adverse consequences, albeit in a minority of individuals. Testing for *H. pylori* by noninvasive means is reasonably accurate and widely available. Intervention to eradicate *H. pylori* is also available and relatively cheap. Is screening and eradication of *H. pylori* therefore a practical proposition?

The arguments against screening and eradication are:

☐    the cost-benefit balance

☐    induction of resistant organisms by widespread use of antibiotics

☐    side effects of antibiotic therapy, and

☐    declining prevalence of *H. pylori* and declining incidence of
     *H. pylori*-associated diseases.

Cost-benefit analysis, focused on the prevention of gastric cancer, has been conducted in the US.[15] Overall screening and eradication could barely be justified, but in subpopulations with a substantially higher incidence of gastric cancer than the general population this intervention would be warranted on both clinical and economic grounds. Thus, screening and eradication of *H. pylori* could be considered in the Japanese-American and African-American groups.

## REFERENCES

1    Marshall BJ, Warren JR. Unidentified curved bacilli in the stomach of patients with gastritis and peptic ulceration. *Lancet* 1984;i:1311–5.
2    Marshall BJ, Goodwin CS, Warren JR, Murray R *et al.* Prospective double-blind trial of duodenal ulcer relapse after eradication of Campylobacter pylori. *Lancet* 1988;ii:1437–42.
3    Gibbons AH, Legon S, Walker MM, Ghatei M, Calam J. The effect of gastrin-releasing peptide on gastrin and somatostatin messenger RNAs in humans infected with *Helicobacter pylori*. *Gastroenterology* 1997;112:1940–7.

4    Wyatt JI, Rathbone BJ, Sobala GM, Shallcross T *et al.* Gastric epithelium in the duodenum: its association with *Helicobacter pylori* and inflammation. *J Clin Pathol* 1990;**43**:981–6.

5    Covacci A, Falkow S, Berg DE, Rappuoli R. Did the inheritance of a pathogenicity island modify the virulence of *Helicobacter pylori?* Review. *Trends Microbiol* 1997;**5**:205–8.

6    Crabtree JE, Covacci A, Farmery SM, Xiang Z *et al. Helicobacter pylori* induced interleukin-8 expression in gastric epithelial cells is associated with CagA positive phenotype. *J Clin Pathol* 1995;**48**:41–5.

7    Atherton JC, Cao ·P, Peek RM Jr, Tummuru MK *et al.* Mosaicism in vacuolating cytotoxin alleles of *Helicobacter pylori.* Association of specific vacA types with cytotoxin production and peptic ulceration. *J Biol Chem* 1995;**270**:17771–7.

8    Watanabe T, Tada M, Nagai H, Sasaki S, Nakao M. *Helicobacter pylori* infection induces gastric cancer in mongolian gerbils. *Gastroenterology* 1998;**115**:642–8.

9    Correa P. A human model of gastric carcinogenesis. Review. *Cancer Res* 1988;**48**:3554–60.

10   El-Omar EM, Carrington M, Chow WH, McColl KE *et al.* Interleukin-1 polymorphisms associated with increased risk of gastric cancer. *Nature* 2000;**404**:398–402.

11   Neubauer A, Thiede C, Morgner A, Alpen B *et al.* Cure of *Helicobacter pylori* infection and duration of remission of low-grade gastric mucosa-associated lymphoid tissue lymphoma. *J Natl Cancer Inst* 1997;**89**:1350–5.

12   Hawkey CJ, Tulassay Z, Szczepanski L, van Rensburg CJ *et al.* Randomised controlled trial of *Helicobacter pylori* eradication in patients on non-steroidal anti-inflammatory drugs: HELP NSAIDs study. Helicobacter Eradication for Lesion Prevention. *Lancet* 1998;**352**:1016–21.

13   Veldhuyzen van Zanten SJ, Talley NJ, Blum AL, Bolling-Sternevald E *et al.* Combined analysis of the ORCHID and OCAY studies: does eradication of *Helicobacter pylori* lead to sustained improvement in functional dyspepsia symptoms? Gut 2002;**50**(Suppl 4):iv26–30; discussion iv31–2.

14   Labenz J, Blum AL, Bayerdorffer E, Meining A *et al.* Curing *Helicobacter pylori* infection in patients with duodenal ulcer may provoke reflux esophagitis. *Gastroenterology* 1997;**112**: 1442–7.

15   Parsonnet J, Harris RA, Hack HM, Owens DK. Modelling cost-effectiveness of *Helicobacter pylori* screening to prevent gastric cancer: a mandate for clinical trials. *Lancet* 1996;**348**:150–4.

# Medically unexplained gastrointestinal symptoms

Roland Valori

## ☐ INTRODUCTION

A large proportion of patients with gastroenterological symptoms attending their general practitioner (GP) or hospital outpatients will not have an identifiable underlying gastroenterological disorder. Even patients with well documented disease such as chronic pancreatitis or Crohn's may have symptoms that either cannot be explained by the disease process or are out of proportion to the severity of the disease.

## ☐ TERMINOLOGY

There is a great variety of unexplained gastrointestinal symptoms. To describe them, doctors use either generic terms such as 'functional symptoms', 'non-organic disease' and 'somatisation disorder' or more specific labels such as 'irritable bowel syndrome' (IBS) and 'nonulcer dyspepsia'. Most patients are confused by these terms and this confusion can adversely affect the outcome of the consultation. In contrast, the term 'medically unexplained gastrointestinal symptoms' conveys meaning to the patient. If they understand and accept this meaning, the need for diagnostic tests is reduced and the outcome of the consultation improves.

Considerable effort has been expended by doctors and scientists defining and subcategorising discrete symptomatic groups. The aim of this process is twofold:

1   To make unexplained symptoms fit into the classic medical model to enable patients to be managed in a conventional medical way (ie to deliver a treatment targeted at an underlying pathological process).

2   To improve patient selection into randomised clinical trials.

To date, this effort has failed to identify a discrete pathological process for any of these discrete symptomatic groups. Research has identified changes in functioning of the gut and an increase in its sensitivity. The pharmaceutical industry has produced drugs that can modify function and, to some degree, improve symptoms. Furthermore, some labels such as IBS have passed into common usage. For some patients, an IBS label has meaning and is helpful to convey to others the problem they suffer. However, applying labels that have no definite physiological basis is, in general, not helpful to the patient. Patients often fall into more than one group or have a multitude of other symptoms that do not fit into any group. Applying such a label can distract both doctor and patient from the real issues underpinning medically unexplained symptoms.

## ☐ MANAGING THE PATIENT

Successful management of patients with unexplained symptoms requires a mixture of a conventional medical and a patient-focused approach. Patients have expectations of how a doctor will approach their symptoms and often have reasonable concerns about their cause. Thus, to explore their symptoms in a conventional way is appropriate and reassuring. However, the conventional medical approach flounders when no abnormality is found and a different approach is required. The key here is to understand the patient's perspective.

Understanding what patients want from their doctor (whether in primary or secondary care) provides a focus for the consultation and leads to a higher chance of a satisfactory outcome. Most patients with unexplained symptoms desire:

☐  unambiguous, but realistic, reassurance that nothing serious underlies their symptoms

☐  a simple explanation for the physiological mechanism of symptoms

☐  a plausible cause for this disturbance in physiology, and

☐  advice on treatment.

**Unambiguous but realistic reassurance**

Most experienced doctors know within a few moments of questioning a patient whether or not they have unexplainable symptoms. It is, however, difficult for the patient to understand how such a quick exploration enables the doctor to be certain there is no underlying organic disease. To provide effective reassurance, more than a cursory history and an appropriate examination are needed before concluding that there is no medical explanation for the symptoms.

*Investigation*

The next step is to decide whether investigation is necessary. An investigation is a powerful way of reassuring a patient, but in certain situations can reinforce beliefs that there is an underlying disease to be found. Moreover, performing investigations for reassurance consumes valuable healthcare resource, particularly in gastro-enterology when either endoscopy or radiology is required. To achieve a fair balance between objective reassurance and overconsumption of resource, it is helpful to understand what determines investigation decisions when there is a low likelihood of underlying disease.

Using a history, examination and tests, probabilities of a short list of disorders (the differential diagnosis) are adjusted according to the verbal responses, physical signs and results of tests. Some symptoms such as abdominal bloating, knife-like pains in the abdomen or relief of abdominal cramping pain with passage of wind or stool, strongly suggest that there is not an underlying disease process (Fig 1). On the other hand, symptoms such as bloody diarrhoea are highly predictive of pathology. Thus, probabilities are adjusted as the diagnostic process is continued. With patients with unexplained symptoms, in most circumstances it is quickly concluded that there is a very low probability of underlying disease.

At this stage, the principal question for both doctor and patient is what level of certainty is needed before tests are stopped, or when is an acceptable threshold of certainty that nothing will be found reached?

This threshold (Fig 1) varies according to several different factors. First, some patients and doctors tolerate a high degree of uncertainty (ie a relatively high probability of missing something) whereas others tolerate only a low or no chance of missing something. Thus, in some situations, further investigations are necessary to satisfy an unduly anxious patient or doctor, while in others the patient might be happy to accept reassurance without further tests.

Secondly, the possible underlying diagnosis and the consequences of missing it. The consequences of delaying a diagnosis of colorectal cancer are much greater than a delayed diagnosis of IBS. An acceptable threshold of certainty depends on the doctor, the patient and the possible underlying disease process.

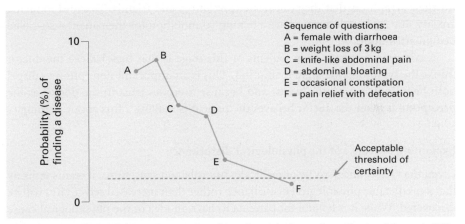

**Fig 1** Making a diagnosis of no disease: the effect of questioning on the estimate of the probability of disease.

*Key points in reassurance*

In summary, there are five key points to consider when reassuring patients with unexplained symptoms:

1   Be careful to make a clinical assessment that the patient will find convincing.

2   If it is thought that there is no underlying organic disease, the patient should be told before discussing further tests.

3    Be realistic and explicit about uncertainty.

4    Ask the patient what degree of certainty they would find acceptable.

5    Negotiate about further investigations.

If, after a series of tests, a patient continues to harbour a belief that the symptoms have a pathological basis, it is effectively impossible to proceed to the next stage of explanation and treatment. Preparing them for the likely outcome well before investigation is a critical part of this process. Informing the patient early that their symptoms are believed to be medically unexplained is particularly important. When the test outcome matches the patient's expectations the need for further tests is diminished. If there is an unexpected abnormal result, both patient and doctor are relieved the test was done. Either way it is a win-win situation for both parties.

### Physiological explanation for symptoms

Most patients with unexplained symptoms experience genuine symptoms and do not exaggerate them. There are cultural differences in their expression, but probably little difference in the way they are experienced. Acknowledging the nature and severity of symptoms, and providing an understandable explanation for them, are both important for the patient. It is important for the patient to have an explanation for their symptoms that they can relate to relatives and friends. To avoid inducing anxiety, any explanation must have a benign connotation for the patient – so-called benign attribution.

A common response from patients at this stage is that they believe the doctor thinks the symptoms are all in their mind. This is an important perception to dispel both because it is not usually true and because it erodes trust in the doctor as the perception implies the doctor believes the patient is making a fuss about nothing.

### Explaining the cause of the physiological disturbance

Given the variety and severity of medically unexplained symptoms, it seems unlikely that a predictable physiological disturbance (other than increased sensitivity) will be discovered. While it is helpful for patients to have an idea of the physiological cause of their symptoms, it is particularly important to go one step back in the causative process and ask what caused the physiological disturbance in the first place. Identifying and rectifying this is likely to achieve the best outcome.

*Stress*

The conventional view is that the physiological disturbance is caused by stress, anxiety or depression. Patients are often labelled as being 'mad' and are sometimes referred to psychiatrists. Psychiatric referral is usually unhelpful unless the psychiatrist has an interest in patients with unexplained symptoms. The usual response is 'no psychiatric diagnosis, are you sure you have excluded organic disease?'. This is because most patients with unexplained symptoms do not have conventional psychiatric diagnoses and many psychiatrists feel uncomfortable with patients expressing unpleasant symptoms.

The few patients who are clinically depressed or very anxious require specific treatment that may need the expertise of a psychiatrist. However, such levels of anxiety and depression are unusual. Stress may be a factor, but stress is a difficult concept to define and it is clear that stress can have both positive and negative effects on patients.

### Quality of life

Much more important is their quality of life (QoL) (Fig 2). A high QoL is invariably associated with wellness and vigour, while a poor QoL is often associated with symptoms and malaise. QoL is a difficult concept to define. In a systematic review of health-related QoL, four of seven definitions referred to QoL as being a function of the gap between an individual's aspirations and achievements. The greater the gap, the lower the quality of life (Figs 3 and 4).

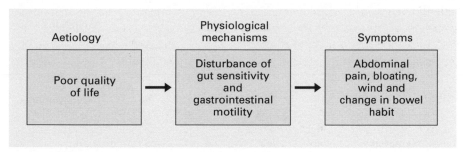

**Fig 2** The aetiology and physiology of medically unexplained gastrointestinal symptoms.

Such a concept does not explain the basis of all unexplained symptoms. An additional dimension affects the point (or threshold) at which a QoL gap will cause symptoms (Figs 4 and 5). Several potential factors will influence the development of symptoms for a given QoL:

☐ genetics and/or learned behaviour

☐ coping strategies

☐ previous psychological trauma

☐ exhaustion.

For example, many patients with unexplained symptoms have taken little rest or recreation in the preceding months and years. Even though the gap between their aspirations and achievements is small, they quickly develop unexplained symptoms (Fig 6); they become mentally and physically exhausted (otherwise known as 'burn out' or 'vital exhaustion'). Reasonable and regular periods of rest are often all that is required to restore a normal response to a given QoL gap (Fig 6).

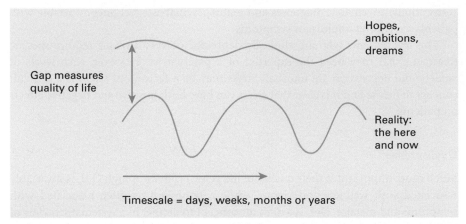

**Fig 3** The gap between aspirations and achievements is a measure of quality of life (adapted from Calman, 1984).

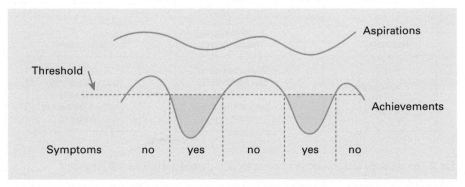

**Fig 4** Symptoms develop when there is a large gap between aspirations and achievements (ie when a threshold of sufficiently low quality of life is reached).

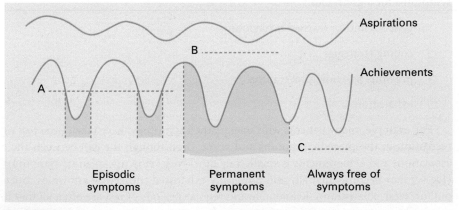

**Fig 5** Different people have different thresholds (A, B and C) at which they develop symptoms.

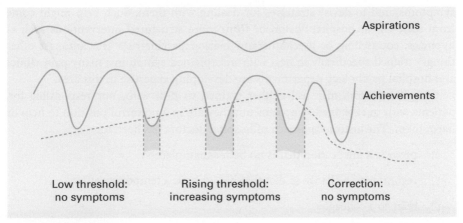

**Fig 6** Effect of exhaustion on the threshold at which a given poor quality of life will lead to symptoms.

Clearly, there are many different dimensions to QoL, and the gap for each dimension will vary over time. The effect is probably summative. There are four broad categories to QoL:

☐ health

☐ professional or occupational life

☐ hobbies and recreation, and

☐ personal life.

## ☐ TARGETS FOR TREATMENT

With this concept of the underlying cause of unexplained symptoms it is possible to generate three possible targets for treatment:

☐ an individual's aspirations

☐ their achievements

☐ the various factors that determine the threshold at which a given QoL causes symptoms.

For example, if a person's aspirations are reduced to a realistic level, the gap between aspirations and achievements will narrow. Alternatively, if their functioning has improved so that their achievements match their aspirations (eg an improved marital relationship), they will achieve a better QoL. If the problem is exhaustion, clearly enforced holidays or rest periods will invariably provide a solution (Fig 6).

In most circumstances, pointing out the relationship of symptoms to QoL, with recommendations of what a patient might consider changing, will enable that patient to achieve control of their symptoms through lifestyle modification. The patient may need more support to understand the factors that underpin their symptoms, and to devise strategies for dealing with them. Such help might come from their GP or hospital doctor, or from more structured interventions such as hypnosis, counselling or psychotherapy. Liaison psychiatrists are (amongst other things) trained specifically to deal with unexplained symptoms; many pain clinics and hospital psychology departments are developing expertise in this area.

Hospital doctors may feel neither trained to deal with, nor responsible for, patients with unexplained symptoms but they are in a powerful position to help or harm them. The historic approach of hospital doctors has been to:

- [ ] provide a medication that is no better than placebo

- [ ] recommend a change in diet that has, at best, a temporary effect

- [ ] refer to a colleague

- [ ] arrange follow-up with a trainee doctor (usually the most inexperienced of the team)

- [ ] refer back to the GP.

Most of these options (except the final one) may cause more harm than good. Fortunately, there is an alternative approach. It may take more time initially but, overall, time will be saved and the outcome for the patient better. This alternative approach might include:

- [ ] asking what the patient expects to achieve from the consultation

- [ ] exploring the patient's beliefs about the symptoms

- [ ] open-ended questions about family life, work, hobbies and leisure time and how the symptoms affect them

- [ ] pointing out the link between symptoms and adverse lifestyle, life events or poor QoL

- [ ] advising the patient to consider this link, and make appropriate changes to their lifestyle.

Such an approach invariably leads to a more satisfied patient who will consult less and require fewer investigations.

However, such an approach does not help some patients or the disturbance to QoL is so severe that the symptoms become self-perpetuating. In this circumstance, the symptoms prevent the patient functioning normally so that the gap between aspirations and achievements cannot be closed. Unless the patient is given temporary relief from their symptoms to enable them to re-establish their achievements, they will continue to have symptoms.

Most medications used for medically unexplained gastrointestinal symptoms are no better than placebo. The exception is low-dose antidepressants, with which three patients need to be treated to achieve one extra favourable outcome. Because of the stigma attached to antidepressants, patients are often resistant to taking them or fail to comply with treatment. However, their use for temporary relief of symptoms may enable the patient to restore their QoL. Other options are hypnosis and formal psychotherapy. Both these interventions have been shown in randomised controlled trials to benefit patients with IBS, but the NHS does not currently fund them.

## □ SUMMARY

'Medically unexplained gastrointestinal symptoms' is the preferred terminology for patients who have gut symptoms without an underlying disease process. Such patients require a careful clinical assessment supported by limited or no investigation. They often respond well to unambiguous reassurance combined with a careful explanation of the cause of the symptoms and the causal link between symptoms and lifestyle. Some patients require more targeted treatment aimed at supporting self-management of contributing psychological factors. A few will benefit from a limited course of low-dose antidepressants to enable them to re-establish a normal pattern of behaviour to achieve a better QoL. Only a tiny proportion requires formal psychiatric evaluation and support.

## FURTHER READING

1   Calman KC. Quality of life in cancer patients – an hypothesis. *J Med Ethics* 1984;**10**:124–7.
2   Thompson WG. Gut reactions. Understanding symptoms of the digestive tract. New York: Plenum Press, 1989.
3   Creed F, Mayou RA, Hopkins A (eds). *Medical symptoms not explained by organic disease.* London: The Royal College of Psychiatrists and the Royal College of Physicians of London, 1992.
4   Salmon P, Sharma N, Valori R, Bellenger N. Patients' intentions in primary care: relationship to physical and psychological symptoms, and their perception by general practitioners. *Soc Sci Med* 1994;**38**:585–92.
5   Mayou R, Bass C, Sharpe M (eds). *Treatment of functional somatic symptoms.* Oxford: Oxford University Press, 1995.
6   Salmon P, Peters S, Stanley I. Patients' perceptions of medical explanations for somatisation disorders: qualitative analysis. *BMJ* 1999;**318**:372–6.
7   Camilleri M, Spiller RC. *Irritable bowel syndrome: diagnosis and treatment.* Edinburgh: WB Saunders, 2002.

# Advances in inflammatory bowel disease

Jonathan Rhodes

## ☐ PATHOGENESIS: GENES AND ENVIRONMENT

### *NOD2/CARD15* and sick phagocytes

It has long been recognised that genetic factors contribute to the risk for inflammatory bowel disease (IBD). An individual whose identical twin has Crohn's disease has an approximately 50% chance of developing the disease, with a lower risk (probably around 15%) for ulcerative colitis. The first IBD gene has now been identified, initially called nucleotide-binding oligomerisation protein 2 (*NOD2*) but now renamed caspase activation and recruitment domain (*CARD15*) (Fig 1). It contains three mutation sites associated with increased risk for Crohn's disease.[1,2] Heterozygotes for one of these mutations have a 2–4 fold relative risk for Crohn's disease, whilst homozygotes or compound heterozygotes have a 20–40 fold relative risk compared with the background risk in the western population of about one per 1,000 – which implies that the overwhelming majority of individuals with the gene mutation do not have Crohn's disease. Moreover, the *CARD15* abnormality

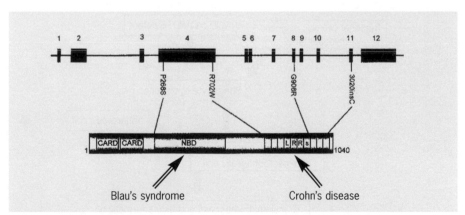

**Fig 1** The first identified inflammatory bowel disease gene, nucleotide-binding oligomerisation protein 2 (*NOD2*)/caspase activation and recruitment domain (*CARD15*). It is selectively expressed in macrophages, neutrophils and epithelial cells, abnormal in about 29% of Crohn's disease patients (homozygous or compound heterozygous abnormality ca 8%) and 7% of controls, and is associated with ileal or ileo-colonic but not isolated colonic Crohn's disease. Mutations in the nucleotide binding domain (NBD) of *NOD2* are associated with the rare granulomatous condition, Blau's syndrome, which is not associated with intestinal disease. Mutations in the leucine-rich region (LRR), which acts as a receptor for bacterial cell wall proteoglycan, are associated with Crohn's disease and affect intracellular killing of bacteria.

contributes only about 15% of the attributable risk for familial Crohn's disease and rather less of the risk for the commoner sporadic Crohn's disease.

**Mechanisms underlying Crohn's disease** (Fig 2)

The main achievement of the *CARD15* discovery is likely to be the insight it gives into the pathogenic mechanisms that underlie the disease. Here rapid progress is being made. *CARD15* is expressed particularly within the cytoplasm of macrophages and activated neutrophils, and to a lesser extent within epithelial cells. The leucine-rich region that is the site of the Crohn's disease-associated mutations functions as a binding domain for bacterial cell wall proteoglycan,[3] and the mutations have been shown to diminish the ability of the affected cells to kill intracellular bacteria.[4] This is in keeping with immunohistochemical studies showing *Escherichia coli*, Listeria and other bacteria within macrophages in Crohn's disease tissue.[5] It also fits in with evidence that rare genetic disorders such as chronic granulomatous disease and glycogen storage disease type 1b, that are also associated with defects in phagocyte killing of bacteria, are associated with intestinal disease that closely mimics Crohn's disease.[6,7] The *NOD2/CARD15* abnormalities have been shown to be associated with ileal or ileo-colonic Crohn's disease but not with isolated colonic disease, raising the possibility that the latter is not in fact Crohn's disease.

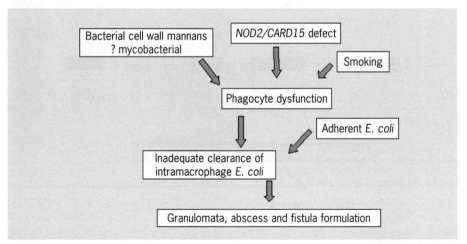

**Fig 2** A hypothesis for Crohn's disease as a defective phagocytic disorder (*CARD15* = caspase activation and recruitment domain; *NOD2* = nucleotide-binding oligomerisation protein 2; *E. coli* = *Escherichia coli*).

**Smoking**

In 'mixed disease' families, in which one member has ulcerative colitis and another Crohn's disease, the individual with Crohn's disease usually has isolated colonic disease and is nearly always a smoker.[8] It is plausible that the ulcerative colitis genotype can be converted to the 'isolated colonic Crohn's' phenotype by smoking.

Smoking is much the strongest environmental factor for Crohn's disease so far identified. About two-thirds of patients with Crohn's disease smoke, compared with about one-third of the general population. Smoking is associated with an increased risk for 'perforating' Crohn's disease – formation of abscesses or fistulae, with greater risk of relapse after surgical resection.[9] Indeed, evidence suggests that smoking cessation probably has a substantially greater impact on likelihood of remission than any currently available maintenance therapy (Fig 3).[10]

The mechanism for the harmful effect of smoking is unclear, but there is some evidence that it could act via suppression of the ability of macrophages to kill intracellular bacteria.[11]

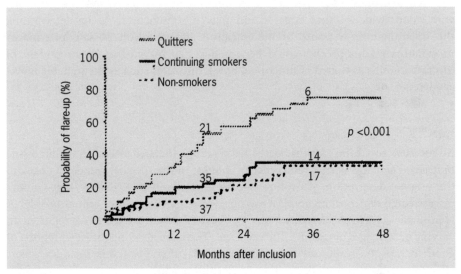

**Fig 3** The beneficial effect of smoking cessation on the course of Crohn's disease[10] (p value is for comparison between quitting and continuing smokers).

## Autoimmunity and p-antineutrophil cytoplasmic antibody

Rather less progress has been made in understanding the pathogenesis of ulcerative colitis. There is evidence of HLA class 2 associations, with HLA DRB1*0103 conferring an approximately 10-fold relative risk for severe disease. There is more evidence to support autoimmunity as a central mechanism for ulcerative colitis than for Crohn's disease, with about two-thirds of ulcerative colitis patients possessing a circulating antineutrophil antibody, an atypical p-antineutrophil cytoplasmic antibody (pANCA). Unlike the pANCA found in association with vasculitis, myeloperoxidase is not a major antigen for colitis-associated pANCA. The antigen or antigens have proved hard to define and may include a range of neutrophil nuclear antigens. There is also evidence of cross-reactivity with bacterial antigens. Given recent evidence that the antimyeloperoxidase pANCA of vasculitis may have a central role in the pathogenesis of vasculitis mediated via activation of neutrophils,[12] it is feasible that ulcerative colitis could also be an autoimmune condition mediated by pANCA.

## Stress

The striking association between ulcerative colitis and nonsmoking or ex-smoking (only about 5% of patients with ulcerative colitis are current smokers) is hard to explain. The argument that smoking simply changes the phenotype from ulcerative colitis to Crohn's disease makes it hard to explain the impressive anecdotes of patients who have deteriorated after cessation of smoking and been 'cured' by going back to their cigarettes. Many patients notice that their colitis is worse at times of stress, and a New World monkey, the cotton-top tamarin, develops what seems to be the same disease in captivity.

Good progress is being made in understanding the complex interactions between neurones, epithelial cells and inflammatory cells within the intestine, with good evidence that stress could play a significant role in determining the inflammatory response of the intestine. Identification of safe pharmaco-modulators of this process could be a major step forward in the treatment of ulcerative colitis as well as of functional bowel disorders such as the irritable bowel syndrome.

## Mycobacteria

About 70% of Crohn's disease cases have granulomata identifiable within tissue biopsies. There has been a resurgence of interest in the speculation, dating back to the original description of Crohn's disease in Scotland by Dalziel,[13] that Crohn's disease could represent an atypical mycobacterial infection. Trace amounts of DNA identifiable as *Mycobacterium avium var paratuberculosis* have been reported in varying percentages of Crohn's disease tissue. There are also uncontrolled reports of good therapeutic responses to antimycobacterial therapy if this includes agents effective against this mycobacterium (eg clarithromycin).

The story is far from clear because mycobacteria have been cultured from only a very few Crohn's disease tissue samples. Moreover, the antitumour necrosis factor α (TNFα) antibody, infliximab (see later), is good for Crohn's disease but bad for tuberculosis. An intriguing study has demonstrated that *M. paratuberculosis* DNA can be identified using polymerase chain reaction amplification on tissue microdissected from Crohn's disease granulomas using laser dissecting microscopy.[14]

We are investigating the possibility that microbial cell wall mannans might be able to induce a defect in macrophage function within the intestinal mucosa similar to the alterations that occur genetically in the genetic forms of Crohn's disease. The same mannans might also be candidates for the antigen identified by the anti-*Saccharomyces cerevesiae* (Baker's yeast) antibody present in about 60% of Crohn's disease patient sera. This antibody is directed against a cell wall mannan with a specific (1–3) linkage also found in some forms of mycobacteria. It is feasible that low level mycobacterial infection might depress intramucosal macrophage function allowing secondary infection with a range of intestinal bacteria. Trials of antimycobacterial therapy that include agents effective against atypical mycobacteria are currently underway.

# ☐ IMPLICATIONS FOR THERAPY

## Crohn's disease

### *Corticosteroids*

If Crohn's disease is due to disordered phagocyte function, corticosteroids are not appropriate therapy. However, corticosteroids remain the most popular and best tested choice for induction of remission, despite the clear evidence that they are not effective at preventing relapse and do not induce mucosal healing. They achieve rapid, effective short-term (ie three months) symptomatic benefit. There is increasing recognition that in probably no other condition are high-dose corticosteroids used to obtain only short-term symptomatic relief with no expectation of affecting the natural history.

When steroids are the preferred option, budesonide, which has rapid first-pass metabolism by the liver, can be used in a preparation formulated to allow delivery to the terminal ileum. In comparison with prednisolone, this achieves approximately 50% reduction in steroid-related side effects for a similar therapeutic response.

### *Alternative treatments*

Alternatives to steroids include:

- ☐ antibiotics

- ☐ immunosuppressives

- ☐ dietary therapy

- ☐ antiTNFα antibody, and

- ☐ surgery.

*Antibiotics.* It might be logical to use antibiotics which achieve good penetration within macrophages. Clarithromycin has been shown to be effective in uncontrolled studies. Metronidazole is effective in colonic Crohn's disease: in a dose of 400 mg three times daily for three months it reduces postoperative relapse in the first year after resective surgery. Further controlled trials are needed.

*Immunosuppressives.* The immunosuppressive agents azathioprine, its metabolite 6-mercaptopurine and methotrexate have all been shown to be effective in Crohn's disease. Although initially used as 'steroid-sparing' agents, they have efficacy in their own right. Unlike corticosteroids, azathioprine (usually 2–2.5 mg/kg/day) heals mucosal ulceration.

The use of immunosuppressive agents requires close monitoring of blood counts and hepatic function, but side effects seem somewhat less frequent in Crohn's disease than in rheumatoid arthritis. Use of azathioprine for up to five years is not associated with any increased risk of cancer in IBD. Methotrexate (eg 25 mg intramuscularly weekly plus folic acid 5 mg/day) is currently usually reserved for the 10% of patients who cannot tolerate azathioprine.

*Dietary therapy.* Enteral feeding with specially formulated feeds as the sole therapy usually induces remission within about three weeks in about two-thirds of Crohn's disease patients, particularly if there is small intestinal involvement. Some, but not all, whole protein feeds are effective.

It remains unclear how enteral feeding works. Much of its effect may be due to reducing the quantity of the intestinal flora. Although unequivocally safe and effective, it is relatively expensive and inconvenient, and requires a well-motivated patient. It is particularly useful in achieving remission in the complex septic patient, perhaps as a prelude to resective surgery.

*Antitumour necrosis factor α antibody (infliximab).* TNFα is central to inflammation, but it is nevertheless impressive and surprising that a single infusion of humanised antibody against TNFα has such a profound clinical effect, with mucosal healing persisting for two months or longer. The mechanism of its effect in Crohn's disease is still uncertain. Recombinant TNFα receptor (etanercept) seems to be ineffective, and it has been suggested that the prolonged effect of infliximab is probably the result of apoptosis of a subclass of T lymphocytes and macrophages which express transmembrane TNFα. Although 'humanised', the antibody still contains about 10% mouse immunoglobulin, and antibodies develop against it which can render repeated infusions difficult. This antibody formation is largely prevented if the patient is already receiving either azathioprine or methotrexate. All patients should arguably have relapsed on one of those immunosuppressive therapies before infliximab is considered.[15]

Infliximab therapy has been approved by the National Institute for Clinical Excellence (NICE) for patients with severe disease who have failed with conventional immunosuppressive therapy, who have failed or are intolerant of steroids, and those in whom surgery is inappropriate. It is contraindicated in patients who have sepsis (those with significant perineal disease are likely to need magnetic resonance scanning before starting therapy) and also in patients with strictures that are causing obstruction (eg proximal dilatation on barium radiology). Repeated dosing 'maintenance' therapy has been shown to be effective for at least four doses (Fig 4),[16] but infliximab is currently approved by NICE only for repeated treatment in cases of symptomatic relapse. It may promote fistula closure, but usually only temporarily. The presence of fistulae in the absence of other features of severe disease is not currently considered sufficient indication for infliximab. All patients should have a chest X-ray to exclude tuberculosis which has been shown to be markedly reactivated by infliximab therapy. Short-term safety seems excellent with only fairly minor infusion reactions, but long-term safety is still not well established.

*Surgery.* About 80% of patients with Crohn's disease require surgery at some time, usually because of stricturing. It should not be thought of only as a 'last resort'. Surgical resection in patients with a short ileal stricture, increasingly performed by laparoscope-assisted right hemicolectomy, achieves complete symptomatic remission for an average period of five years and may often be an appropriate initial option.

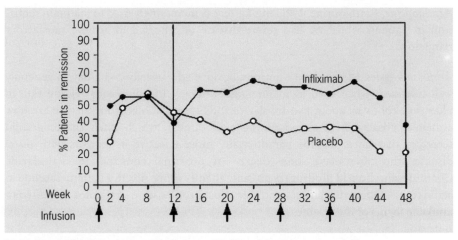

**Fig 4** Beneficial effect of repeated infusions of infliximab in Crohn's disease.[16]

### Ulcerative colitis

There was a high mortality from ulcerative colitis before the introduction of corticosteroids and safer colectomy in the 1950s. It remains important to recognise when colitis has become severe. Severe colitis is a systemic illness, characterised by any one of the following:

- tachycardia (>90 beats/min)

- fever (>37.5°)

- anaemia (<10.0 g/dl)

- hypoalbuminaemia (<30 g/dl), or

- severe abdominal pain in association with bloody diarrhoea (usually six or more times per 24 hours).

*Treatment*

*Corticosteroids/ciclosporin.* Any of the features listed above is an indication for immediate hospital admission and high-dose corticosteroid therapy (usually intravenous (iv) hydrocortisone 100 mg four times daily). About one in three such cases will require colectomy (one-quarter of patients with ulcerative colitis will need a colectomy at some time). Plain abdominal X-ray is helpful, not only to exclude toxic dilatation (transverse colon diameter >5 cm), but also as an approximate guide to disease extent (severely ulcerated colon usually contains no faeces). If the serum C-reactive protein remains above 45 g/l after three days of therapy, the chance of a successful response to corticosteroids is small and ciclosporin (4 mg/kg/day iv) is now increasingly being started. It is still controversial therapy as the overall reduction in colectomy rate achieved with ciclosporin is probably less than 50% and a small, but definite, mortality (probably about 2%) is associated with its use – arguably greater than the mortality associated with severe colitis (<1% in specialist centres).[17]

*Azathioprine.* Azathioprine, 2–2.5 mg/kg/day, is increasingly used to maintain remission in patients who have had severe disease or who fail to achieve satisfactory remission.

*Aminosalicylates.* Mesalazine (5-aminosalicylic acid), usually 2–3 g/day, is generally well tolerated; when used as maintenance therapy it reduces the relapse rate in ulcerative colitis by about two-thirds. Various formulations of mesalazine are now available. Olsalazine (5-aminosalicylic acid dimer), which often causes a mild secretory diarrhoea, may be paradoxically more effective in patients with distal disease who often have some degree of proximal constipation. Balsalazide (5-aminosalicylic acid prodrug) is possibly slightly more effective than mesalazine in acute colitis. Otherwise, efficacy and side effect profiles seem similar for the different available forms of mesalazine.

## Pouchitis

Most patients undergoing colectomy for ulcerative colitis are offered a pouch reconstruction as an alternative to a permanent ileostomy. The pouch is constructed from a 'J' of ileum doubled back on itself with the apex of the J anastomosed to the anal mucosa. This usually requires at least one further operation, generally leaving the patient with symptoms equivalent to those of mild colitis (ca 4 semi-formed bowel actions per day and one during the night), usually needing continued antidiarrhoeal therapy such as loperamide. Most patients find this manageable and preferable to ileostomy. The pouch becomes significantly inflamed in about 10% of patients and some degree of histological inflammation is almost universal. Curiously, this inflammation (pouchitis) does not occur in patients with familial polyposis undergoing the same operation, so it seems to imply a latent abnormality in the ileal mucosa in patients with ulcerative colitis.

Ulcerative colitis does not usually respond to antibiotics, but pouchitis responds well to metronidazole, ciprofloxacin or clarithromycin. Only a short course of antibiotics is usually required, but some patients have more troublesome chronic symptoms. In this situation, a cocktail of eight 'probiotic' bacteria is effective.[18] This is one of the first examples of controlled evidence showing a beneficial effect of probiotic bacteria. It is still unclear how they work. Some experimental evidence suggests it may be via an effect of bacterial DNA, particularly unmethylated cytosine guanine (CpG) islands, acting via interaction with Toll-like receptor 9 which exerts an anti-inflammatory role in the innate immune response to bacteria (in which case dead bacteria might work just as well). This has opened up another promising avenue of research.

## REFERENCES

1    Hugot JP, Chamaillard M, Zouali H, Lesage S *et al.* Association of NOD2 leucine-rich repeat variants with susceptibility to Crohn's disease. *Nature* 2001;411:599–603.
2    Ogura Y, Bonen DK, Inohara N, Nicolae DL *et al.* A frameshift mutation in NOD2 associated with susceptibility to Crohn's disease. *Nature* 2001;411:603–6.

3    Girardin SE, Boneca IG, Viala J, Chamaillard M *et al.* Nod2 is a general sensor of peptidoglycan through muramyl dipeptide (MDP) detection. *J Biol Chem* 2003;**278**:8869–72.

4    Hisamatsu T, Suzuki M, Reinecker HC, Nadeau WJ *et al.* CARD15/NOD2 functions as an antibacterial factor in human intestinal epithelial cells. *Gastroenterology* 2003;**124**:993–1000.

5    Liu Y, van Kruiningen HJ, West AB, Cartun RW *et al.* Immunocytochemical evidence of Listeria, *Escherichia coli*, and Streptococcus antigens in Crohn's disease. *Gastroenterology* 1995;**108**:1396–404.

6    Isaacs D, Wright VM, Shaw DG, Raafat F, Walker-Smith JA. Chronic granulomatous disease mimicking Crohn's disease. *J Pediatr Gastroenterol Nutr* 1985;**4**:498–501.

7    Couper R, Kapelushnik J, Griffiths AM. Neutrophil dysfunction in glycogen storage disease Ib: association with Crohn's-like colitis. Review. *Gastroenterology* 1991;**100**:549–54.

8    Bridger S, Lee JC, Bjarnason I, Jones JE, Macpherson AJ. In siblings with similar genetic susceptibility for inflammatory bowel disease, smokers tend to develop Crohn's disease and non-smokers develop ulcerative colitis. *Gut* 2002;**51**:21–5.

9    Picco MF, Bayless TM. Tobacco consumption and disease duration are associated with fistulizing and stricturing behaviors in the first 8 years of Crohn's disease. *Am J Gastroenterol* 2003;**98**:363–8.

10   Cosnes J, Beaugerie L, Carbonnel F, Gendre JP. Smoking cessation and the course of Crohn's disease: an intervention study. *Gastroenterology* 2001;**120**:1093–9.

11   King TE Jr, Savici D, Campbell PA. Phagocytosis and killing of Listeria monocytogenes by alveolar macrophages: smokers versus nonsmokers. *J Infect Dis* 1988;**158**:1309–16.

12   Xiao H, Heeringa P, Hu P, Liu Z *et al.* Antineutrophil cytoplasmic autoantibodies specific for myeloperoxidase cause glomerulonephritis and vasculitis in mice. *J Clin Invest* 2002;**110**:955–63.

13   Dalziel TK. Chronic interstitial enteritis. *BMJ* 1913;**2**:1068–70.

14   Ryan P, Bennett MW, Aarons S, Lee G *et al.* PCR detection of *Mycobacterium paratuberculosis* in Crohn's disease granulomas isolated by laser capture microdissection. *Gut* 2002;**51**:665–70.

15   Sandborn WJ. Strategies for targeting tumour necrosis factor in IBD. *Best Pract Res Clin Gastroenterol* 2003;**17**:105–17.

16   Rutgeerts P, D'Haens G, Targan S, Vasiliauskas E *et al.* Efficacy and safety of treatment with anti-tumour necrosis factor antibody (infliximab) to maintain remission in Crohn's disease. *Gastroenterology* 1999;**117**:761–9.

17   Hawthorne AB. Ciclosporin and refractory colitis. *Eur J Gastroenterol Hepatol* 2003;**15**:239–44.

18   Gionchetti P, Amadini C, Rizzello F, Venturi A, Campieri M. Review article: treatment of mild to moderate ulcerative colitis and pouchitis. *Aliment Pharmacol Ther* 2002;**16**(Suppl 4):13–19.

# ☐ GASTROENTEROLOGY SELF ASSESSMENT QUESTIONS

*Helicobacter pylori*

1   Eradication of *H. pylori* is effective in the treatment of:
   (a)  Duodenal ulcer
   (b)  Gastric adenocarcinoma
   (c)  Low-grade MALT lymphoma of the stomach
   (d)  Gastro-oesophageal reflux disease
   (e)  Cirrhosis

2   Current therapy for *H. pylori* includes:
   (a)  Lansoprazole, clarithromycin and amoxycillin
   (b)  Celecoxib
   (c)  Bismuth salts, omeprazole, metronidazole and amoxycillin
   (d)  Oral vaccine
   (e)  Omeprazole, tetracycline, metronidazole

3   The following diagnostic methods are appropriate:
   (a)  Faecal antigen test in patients with dyspepsia aged below 50
   (b)  Serum antibody test after attempted eradication
   (c)  $^{13}$C urea breath test on the last day of an eradication course
   (d)  Biopsy and urease test on asymptomatic children of *H. pylori* infected parents
   (e)  Biopsy and culture after initial treatment failure in a patient with complicated duodenal ulcer

## Medically unexplained gastrointestinal symptoms

1   In an otherwise healthy individual the following symptoms  predict underlying gastrointestinal (GI) disease:
   (a)  Severe knife-like abdominal pain
   (b)  Changing bowel habit
   (c)  Bloody diarrhoea
   (d)  Abdominal bloating
   (e)  Relief of abdominal pain with defecation

2   Medically unexplained GI symptoms are usually caused by:
   (a)  A vivid imagination
   (b)  A change in gut sensitivity
   (c)  Psychiatric disorder
   (d)  Poor quality of life
   (e)  Medications

3   Medically unexplained GI symptoms are best managed by:
   (a)  Unambiguous reassurance and an explanation of the symptoms
   (b)  Multiple investigations

   (c) Psychiatrists
   (d) Hypnotherapy
   (e) Antispasmodic medications

## Advances in inflammatory bowel disease

1   Crohn's disease:
   (a) Is more likely to be complicated by abscess or fistula in a smoker
   (b) Is more likely to relapse after surgery in a smoker
   (c) Is usually associated with mutations in the *Nod2/Card15* gene
   (d) Undergoes mucosal healing in response to azathioprine and infliximab but not corticosteroids
   (e) Is improved by conventional antituberculosis therapy

2   Ulcerative colitis:
   (a) Is commonly associated with the presence of a circulating antineutrophil antibody (pANCA)
   (b) Usually occurs in nonsmokers or ex-smokers
   (c) Is associated with a lifetime colectomy rate of about 50%
   (d) Warrants admission to hospital if bloody diarrhoea is accompanied by a pulse rate above 90 per min
   (e) Is complicated by toxic dilatation if the transverse colon diameter is at least 3 cm

3   Infliximab therapy:
   (a) Should be used in Crohn's disease only after failure of therapy with azathioprine, 6-mercaptopurine or methotrexate
   (b) Is contraindicated in patients with radiological evidence of obstruction
   (c) Is contraindicated in patients with perianal disease
   (d) Should always be preceded by a chest X-ray to exclude tuberculosis
   (e) Is less likely to be effective in colonic disease

# Prevention of
# Coronary Artery Disease

# Therapeutic intervention to prevent coronary heart disease and stroke

Peter Sever

## ☐ INTRODUCTION

Mortality from cardiovascular disease (CVD), including coronary heart disease (CHD) and stroke, in the UK remains the commonest cause of death (Table 1) and the rates are amongst the highest in the world. Rates for coronary disease are exceeded only by the former Eastern bloc countries. These high rates are partly explained by inadequate intervention strategies to reduce high levels of major risk factors including hypertension and dyslipidaemia. In the recent Health Survey for England, only 12% of patients with hypertension had blood pressure controlled to levels recommended by contemporary guidelines. The use of lipid-lowering therapy to reduce cardiovascular risk is less prevalent in the UK than in most European countries.[1]

**Table 1** UK mortality from cardiovascular disease, coronary heart disease and stroke, 2000.

|  | No. of deaths |
| --- | --- |
| Cardiovascular disease | 235,000 |
| Coronary heart disease | 125,000 |
| Stroke | 60,000 |

## ☐ BLOOD PRESSURE TREATMENT

### Coronary heart disease prevention

Despite a clear log-linear relationship between increasing levels of blood pressure (both systolic and diastolic) and coronary risk, the results of earlier intervention trials of blood pressure lowering produced fewer benefits than predicted from the magnitude of blood pressure lowering.[2] In early trials, such as the Medical Research Council (MRC) trial of the treatment of mild hypertension,[3] active treatment conferred no benefit compared with placebo on coronary event rates, despite a reduction in stroke incidence. Several of these early trials were underpowered; pooled analyses of all the placebo-controlled trials undertaken before 1990 showed an overall reduction in coronary event rates of around 16% (Fig 1), somewhat less

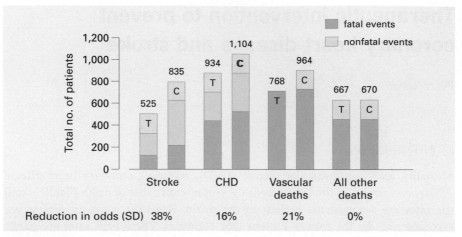

**Fig 1** Meta-analysis of blood pressure lowering trials (17 trials, 47,653 patients, blood pressure differences: systolic 10–12 mmHg, diastolic 5–6 mmHg) (C= control; CHD = coronary heart disease; SD = standard deviation; T = treatment).[2]

than the 20–25% reduction predicted from observational studies.[2] In some of the more recently reported trials in elderly hypertensive patients, notably the diuretic treated group in the MRC elderly trial,[4] and in two trials of treatment of isolated systolic hypertension (SHEP[5] and SYST-EUR[6]) (see end of text for explanation of studies), there were significant reductions (ca 30%) in coronary disease events.

Recent attempts have been made to differentiate particular drug treatment strategies in their impact on coronary disease. Pooled analyses of the data (Tables 2 and 3)[13] and the recent large ALLHAT study[14] have failed to identify any treatment benefits attributable to a particular class of agent. Uncontrolled observational studies, which are less reliable than randomised controlled trials, had suggested an adverse impact on coronary disease of drug regimens which included a calcium-channel blocker. However, it is important that no such adverse impact was reported in the most recent ALLHAT study. The ongoing ASCOT study[15] in almost 20,000 patients is also investigating different combination treatments. An older regimen of a beta-blocker, alone or in combination, and a diuretic is being compared

**Table 2** Meta-analysis from the Blood Pressure Lowering Treatment Trialists' Collaboration, 2000 (STOP-2,[7] UKPDS,[8] CAPPP[9]): angiotensin-converting enzyme inhibitors vs diuretic or beta-blocker.

|  | Odds ratio | Confidence interval |
|---|---|---|
| Stroke | 1.01 | 0.92–1.19 |
| Coronary heart disease | 1.00 | 0.88–1.14 |
| Heart failure | 0.92 | 0.77–1.09 |
| All cardiovascular events | 1.00 | 0.93–1.08 |
| Mortality | 1.03 | 0.93–1.14 |

**Table 3** Meta-analysis from the Blood Pressure Lowering Treatment Trialists' Collaboration, 2000 (INSIGHT,[10] NICS-EH,[11] STOP-2,[7] NORDIL[12]): calcium-channel blockers vs diuretic or beta-blocker.

|  | Odds ratio | Confidence interval |
|---|---|---|
| Stroke | 0.87 | 0.77–0.98 |
| Coronary heart disease | 1.12 | 1.00–1.26 |
| Heart failure | 1.12 | 0.95–1.33 |
| All cardiovascular events | 1.02 | 0.95–1.10 |
| Mortality | 1.01 | 0.92–1.11 |

with a newer regimen of a calcium-channel blocker with or without an angiotensin-converting enzyme (ACE) inhibitor. The results will be available within the next couple of years.

The HOPE study,[16] which was not designed as a blood pressure study, investigated the use of the ACE inhibitor ramipril compared with placebo in high risk cardiovascular patients. There were significant reductions in the incidence of many cardiovascular end-points, including myocardial infarction (MI). This was most likely due to a blood pressure lowering effect of ramipril; this was observed in a small ambulatory blood pressure monitoring substudy in contrast to the much smaller blood pressure differences obtained by casual measurements and reported in the main HOPE paper.

### Stroke prevention

Highly consistent benefits in stroke prevention have been seen in individual hypertension trials and in pooled analyses of the trial outcome data. Compared with observational studies, the size of the reduction was similar to that predicted for the difference in blood pressure achieved in the trials. Two trials have suggested that stroke outcome may be influenced by individual drug classes. Both the MRC trial of mild hypertension in the elderly[4] and the LIFE study[17] indicated that beta-blocker based treatment is less likely to confer the full benefit than either a diuretic-based regimen or one based on an angiotensin-receptor blocker.

PROGRESS,[18] a recent trial carried out in stroke survivors, has clearly demonstrated a substantial reduction in the incidence of recurrent stroke with a treatment regimen based on the ACE inhibitor perindopril and indapamide. Many will view this as persuasive evidence that stroke survivors will benefit from blood pressure lowering. However, it is not clear whether blood pressure lowering would be beneficial or harmful in the context of acute stroke. This is an area that requires further research.

### ☐ LIPID LOWERING

### Coronary disease prevention

Early trials of the secondary prevention of coronary disease in patients who have survived an MI, including 4S,[19] CARE[20] and LIPID,[21] clearly demonstrated that cholesterol lowering with statins reduced the incidence of recurrent MI and fatal CHD by about 30% over a five-year follow-up period (Fig 2). More recent studies involving high risk patients, but with lower levels of initial cholesterol, have shown a similar magnitude of benefit.

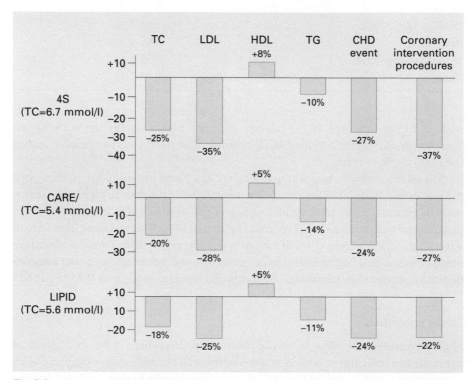

**Fig 2** Percentage reduction in lipids and events in the early secondary prevention trials of coronary disease (CHD = coronary heart disease; HDL = high-density lipoprotein; LDL = low-density lipoprotein; TC = total cholesterol; TG = triglycerides) (for explanation of studies see end of text).

In primary intervention, evidence of benefit from lipid lowering was seen in the earliest trials with cholestyramine and gemfibrozil. These results have been confirmed and extended with the introduction of statins in the WOSCOPS[22] and AFCAPS/TexCAPS[23] studies in which a 20% reduction in cholesterol was associated with a 30–40% reduction in the incidence of CHD (Fig 3). The ASCOT-LLA[24] was stopped early after 3.3 years of follow-up because there were 36% and 27% reductions in the incidence of CHD and stroke, respectively, in the active treatment arm (atorvastatin). In both ASCOT-LLA and AFCAPS/TexCAPS, patients were recruited with lower cholesterol levels than those usually recommended for lipid-lowering therapy.

The results of these lipid-lowering trials with reference to the absolute reduction in CHD events over the range of low-density lipoprotein cholesterol reduction are summarised in Fig 4.

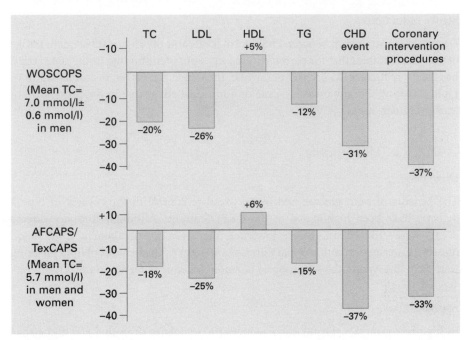

**Fig 3** Percentage reduction in lipids and events in the early primary prevention trials of coronary disease (CHD = coronary heart disease; HDL = high-density lipoprotein; LDL = low-density lipoprotein; TC = total cholesterol; TG = triglycerides) (for explanation of studies see end of text).

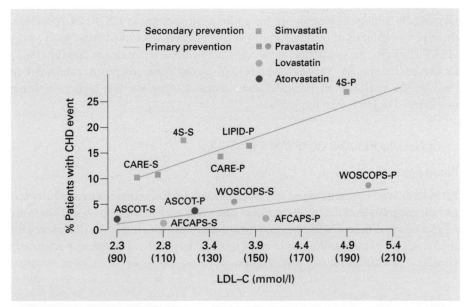

**Fig 4** Overview of landmark statin trials: low-density lipoprotein cholesterol (LDL-C) vs events (CHD = coronary heart disease; P = placebo treated; S = statin treated) (for explanation of studies see end of text).

## Stroke reduction

Despite the relationship between cholesterol levels and the risk of subsequent stroke being less clear than that for coronary disease, a consistent finding in the statin trials has been reduction in ischaemic stroke incidence (25–50% in some studies). Lipid-lowering therapy provides a major additional advantage in the prevention of cardiovascular disease (CVD).

## □ OTHER INTERVENTIONS

### Diabetes

The benefits of both glucose and blood pressure control in the context of type 2 diabetes have been highlighted in the UKPDS study.[8] Although coronary disease events were reduced by glucose lowering, there was greater benefit from blood pressure lowering for both coronary disease and stroke. The benefits of lipid lowering were also observed in the subgroup of normolipidaemic diabetics in ASCOT.

### Aspirin

In high risk groups, aspirin clearly reduces the incidence of both CHD and stroke events by approximately 25%. In low risk patients, however, the coronary disease risk reduction is offset by an increased risk of gastrointestinal bleeding and haemorrhagic stroke.

### Antioxidants

Despite the biological plausibility for antioxidant therapy in CVD risk reduction, there is no evidence of benefit in prospective placebo-controlled trials such as the HPS.[25] Similarly, the theoretical advantages of hormone replacement therapy (HRT) in the prevention of coronary disease and stroke have not been confirmed in randomised trials. If anything, cardiovascular end-points are higher in those randomised to HRT than to placebo.

## □ CONCLUSIONS AND OUTSTANDING ISSUES

### Blood pressure

Early trials were underpowered to detect advantages in coronary disease outcome, and the magnitude of the benefit remains uncertain even in meta-analyses. There are no clear drug differences in outcome for coronary disease, but some differences for stroke. A crucial outstanding issue is the optimal target blood pressure, particularly systolic; this requires further investigation.

### Lipid lowering

Consistent benefits on coronary disease and stroke have been found in the lipid-lowering trials, with the size of the benefit related to the degree to which cholesterol levels have been reduced. Recent studies in high risk individuals (eg those with diabetes but relatively normal lipid levels) confirm the benefits of lipid lowering. The most critical outstanding issue is *how* low to go. Observational studies clearly indicate that there is no threshold for risk and it is likely that there is no level below which benefit is not observed. The issue relating to treatment of patients with lower levels of cholesterol then becomes an economic argument rather than one demanding an evidence base.

### Guidelines for intervention

Given the generally available evidence from observational studies and intervention trials, it is remarkable that international guidelines are inconsistent in their recommendations on thresholds for intervention to prevent CHD and CVD.

*Blood pressure reduction*

In recent years, however, the following recommendations have been made:[26]

☐ Systolic and diastolic thresholds of 160 mmHg and 100 mmHg, respectively, are clear indications for drug treatment when nonpharmacological measures have failed.

☐ In the range of 140–159 mmHg systolic and 90–99 mmHg diastolic pressures, treatment is indicated if there is evidence of target organ damage, for example:
  – left ventricular hypertrophy
  – concomitant disease such as diabetes
  – older age, or
  – an estimated 10-year coronary risk of 15% (equivalent to a CVD risk of 20%).

Guidelines for lipid lowering formerly set higher thresholds of global risk for intervention. In the UK, a threshold of a 30% 10-year coronary risk (40% cardio-vascular risk) has been recommended.[27] However, the evidence for the benefits at lower levels of risk is overwhelming. Lower thresholds have been recommended by many other guidelines in Europe and the USA.[28] Current joint British Guidelines will bring down global risk indications for lipid lowering to the levels proposed for intervention on blood pressure – that is, a 10-year 15% risk of CHD or 20% CVD.

The major problem with implementing policies based on global estimates of risk is that they are dominated by age. Most elderly people will exceed the threshold for intervention both on blood pressure and lipid lowering. In contrast, younger people, notably women, may have high levels of blood pressure or cholesterol which, when projected throughout their lifetime, would reduce life expectancy but under current guidelines would not warrant therapeutic intervention. Health economists will need to take into account not only the short-term risk reductions from treatment, but also the longer-term benefits in terms of life-years saved and estimates of prevention of disability and impaired quality of life.

## ☐ TRIAL ACRONYMS

| | |
|---|---|
| 4S | Scandinavian Simvastatin Survival Study |
| AFCAPS/TexCAPS | |
| | Air Force/Texas Coronary Atherosclerosis Prevention Study |
| ALLHAT | Antihypertensive and Lipid-Lowering Trial to Prevent Heart Disease |
| ASCOT | Anglo-Scandinavian Cardiac Outcomes Trial |
| ASCOT-LLA | Anglo-Scandinavian Cardiac Outcomes Trial-Lipid Lowering Arm |
| CAPPP | Captopril Prevention Project |
| CARE | Cholesterol and Recurrent Events |
| HOPE | Heart Outcomes Prevention Evaluation |
| HPS | Heart Protection Study |
| INSIGHT | International Nifedipine Study: Intervention as a Goal in Hypertension Treatment |
| LIFE | Losartan Intervention For End-point Reduction in Hypertension |
| LIPID | Long-term Intervention with Pravastatin in Ischaemic Disease |
| NICS-EH | National Intervention Co-operative Study in Elderly Hypertensives |
| NORDIL | Nordic Diltiazem |
| PROGRESS | Perindopril Protection Against Recurrent Stroke Study |
| SHEP | Systolic Hypertension in the Elderly Program |
| STOP-2 | Swedish Trial in Old Patients with Hypertension-2 |
| SYST-EUR | Systolic Hypertension in Europe |
| UKPDS | UK Prospective Diabetes Study |
| WOSCOPS | West Of Scotland Coronary Prevention Study |

## REFERENCES

1   *Coronary heart disease statistics.* British Heart Foundation Statistics Database, 2002.

2   Collins R, Peto R. Antihypertensive drug therapy: effects on stroke and coronary heart disease. In: Swales JD (ed). *Textbook of hypertension.* Oxford: Blackwell Scientific Publications, 1994:1156–64.

3   Medical Research Council trial of treatment of mild hypertension: principal results. MRC Working Party. *BMJ (Clin Res Ed)* 1985;291:97–104.

4   Report by the Management Committee. MRC trial of mild hypertension in the elderly. *Med J Aust* 1981;2:398–402.

5   Prevention of stroke by antihypertensive drug treatment in older persons with isolated systolic hypertension. Final results of the Systolic Hypertension in the Elderly Program (SHEP). SHEP Co-operative Research Group. *JAMA* 1991;265:3255–64.

6   Staessen JA, Fagard R, Thijs L, Celis H *et al.* Randomised double-blind comparison of placebo and active treatment for older patients with isolated systolic hypertension. The Systolic Hypertension in Europe (Syst-Eur) Trial Investigators. *Lancet* 1997;350:757–64.

7   Hansson L, Lindholm LH, Ekborn T, Dahlof B *et al.* Randomised trial of old and new antihypertensive drugs in elderly patients: cardiovascular mortality and morbidity. The Swedish Trial in Old Patients with Hypertension-2 study. *Lancet* 1999;354:1751–6.

8   Tight blood pressure control and risk of macrovascular and microvascular complications in type 2 diabetes: UKPDS 38. UK Prospective Diabetes Study Group. *BMJ* 1998;317:703–13.

9   Hansson L, Lindholm LH, Niskanen L, Lanke J et al. Effect of angiotensin-converting-enzyme inhibition compared with conventional therapy on cardiovascular morbidity and mortality in hypertension: the Captopril Prevention Project (CAPPP) randomised trial. *Lancet* 1999; 353:611–6.

10  Brown MJ, Palmer CR, Castaigne A, de Leeuw PW et al. Morbidity and mortality in patients randomised to double-blind treatment with a long-acting calcium-channel blocker or diuretic in the International Nifedipine GITS study: Intervention as a Goal in Hypertension Treatment (INSIGHT). *Lancet* 2000;**356**:366–72.

11  Randomized double-blind comparison of a calcium antagonist and a diuretic in elderly hypertensives. National Intervention Cooperative Study in Elderly Hypertensives Study Group. *Hypertension* 1999;**34**:1129–33.

12  Hansson L, Hedner T, Lund-Johansen P, Kjeldsen SE et al. Randomised trial of effects of calcium antagonists compared with diuretics and beta-blockers on cardiovascular morbidity and mortality in hypertension: the Nordic Diltiazem (NORDIL) study. *Lancet* 2000;**356**: 359–65.

13  Neal B, MacMahon S, Chapman N. Blood Pressure Lowering Treatment Trialists' Collaboration. Effects of ACE inhibitors, calcium antagonists, and other blood-pressure-lowering drugs: results of prospectively designed overviews of randomised trials. *Lancet* 2000;**356**:1955–64.

14  ALLHAT Officers and Coordinators for the ALLHAT Collaborative Research Group. Major outcomes in high-risk hypertensive patients randomized to angiotensin-converting enzyme inhibitor or calcium channel blocker vs diuretic. The Antihypertensive and Lipid-Lowering Treatment to Prevent Heart Attack Trial (ALLHAT). *JAMA* 2002;**288**:2981–97.

15  Sever PS, Dahlof B, Poulter NR, Wedel H et al. Rationale, design, methods and baseline demography of participants of the Anglo-Scandinavian Cardiac Outcomes Trial. ASCOT investigators. *J Hypertens* 2001;**19**:1139–47.

16  Yusuf S, Sleight P, Pogue J, Bosch J et al. Effects of an angiotensin-converting-enzyme inhibitor, ramipril, on cardiovascular events in high-risk patients. The Heart Outcomes Prevention Evaluation Study Investigators. *N Engl J Med* 2000;**342**:145–53.

17  Dahlof B, Devereux RB, Kjeldsen SE, Julius S et al. Cardiovascular morbidity and mortality in the Losartan Intervention For Endpoint reduction in hypertension study (LIFE): a randomised trial against atenolol. *Lancet* 2002;**359**:995–1003.

18  PROGRESS Collaborative Group. Randomised trial of a perindopril-based blood-pressure-lowering regimen among 6,105 individuals with previous stroke or transient ischaemic attack. *Lancet* 2001;**358**:1033–41.

19  Randomised trial of cholesterol lowering in 4444 patients with coronary heart disease: the Scandinavian Simvastatin Survival Study (4S). *Lancet* 1994;**344**:1383–9.

20  Sacks EM, Pfeffer MA, Moye LA, Rouleau JL et al. The effect of pravastatin on coronary events after myocardial infarction in patients with average cholesterol levels. Cholesterol and Recurrent Events Trial Investigators. *N Engl J Med* 1996;**335**:1001–9.

21  Prevention of cardiovascular events and death with pravastatin in patients with coronary heart disease and a broad range of initial cholesterol levels. The Long-Term Intervention with Pravastatin Group in Ischaemic Disease (LIPID) Study Group. *N Engl J Med* 1998;**339**: 1349–57.

22  Shepherd J, Cobbe SM, Ford I, Isles CG et al. Prevention of coronary heart disease with pravastatin in men with hypercholesterolemia. West of Scotland Coronary Prevention Study Group. *N Engl J Med* 1995;**333**:1301–7.

23  Downs JR, Clearfield M, Weis S, Whitney E et al. Primary prevention of acute coronary events with lovastatin in men and women with average cholesterol levels: results of AFCAPS/TexCAPS. Air Force/Texas Coronary Atherosclerosis Prevention Study. *JAMA* 1998;**279**: 1615–22.

24  Sever PS, Dahlof B, Poulter NR, Wedel H et al. Prevention of coronary and stroke events with atorvastatin in hypertensive patients who have average or lower-than-average cholesterol concentrations, in the Anglo-Scandinavian Cardiac Outcomes Trial-Lipid Lowering Arm (ASCOT-LLA): a multicentre randomised controlled trial. *Lancet* 2003;**361**:1149–58.

25    Heart Protection Study Collaborative Group. MRC/BHF Heart Protection Study of antioxidant vitamin supplementation in 20,536 high-risk individuals: a randomised placebo-controlled trial. *Lancet* 2002;**360**:23–33.

26    Ramsay L, Williams B, Johnston G, MacGregor G *et al.* Guidelines for management of hypertension: report of the third working party of the British Hypertension Society. Review. *J Hum Hypertens* 1999;**13**:569–92.

27    Joint British recommendations on prevention of coronary heart disease in clinical practice. British Cardiac Society, British Hyperlipidaemia Association, British Hypertension Society, endorsed by the British Diabetic Association. *Heart* 1998;**80**(Suppl 2):S1–29.

28    De Backer G, Ambrosioni E, Borch-Johnsen K, Brotons C *et al.* European guidelines on cardiovascular disease prevention in clinical practice. Third Joint Task Force of European and Other Societies on Cardiovascular Disease Prevention in Clinical Practice. *Eur Heart J* 2003; 24:1601–10.

# Cardiovascular disease in UK Indian Asians

Jaspal Kooner and John Chambers

## ☐ EPIDEMIOLOGY OF VASCULAR DISEASE IN INDIAN ASIANS

Cardiovascular disease (CVD) mortality is higher amongst Indian Asians than other ethnic groups.[1] The World Health Organization reported that India accounted for one-fifth of the 14 million cardiovascular deaths worldwide in 1990 (Fig 1).[1] Furthermore, CVD mortality is expected to double in India by the year 2015, in contrast to the falling cardiovascular mortality rates in North America and Europe.[1] Indian Asians are on course to becoming the largest single contributor to global coronary heart disease (CHD) mortality and morbidity.

Previous studies show that the burden of CVD is greatest amongst Indian Asians living in urban areas and overseas. Based upon analysis of ECG Q waves, the prevalence of CHD is 4–5 fold higher in urban India than rural India. National mortality registries also show that CHD mortality is higher amongst Indian Asians living overseas in the UK, Canada, Singapore, South Africa, Uganda, Fiji and Trinidad than in the respective indigenous populations.[2]

Indian Asians represent the largest ethnic minority group in the UK. Mortality from CHD amongst UK Indian Asians is 40% higher,[2] and admission rates with myocardial infarction (MI) twofold higher[3] than for European whites. The increase in CHD risk is evident in each of the major Asian cultural subgroups,[4] and is most

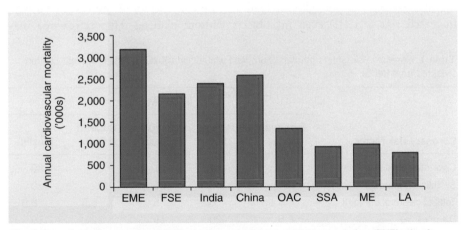

**Fig 1** Annual cardiovascular mortality in the established market economies (EME), the former socialist economies (FSE), India, China, other Asian Countries (OAC), sub-Saharan Africa (SSA), Middle East (ME) and Latin America (LA) (adapted from Ref 1).

striking in young men whose CHD mortality is at least twofold higher than Europeans.[2] There is also loss of immunity from CHD in Indian Asian women.

## ☐ RISK FACTORS UNDERLYING CORONARY HEART DISEASE IN INDIAN ASIANS

### Diabetes and insulin resistance

Population studies have consistently identified a high prevalence of non-insulin dependent diabetes mellitus (NIDDM) amongst urban and overseas Indian Asians. It is reported to be 2–5% in rural Indians, 5–10% in urban Indians and almost 20% in UK Indian Asians, compared with 4% in European white men.[5,6] Indian Asians in the UK develop diabetes, on average, 10 years earlier than Europeans, and those with diabetes show a markedly increased predisposition to CVD. In a large prospective study, cardiovascular and CHD mortality was twofold higher amongst Indian Asians with diabetes than in Europeans.[7] Furthermore, circulatory disease accounted for 77% of deaths amongst Indian Asians compared with 46% amongst Europeans.[7]

In addition to the high prevalence of diabetes, insulin resistance and its related metabolic abnormalities (central obesity, glucose intolerance, elevated plasma insulin, increased triglycerides, raised plasminogen activator inhibitor type 1 (PAI-1), and reduced high-density lipoprotein (HDL) cholesterol) are more common amongst Indian Asians than European white populations (Table 1).[5,6,8] It is estimated that diabetes and insulin resistance may account for up to 70% of major Q wave ECG abnormalities in UK Indian Asians.[9]

The mechanisms underlying the relationship between insulin resistance and CHD are not established. Hyperglycaemia, hyperinsulinaemia, dyslipidaemia, a prothrombotic state and hypertension may each make a separate contribution.[10] Elevated fasting and post-glucose load glucose concentrations are associated with increased risk of CHD even in subjects without diabetes. Hyperglycaemia may

**Table 1**. Coronary risk factors amongst European whites and UK Indian Asians in West London (adapted from Ref 5).

| | | UK Indian Asians | | | |
|---|---|---|---|---|---|
| **Coronary risk factor** | **European whites** | **Punjabi Sikh** | **Punjabi Hindu** | **Gujarati Hindu** | **Muslim** |
| Cigarette smoking (%) | 30 | 4 | 21 | 33 | 30 |
| Systolic BP (mmHg) | 121 | 128 | 126 | 122 | 120 |
| Total cholesterol (mmol/l) | 6.1 | 6.1 | 5.9 | 5.5 | 6.0 |
| Diabetes (%) | 5 | 20 | 19 | 22 | 19 |
| Waist-hip girth ratio | 0.93 | 0.98 | 0.98 | 0.98 | 0.97 |
| 2-hour insulin (mU/l) | 19 | 39 | 42 | 49 | 43 |
| Fasting triglycerides (mmol/l) | 1.48 | 1.73 | 1.74 | 1.49 | 1.85 |
| HDL cholesterol (mmol/l) | 1.24 | 1.22 | 1.17 | 1.14 | 1.04 |

BP = blood pressure; HDL = high-density lipoprotein.

contribute to accelerated atherosclerosis through glycation of collagen and lipoproteins, generation of reactive oxygen species and impaired vascular endothelial function. Hyperinsulinaemia may promote atherosclerosis through increasing blood pressure, smooth muscle cell proliferation, release of PAI-1, and inhibition of fibrinolysis. However, the beneficial effects of insulin therapy on the risk of CHD events in patients with type 2 diabetes argue against hyperinsulinaemia as the primary atherogenic defect in insulin resistant states. A reduction in insulin mediated adipocyte lipogenesis secondary to insulin resistance may be more important.[10] Insulin resistance is associated with increased levels of free fatty acids, which lead to increased hepatic very low-density lipoprotein synthesis, hyper-triglyceridaemia, a reduction in HDL cholesterol and an increase in atherogenic small dense low-density lipoprotein (LDL) cholesterol.[10] This pattern of dyslipidaemia is associated with increased entry of cholesterol into, and reduced clearance of cholesterol from, the arterial wall. Observations that CHD mortality is low in African-Caribbeans, who have a high prevalence of insulin resistance and hypertension but a favourable lipoprotein profile, suggest that the dyslipidaemia associated with insulin resistance may underlie CHD.

### Conventional risk factors

High CHD mortality is shared by Hindu, Sikh and Muslim Asians.[4] In contrast, levels of cigarette smoking, blood pressure and cholesterol are not consistently raised in all Indian Asian groups (Table 1).[5] This has led to the belief that conventional risk factors do not contribute to high CHD mortality rates in Asians,[5] but this is open to debate. As a group, serum cholesterol concentrations are similar but mean blood pressure levels are higher in UK Indian Asians than in European whites.[6,8] Furthermore, cigarette smoking is twice as common in Bangladeshis and the prevalence of hypertension is twofold higher in Sikhs[5,6] than in Europeans. It is therefore not unreasonable to propose that hypertension, hypercholesterolaemia and cigarette smoking make an important contribution to CHD mortality in UK Indian Asians.

The importance of conventional risk factors underlying increased CHD risk in urban and overseas Indian Asians is further illustrated by comparisons of risk factors between migrant and non-migrant Asians. Serum cholesterol, blood pressure, smoking rates and body mass index (BMI) are all substantially higher in urban than in rural Indians. Similar differences exist between overseas Indian Asians and their non-migrant siblings (Table 2).[11] These observations support the view that classic risk factors impact on the high CHD rates in urban and overseas Indian Asians, although the precise extent to which each contributes to increased CHD risk in Asians remains to be determined.

### Other risk factors

A key question is whether diabetes, insulin resistance and the established CHD risk factors account for the increased risk of CHD amongst Indian Asians compared with

**Table 2** Coronary risk factors amongst UK Indian Asian men in West London and their nonmigrant male siblings in India (adapted from Ref 11).

| Coronary risk factor | West London | Punjab | p |
|---|---|---|---|
| Age (years) | 46.0 ± 10.6 | 44.4 ± 9.4 | NS |
| Body mass index (kg/m$^2$) | 26.8 ± 5.2 | 22.9 ± 4.7 | <0.001 |
| Systolic BP (mmHg) | 146 ± 23 | 132 ± 22 | <0.001 |
| Diastolic BP (mmHg) | 93 ± 14 | 87 ± 12 | <0.001 |
| Total cholesterol (mmol/l) | 6.6 ± 1.4 | 4.9 ± 1.1 | <0.001 |
| HDL cholesterol (mmol/l) | 1.12 ± 0.45 | 1.21 ± 0.43 | NS |
| Triglycerides (mmol/l) | 2.10 (1.88–2.35) | 2.06 (1.78–2.38) | NS |
| Fasting glucose (mmol/l) | 5.7 ± 1.4 | 4.5 ± 1.0 | <0.001 |
| Fasting insulin (mU/l) | 8.4 (7.2–9.8) | 6.7 (5.4–8.4) | NS |

BP = blood pressure; HDL = high-density lipoprotein.

other populations. To date, no large-scale prospective study has examined CHD mortality in Indian Asians or its relationship to CHD risk factors. Much of the evidence is based upon the results of cross-sectional studies comparing risk factors between Indian Asians and other population groups. In West London, there was a 1.4-fold excess of pathological Q waves (a surrogate marker of CHD) amongst Indian Asians compared with Europeans; this became a 1.5-fold excess after adjustment for age, smoking, cholesterol, fasting and two-hour insulin, waist-hip girth ratio and glucose intolerance.[9] Similarly in Canada, Indian Asian ethnicity is associated with an excess of CHD not accounted for by conventional risk factors, diabetes, HDL cholesterol, PAI-1 or fibrinogen.[8] The results of these studies suggest that other risk factors contribute to the excess CHD mortality amongst Indian Asians.

## Inflammation

Inflammation is now widely recognised as a central feature of atherogenesis; in particular, it seems to play a critical role in destabilisation of the fibrous cap tissue, predisposing to the plaque rupture which triggers most episodes of coronary thrombosis. C-reactive protein (CRP), the classical acute-phase reactant, is an extremely sensitive systemic marker of inflammation. Increased CRP concentrations have been shown in both clinical and epidemiological studies to be associated with atherothrombotic events. In healthy subjects and patients with CHD, raised CRP is a predictor of future risk of cardiovascular events.

Recent studies indicate that CRP concentrations are higher in healthy asymptomatic Indian Asians than in European whites (Fig 2)[12] and closely associated with central obesity and markers of insulin resistance (Fig 3).[12] This is consistent with experimental studies suggesting that abdominal adipose tissue is a major source of cytokines, including interleukin-6, an important determinant of hepatic CRP synthesis. The difference in CRP concentrations between Indian Asians

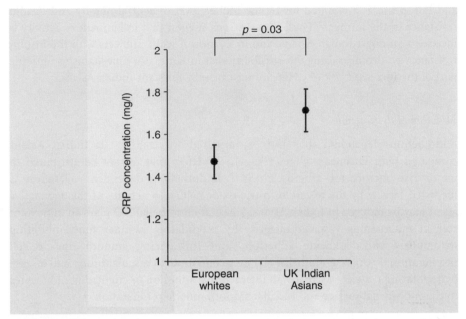

**Fig 2** C-reactive protein (CRP) concentrations in healthy European white and UK Indian Asian men (adapted from Ref 12).

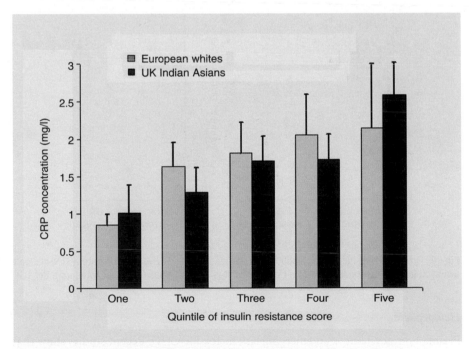

**Fig 3** Mean C-reactive protein (CRP) concentrations according to quintile of insulin resistance score (IRS) in European whites and UK Indian Asians (IRS calculated as the sum of Z-scores for systolic blood pressure, fasting glucose, waist-hip girth ratio, high-density lipoprotein cholesterol and fasting triglycerides) (adapted from Ref 12).

and Europeans is accounted for by the higher level of central obesity and insulin resistance in the former.[12] These observations suggest that inflammatory activity is increased amongst Indian Asians, and in European white subjects with the insulin resistance syndrome, raising the possibility that inflammatory mechanisms underlie part of the increased risk of CHD amongst insulin-resistant Indian Asians.

## Endothelial dysfunction

Endothelium-dependent dilatation is impaired in healthy UK Indian Asians compared with European whites (Fig 4),[13] a defect that cannot be attributed to major risk factors for atherosclerosis.[13] Endothelium-dependent dilatation is mediated largely by the release of nitric oxide (NO), so activity of this vasoactive agent may be reduced in Indian Asians. Vascular endothelial NO plays an important role in maintaining vascular integrity by modulating vascular tone, inhibiting thrombosis and leukocyte adhesion, and influencing smooth muscle cell proliferation. Reduced endothelial NO may contribute to vascular injury and disease by facilitating platelet-vascular wall interactions, adhesion of circulating monocytes to the endothelial surface and vascular smooth muscle proliferation.

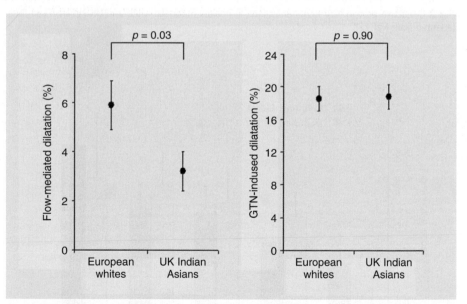

**Fig 4** Flow-mediated dilatation (endothelium dependent) and glyceryl trinitrate (GTN)-induced dilatation (endothelium independent) in European whites and UK Indian Asians (adapted from Ref 13).

## Homocysteine

Plasma homocysteine is an emerging risk factor for CHD. Recent studies show that concentrations are higher in Indian Asians than European whites (Fig 5),[6,13,14] suggesting that elevated homocysteine may contribute to their increased CHD mortality.[6] Elevated homocysteine in Indian Asians is accounted for by reduced

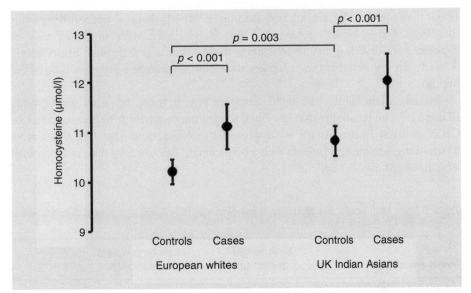

**Fig 5** Fasting plasma homocysteine concentrations in coronary heart disease (CHD) cases and controls amongst European white and UK Indian Asian men. Homocysteine concentrations are higher in UK Indian Asians than European whites; elevated homocysteine is associated with CHD in both populations (adapted from Ref 6).

concentrations of vitamin B12 and folate compared with Europeans.[6] In contrast, the methylenetetrahydrofolate reductase (MTHFR) 677C→T mutation, identified as a major determinant of homocysteine concentrations in Europeans, is less prevalent and does not influence homocysteine concentrations in Asians. It remains to be determined whether the increased CHD risk in this racial group can be reduced by dietary supplementation with homocysteine-lowering B vitamins.

*Lipoprotein(a)*

Lipoprotein(a), formed from the assembly of the protein apolipoprotein A (apoA), has been identified as an independent risk factor for vascular disease including CHD.[15] The mechanism underlying this relationship is uncertain but *in vitro* studies suggest that lipoprotein(a) may influence cholesterol uptake and inhibit fibrinolysis.[15] Serum lipoprotein(a) concentrations are influenced primarily by genetic factors, with over 30 apoA alleles identified to date. They are reported to be higher in Indian Asians than in European whites and Chinese, and may influence CHD risk in this racial group.[8,11]

*Low birth weight*

Observational studies in predominantly white populations show that persons of low birth weight have increased CHD mortality in later life.[16] This increase in risk of future CHD is most marked amongst those with intrauterine growth retardation, rather than prematurity, and greatest amongst those who become obese during adult life. Intrauterine growth retardation has been linked with increased risk of hypertension, diabetes, insulin resistance, dyslipidaemia and elevated fibrinogen.[16] It has been proposed that these changes arise from intrauterine programming of the hypothalamus.

Indian Asian babies are small compared with those of other populations (Table 3).[17] The possibility that low birth weight may contribute to increased risk of CHD amongst Indian Asians is supported by observations that CHD is almost fourfold higher amongst Indians with a birth weight below 2.5 kg than in those with a birth weight over 3.2 kg.

**Table 3** Mean birth weight and incidence of low birth weight (<2,500 g) amongst different ethnic groups in the UK (adapted from Ref 17).

| Ethnic group | Birth weight (mean) (g) | Low birth weight incidence (%) |
|---|---|---|
| Indian Asian | 3,082 ± 527 | 10.1 |
| African-Caribbean | 3,156 ± 604 | 9.4 |
| African | 3,214 ± 617 | 9.2 |
| Oriental | 3,231 ± 532 | 6.6 |
| European white | 3,377 ± 548 | 5.0 |

*Social factors*

Indian Asians are more likely to live in areas with increased social and economic deprivation. In addition, there is evidence that UK Indian Asians have different access to healthcare. Although they are more likely than Europeans to seek medical advice for symptoms suggestive of angina, regional studies suggest that Indian Asians may be less likely to be referred for exercise testing, wait longer to be seen by a cardiologist and for angiography, and be less likely to receive thrombolysis for acute MI.[18] The contribution of socio-economic deprivation and reduced provision of healthcare services to increased CHD mortality in this ethnic group needs wider investigation.

## ☐ MECHANISMS UNDERLYING DIABETES AND INSULIN RESISTANCE IN INDIAN ASIANS

Epidemiological data suggest that diabetes and insulin resistance are major determinants of the increased CHD mortality amongst UK Indian Asians. The reasons for the higher prevalence of insulin resistance in UK Indian Asians are not known. Studies in Europeans indicate that diabetes and insulin resistance may be influenced by both environmental (including reduced physical activity, increased weight and dietary intake) and genetic factors.

## Environmental factors

UK Indian Asians have higher glucose and insulin concentrations, increased prevalence of diabetes and lower HDL cholesterol than nonmigrant Asians (Table 2).[11] Environmental factors must therefore make an important contribution to insulin resistance in this group.

### Obesity

Obesity in Europeans, in particular visceral adiposity, is associated with reduced insulin sensitivity and increased risk of diabetes and CHD. Population studies show that UK Indian Asians have similar BMI to European whites.[5,6,8,19] This might suggest that adiposity does not account for insulin resistance amongst Indian Asians, but it may be misleading since Asians have greater visceral adiposity than Europeans for the same level of BMI.[5,19] The reasons are unknown. Previous studies have shown that visceral adiposity is closely associated with insulin resistance and its related metabolic disturbances, diabetes, inflammation and CHD amongst Indian Asians.[5,12,19]

### Dietary factors

Diet plays an important role in the development of insulin resistance. In North American and European white populations, a diet high in saturated fatty acids is associated with obesity, hyperglycaemia, hyperinsulinaemia[20] and an increased risk of diabetes and CHD.[20,21] In addition, trans fatty acids (TFA), primarily derived from commercial hydrogenation of polyunsaturated oils, have been associated with raised triglycerides, the ratio of total cholesterol to HDL cholesterol and increased postprandial hyperinsulinaemia, suggesting an effect of TFA on insulin sensitivity.

Diet may also have protective factors. Starchy foods producing relatively flat glycaemic responses are associated with weight loss, reduced blood pressure and lower glucose, insulin and lipid levels. Phytoestrogens such as genestein and daidzen may also confer protection from atherosclerosis through an action on the oestrogen receptor. Phytoestrogens raise HDL cholesterol and lower total cholesterol and total to HDL cholesterol ratio, and may improve insulin sensitivity.

The dietary mechanisms underlying the increased prevalence of insulin resistance and related metabolic disturbances amongst UK Indian Asians are not known. A study based upon weighed seven-day food diaries found that they have higher intakes of polyunsaturated fat and carbohydrate, and lower total and saturated fat intakes than European whites (Table 4).[22] Insulin levels were closely correlated with total and saturated fat intake only in Europeans, suggesting that dietary fat may contribute to reduced insulin sensitivity in Europeans but not Asians. These observations have led some to describe the diet of UK Indian Asians as favourable, and to propose that increased insulin resistance in Asians is largely determined by genetic factors.

However, there are important limitations in our understanding of the relationship between environmental factors and insulin resistance in UK Indian Asians. The

**Table 4.** Dietary intake amongst rural and urban Indian Asians, UK Indian Asians and European whites (adapted from Refs 22 and 23).

| Dietary intake | Indian Asians | | | European whites |
| --- | --- | --- | --- | --- |
| | Rural | Urban | UK | |
| Energy (MJ/day) | 9.2 | 8.9 | 9.5 | 10.8 |
| Fat (% energy intake) | 15 | 25 | 37 | 39 |
| Polyunsaturate/saturate ratio | 0.66 | 0.62 | 0.50 | 0.40 |
| Carbohydrates (% energy intake) | 73 | 62 | 46 | 41 |
| Protein (% energy intake) | 12 | 13 | 14 | 15 |
| Fibre (g/day) | 24 | 25 | 29 | 18 |

relationship of dietary intake with levels of HDL cholesterol, triglycerides and glucose (key components of the metabolic syndrome) or with other conventional CHD risk factors has not been investigated. Similarly, the intake of TFA, high glycaemic foods and phytoestrogens is not known in Indian Asians. Furthermore, studies based on seven-day food diaries have important limitations. Food diaries rely upon accurate knowledge of the nutritional content of individual foodstuffs. Some of this information is available from sources such as the UK Food Tables, but nutrient content is not available for many European dishes and non-existent for most Indian Asian foods.

Comparisons between Europeans and Indian Asians also do not address the changes in insulin sensitivity that have occurred with migration from India. Indeed, no study has examined the dietary changes that have occurred with migration and their possible contribution to insulin sensitivity amongst UK Indian Asians. Total fat constitutes less than 15% of energy in rural India but over 30% in the UK (Table 4),[23] suggesting that increased total or saturated fat intake may contribute to reduced insulin sensitivity in UK Indian Asians. Careful studies of the differences in dietary habits between UK and nonmigrant Indian Asians are needed to define the role of diet in determining CHD amongst the former group.

*Physical activity*

Physical inactivity is recognised as a risk factor for diabetes, obesity, CHD and cardiovascular mortality in North American and European white populations. Physical inactivity increases risk of CHD by up to twofold – comparable with the risk associated with conventional CHD risk factors such as cigarette smoking and hypertension. Increasing evidence suggests that the adverse effects of physical inactivity on CHD risk may be mediated by insulin resistance. An increase in physical activity is associated with a reduction in weight, serum insulin, hyperuricaemia, diastolic blood pressure and increased HDL cholesterol. Increased physical activity may also prevent the onset of diabetes.[24]

Few studies have examined physical activity levels amongst UK Indian Asians but the available data suggest they are lower than in both Europeans and nonmigrant Indian Asians.[19,25] A sedentary lifestyle is associated with increased obesity, fasting insulin and raised blood pressure in Indian Asians as in other populations.[25] Physical inactivity may therefore underlie a component of the increased prevalence of diabetes and insulin resistance in UK Indian Asians. However, the validity in Asians of epidemiological tools that quantify physical activity is not known, nor have exercise intervention studies been conducted in this population to examine the benefits of increased physical activity for insulin resistance and risk of CHD.

### Genetic factors

Family studies in other populations have shown that a component of insulin resistance is inherited. In Mexican Americans, insulin resistance segregates as a familial trait and evidence for linkage has been found between chromosome 6q and insulin action. This chromosomal region contains the gene for PC-1, which may be an inhibitor of insulin-receptor tyrosine kinase. In white NIDDM pedigrees, segregation analysis suggests the presence of a major autosomal locus determining 33% of the variance in fasting insulin. Support for the hypothesis that a component of insulin resistance is inherited in Indian Asians comes from the development of hyperinsulinaemia and impaired nonesterified fatty acid suppression after an oral glucose load in nondiabetic first-degree relatives of UK Indian Asian survivors of premature MI (Fig 6).[26] In recent studies, an increase in central and generalised adiposity, both closely associated with insulin sensitivity in cross-sectional studies, have been linked to the −55 C→T mutations of mitochondrial uncoupling protein 3.[27] However, the mutation is associated with obesity only in females and there is no increased prevalence of the mutation amongst Indian Asians compared with Europeans.[27] The genetic factors underlying reduced insulin sensitivity and increased CHD amongst Indian Asians remain to be determined.

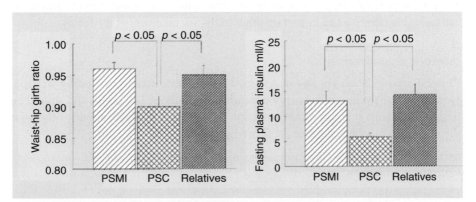

**Fig 6** Waist-hip girth ratios and fasting plasma insulin in Punjabi Sikh survivors of premature myocardial infarction (PSMI), Punjabi Sikh controls (PSC), and relatives of the PSMI patients (adapted from Ref 26).

## ☐ MANAGEMENT OF CORONARY HEART DISEASE RISK FACTORS IN UK INDIAN ASIANS

There is a multifactorial aetiology for CHD, and coronary risk factors have a multiplicative effect. Effective prevention therefore requires identification and treatment of the total burden of risk rather than of single risk factors.

### Diabetes and insulin resistance

The principal cause of death amongst patients with diabetes is CVD.[7] The prevalence of diabetes is fourfold higher in Indian Asians than Europeans[5,6] and diabetes is present in over 50% of Indian Asian CHD patients.[6] Diabetes is therefore of particular importance in this ethnic group. Recent studies amongst Europeans provide unequivocal evidence that the incidence of MI in patients with diabetes can be reduced by 21% through rigorous blood pressure control (target <130/80 mmHg) and by 16% through tight control of blood glucose (target fasting plasma glucose <6.0 mmol/l). Achieving these targets should be a priority in the management and prevention of CHD in UK Indian Asians.

Insulin resistance is the key disturbance underlying increased CHD risk in UK Indian Asians,[5,9] but a major limitation in the treatment of insulin resistance is the lack of solid evidence that improved insulin sensitivity is associated with a reduction in CHD mortality. Nevertheless, weight reduction and increased physical activity are accepted measures to improve insulin sensitivity and may prevent the onset of diabetes.[24] In the future, novel insulin sensitising agents such as thiazolidinediones may have important consequences in Indian Asians.

### *Weight loss*

Weight loss can be achieved by reducing the fat content of the diet without the need for voluntary food intake restriction. In UK Indian Asians, energy intake from fat is twice that of nonmigrants. The most important practical measure is to reduce the quantity of fat/oil used in food preparation. Most Indian Asians live in extended family units and food is generally prepared at home. Targeted education of the 'shopper and cook' can be highly effective and impact on other high-risk members of the family.

### *Increased physical activity*

Physical activity levels are low in Asians.[19,25] Moderate activity, including walking, swimming and cycling have energy expenditures of about 100 kcal/h and should be undertaken daily. It is important to maintain increased physical activity, otherwise the effects on insulin resistance are short-lived.

### Conventional risk factors

### *Cigarette smoking*

Cigarette smoking is one of the most important predictors of MI in Indian Asians. Cigarette smoking rates are higher in Bangladeshi men and similar in Hindu and

Muslim men compared with Europeans.[9] For individuals currently smoking 10 or more cigarettes per day the odds ratio for CHD is estimated at 6.7. Often, success on smoking cessation is greatest after the acute event. Smoking cessation may reduce CHD by about 25% in Indian Asian men (very few Indian Asian women smoke). Health promotion measures must ensure that smoking rates do not rise in second-generation UK Indian Asians.

*Cholesterol reduction*

Primary and secondary prevention studies show that cholesterol lowering reduces CHD risk, even amongst subjects with average cholesterol levels. 'Normal' cholesterol levels, often based on the range 4.0–6.5 mmol/l, should be redefined. Total cholesterol levels have risen by almost 2 mmol/l with migration to the UK from India,[11] and undoubtedly have a major influence on the high CHD rates in UK Indian Asians. Drug therapy to reduce cholesterol should be considered in all high-risk Indian Asians, irrespective of baseline cholesterol level. Many Indian Asians have high triglycerides, low HDL cholesterol and increased small dense LDL cholesterol.[5,6,8,9] Data from clinical and metabolic studies linking mild to moderate hypertriglyceridaemia and low HDL cholesterol to CHD is compelling and favour treatment of this atherogenic phenotype. Ideally, the lipid profile in UK Indian Asians should be similar to nonmigrants: total cholesterol not exceeding 4.5 mmol/l, LDL cholesterol 2.5 mmol/l, triglycerides 1.5 mmol/l and HDL cholesterol higher than 1.0 mmol/l. These values are acceptable because they are similar to rural populations at low risk of CHD.[11]

*Blood pressure*

Raised blood pressure is a strong predictor of CHD. Randomised trials found antihypertensive therapy effective in reducing CHD and stroke rates, while observational studies found over 40% of healthy Indian Asian men have hypertension. Active attempts should be made to detect and control hypertension in these subjects. Blood pressure levels in middle-aged UK Indian Asians, men and women, should probably not exceed the nonmigrant level of 140/85 mmHg.[11]

## ☐ IDENTIFICATION OF INDIAN ASIANS AT INCREASED CORONARY HEART DISEASE RISK

Therapeutic intervention to reduce CHD events should be directed to:

☐ patients with proven CHD

☐ first-degree relatives of patients with premature CHD

☐ asymptomatic individuals at high risk of CHD.

To identify these high-risk persons, the American College of Cardiology, the American Heart Association and the European Society of Cardiology have recommended adoption of the Framingham CHD risk assessment equations.[28] These equations predict CHD risk accurately amongst predominantly white populations in North America and Europe.[29] However, the validity of extrapolating risk functions to populations other than those from which they were derived remains is uncertain.

We have recently evaluated the validity of the Framingham functions amongst UK Indian Asians.[30] The predicted CHD mortality rate in a representative sample was the same as for Europeans, whereas the observed CHD mortality rates were almost twofold higher. The Framingham functions therefore underestimate the risk of CHD amongst Indian Asians by approximately 50% (Fig 7).[30] This may reflect their failure to take account of insulin resistance and related disturbances. A logical solution to this problem might be to lower the threshold for treatment in UK Indian Asians, although this approach has not been validated.

Identification of Indian Asians at increased CHD risk presents a major obstacle for the clinician. Most studies support the view that insulin resistance is the key disturbance underlying their increased CHD risk. The absence of a simple, reproducible marker of insulin resistance presents a further problem to the clinician. In practice, the combination of raised fasting triglycerides (>1.5 mmol/l), low HDL cholesterol (<1.0 mmol/l), raised fasting glucose (>6.0 mmol/l), central obesity (waist-hip girth ratio >1.0 in men, >0.85 in women) and hypertension reliably identifies insulin-resistant subjects who are likely to benefit most from risk factor modification.

## ☐ CONCLUSIONS AND FUTURE DIRECTIONS

Future work is necessary to identify the precise environmental and genetic mechanisms underlying insulin resistance and increased CHD risk in UK Indian

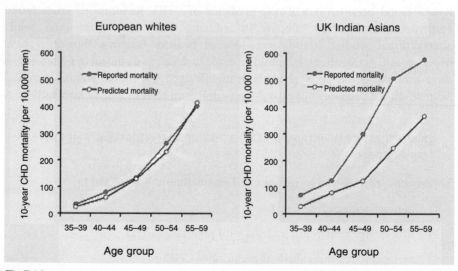

**Fig 7** 10-year coronary heart disease (CHD) mortality rates predicted by the Framingham functions in a representative sample of Indian Asian and European white men living in West London, compared with CHD mortality in West London reported by the Office for National Statistics (adapted from Ref 30).

Asians. Identification of dietary factors, nutrient-gene interactions, underlying insulin resistance and increased risk of CHD amongst Indian Asians will enable formulation of novel strategies for dietary intervention.

Investigation of the heritability of metabolic disturbances within large, extended Indian Asian families may provide important insights into genetic factors determining CHD risk. Key insights into metabolic pathways involved and disease pathogenesis should be provided by large-scale association studies, and ultimately whole genome association studies to discover patterns of genetic variation leading to insulin resistance and atherosclerotic CVD in Indian Asians. The identification of disease-associated genes will have broad implications for management of these disorders in all racial groups.

The failure of the Framingham risk functions to predict increased CHD risk in UK Indian Asians demonstrates the need for prospective population studies in this ethnic group to enable the development of strategies and risk prediction models that identify those at increased CHD risk.

Finally, novel treatment strategies are needed for subjects with insulin resistance, and controlled clinical trials required to assess the effectiveness of treatment specifically in this racial group.

## REFERENCES

1    Reddy KS, Yusuf S. Emerging epidemic of cardiovascular disease in developing countries. Review. *Circulation* 1998;**97**:596–601.

2    Balarajan R. Ethnicity and variations in mortality from coronary heart disease. *Health Trends* 1996;**28**:45–51.

3    Wilkinson P, Sayer J, Laji K, Grundy C et al. Comparison of case fatality in south Asian and white patients after acute myocardial infarction: observational study. *BMJ* 1996;**312**:1330–3.

4    Balarajan R, Bulusu L, Adelstein AM, Shukla V. Patterns of mortality among migrants to England and Wales from the Indian subcontinent. *BMJ (Clin Res Ed)* 1984;**289**:1185–7.

5    McKeigue PM, Shah B, Marmot MG. Relation of central obesity and insulin resistance with high diabetes prevalence and cardiovascular risk in South Asians. *Lancet* 1991;**337**:382–6.

6    Chambers JC, Obeid OA, Refsum H, Ueland P et al. Plasma homocysteine concentrations and risk of coronary heart disease in UK Indian Asian and European men. *Lancet* 2000;**355**:523–7.

7    Mather HM, Chaturvedi N, Fuller JH. Mortality and morbidity from diabetes in South Asians and Europeans: 11-year follow-up of the Southall Diabetes Survey, London, UK. *Diabet Med* 1998;**15**:53–9.

8    Anand SS, Yusuf S, Vuksan V, Devanesen S et al. Differences in risk factors, atherosclerosis, and cardiovascular disease between ethnic groups in Canada: the Study of Health Assessment and Risk in Ethnic groups (SHARE). *Lancet* 2000;**356**:279–84.

9    McKeigue PM, Ferrie JE, Pierpoint T, Marmot MG. Association of early-onset coronary heart disease in South Asian men with glucose intolerance and hyperinsulinemia. *Circulation* 1993;**87**:152–61.

10   Ginsberg HN. Insulin resistance and cardiovascular disease. Review. *J Clin Invest* 2000;**106**:453–8.

11   Bhatnagar D, Anand IS, Durrington PN, Patel DJ et al. Coronary risk factors in people from the Indian subcontinent living in west London and their siblings in India. *Lancet* 1995;**345**:405–9.

12   Chambers JC, Eda S, Bassett P, Karim Y et al. C-reactive protein, insulin resistance, central obesity, and coronary heart disease risk in Indian Asians from the United Kingdom compared with European whites. *Circulation* 2001;**104**:145–50.

13  Chambers JC, McGregor A, Jean-Marie J, Kooner JS. Abnormalities of vascular endothelial function may contribute to increased coronary heart disease risk in UK Indian Asians. *Heart* 1999;81:501–4.

14  Chambers JC, Kooner JS. Homocysteine: a novel risk factor for coronary heart disease in UK Indian Asians. *Heart* 2001;86:121–2.

15  Scanu AM. The role of lipoprotein(a) in the pathogenesis of atherosclerotic cardiovascular disease and its utility as predictor of coronary heart disease events. Review. *Curr Cardiol Rep* 2001;3:385–90.

16  Godfrey KM, Barker DJ. Fetal nutrition and adult disease. Review. *Am J Clin Nutr* 2000;71(5 Suppl):1344S–52S.

17  Steer P, Alam MA, Wadsworth J, Welch A. Relation between maternal haemoglobin concentration and birth weight in different ethnic groups. *BMJ* 1995;310:489–91.

18  Shaukat N, de Bono DP, Cruickshank JK. Clinical features, risk factors, and referral delay in British patients of Indian and European origin with angina matched for age and extent of coronary atheroma. *BMJ* 1993;307:717–8.

19  McKeigue PM, Pierpoint T, Ferrie JE, Marmot MG. Relationship of glucose intolerance and hyperinsulinaemia to body fat pattern in south Asians and Europeans. *Diabetologia* 1992;35:785–91.

20  Ascherio A, Rimm EB, Giovannucci EL, Spiegelman D *et al.* Dietary fat and risk of coronary heart disease in men: cohort follow up study in the United States. *BMJ* 1996;313:84–90.

21  Kushi LH, Lew RA, Stare FJ, Ellison CR *et al.* Diet and 20-year mortality from coronary heart disease. The Ireland-Boston Diet-Heart Study. *N Engl J Med* 1985;312:811–8.

22  Sevak L, McKeigue PM, Marmot MG. Relationship of hyperinsulinemia to dietary intake in south Asian and European men. *Am J Clin Nutr* 1994;59:1069–74.

23  Singh RB, Ghosh S, Niaz AM, Gupta S *et al.* Epidemiologic study of diet and coronary risk factors in relation to central obesity and insulin levels in rural and urban populations of North India. *Int J Cardiol* 1995;47:245–55.

24  Tuomilehto J, Lindstrom J, Eriksson JG, Valle TT *et al.* Prevention of type 2 diabetes mellitus by changes in lifestyle among subjects with impaired glucose tolerance. *N Engl J Med* 2001;344:1343–50.

25  Dhawan J, Bray CL. Asian Indians, coronary artery disease, and physical exercise. *Heart* 1997;78:550–4.

26  Kooner JS, Baliga RR, Wilding J, Crook D *et al.* Abdominal obesity, impaired nonesterified fatty acid suppression, and insulin-mediated glucose disposal are early metabolic abnormalities in families with premature myocardial infarction. *Arterioscler Thromb Vasc Biol* 1998;18:1021–6.

27  Cassell PG, Saker PJ, Huxtable SJ, Kousta E *et al.* Evidence that single nucleotide polymorphism in the uncoupling protein 3 (UCP3) gene influences fat distribution in women of European and Asian origin. *Diabetologia* 2000;43:1558–64.

28  Grundy SM, Pasternak R, Greenland P, Smith S Jr, Fuster V. Assessment of cardiovascular risk by use of multiple-risk-factor assessment equations: a statement for healthcare professionals from the American Heart Association and the American College of Cardiology. Review. *Circulation* 1999;100:1481–92.

29  Leaverton PE, Sorlie PD, Kleinman JC, Dannenberg AL *et al.* Representativeness of the Framingham risk model for coronary heart disease mortality: a comparison with a national cohort study. *J Chronic Dis* 1987;40:775–84.

30  Chambers JC, Wrigley J, Kooner JS. Evaluation of the Joint British Societies coronary heart disease risk calculator in UK Indian Asians. *Heart* 2000;83(Suppl):43A.

# Lifestyle interventions in the prevention of coronary heart disease

Gareth Beevers

## ☐ INTRODUCTION

The striking differences in the prevalence of coronary heart disease (CHD) in international and even intranational comparisons must primarily be due to differences in lifestyle and diet. Most of the differences within genetically similar populations can be explained by the three main cardiovascular risk factors:

- ☐ cigarette smoking

- ☐ plasma lipids, and

- ☐ blood pressure.

A fourth factor, type 2 diabetes, is becoming increasingly important with the rising prevalence of obesity.

The relationship of lifestyle to cardiovascular risk and CHD is well recognised, but the value of lifestyle interventions in reversing these risk factors remains controversial. Many clinicians have become disheartened by the relatively poor impact of attempts to alter cardiovascular risk factors in their patients by means of lifestyle interventions. Thus, whilst a diet low in animal fats should be effective at reducing hyperlipidaemia, trial evidence suggests there is only a small effect. Similarly, attempts to reduce blood pressure by salt restriction or weight reduction have also proved disappointing. This has led to an increasing reliance on drugs that lower lipids and blood pressure to correct the adverse effects of an unhealthy lifestyle.

## ☐ SMOKING CESSATION

There is a close relationship between cigarette smoking and both CHD and stroke. The results of smoking cessation treatments in the primary prevention of CHD have been slightly disappointing, although smoking cessation advice is unsurprisingly more effective for secondary prevention. The prevalence of cigarette smoking has steadily declined in many countries over the last 30 years for many reasons, a change that must in part explain the observed reduction of both CHD and stroke during this time.

The reduction in cigarette smoking is partly the result of public health initiatives and an increasing view that cigarette smoking in public places is unacceptable. There is an almost universal climate of opinion that smoking is dangerous and many people who smoke would sincerely like to stop. The problem is that cigarette smoking has been found to be more addictive than originally thought, and many individuals find it difficult to give up the habit.

## ☐ LIPID LOWERING BY DIETARY MEANS

### Total cholesterol

The effect on plasma total cholesterol levels of alterations of dietary intake of dairy products has been disappointing. For example, a study in the blood pressure clinic at the City Hospital, Birmingham, found no differences between serum total cholesterol levels in patients who claimed to be restricting dairy products compared with those making no restrictions. Similarly, a meta-analysis of several trials of restriction of animal fat intake showed only about a 5% reduction in serum total cholesterol levels from various manoeuvres.[1] At a personal level, this must be regarded as trivial: for example, patients with a serum total cholesterol of 8.0 mmol/l will have a fall of only 0.4 mmol/l to 7.6 mmol/l, which is within the coefficient of replicate variation of serum cholesterol assays. By contrast, on a community based level, a reduction of 5% in the mean serum cholesterol of the whole population would, in theory, bring about a 15% reduction in CHD. This difference between the personal and public health benefits of dietary manoeuvres illustrates the point made by the late Geoffrey Rose that 'a preventive measure which brings much benefit to the population offers little to each individual'.[2]

### Blood pressure

The effects on blood pressure of a reduction of dairy produce intake initially produced inconclusive results in short-term studies. However (as described below), the recent Dietary Approaches to Stop Hypertension (DASH) study showed a significant effect, together with an additive effect of an increased intake of fruit and vegetables and reduced intake of salt.

The disappointing effects of lipid-lowering diets in individual patients is one of the reasons why there has been a widespread reliance on the 3-hydroxy-3-methylglutaryl coenzyme A reductase inhibitors (the statins). These drugs are effective in both primary and secondary prevention of CHD and many studies also showed an unexpected reduction in strokes.

## ☐ LIFESTYLE INTERVENTION AND BLOOD PRESSURE

The topic of blood pressure and lifestyle changes has been well researched and much of the evidence is not controversial. There is, however, a shortage of long-term outcome trials in which the effects of dietary manoeuvres are examined in relation to the hard cardiovascular end-points of CHD and stroke rather than just changes in blood pressure.

## Weight reduction

Epidemiological studies show a close relationship between body mass index (BMI) and blood pressure, and that people who gain weight sustain a rise in blood pressure while those who reduce weight note a fall.[3]

In clinical practice, weight reduction is difficult to achieve in hypertensive patients. There is evidence that referral to a dietitian achieves better weight reduction than clinicians simply giving advice with or without accompanying leaflets.[4]

A weight loss of 1 kg in hypertensive patients would reduce mean arterial pressure by about 1 mmHg – a disappointing result as a 1 mmHg alteration in blood pressure is well within spontaneous variation. It is true, though, that a 10 kg reduction in weight in obese patients with mild hypertension might well normalise blood pressure. In a patient initially weighing 100 kg, the expected results of a 10 kg reduction in body weight are shown in Table 1.

However, these are theoretical considerations and there has been limited research into the benefits of weight restriction. It remains to be seen whether the recently available weight reducing drugs will achieve the results that might be expected from the theoretical considerations.

**Table 1** Expected results of a 10 kg weight reduction in an individual weighing 100 kg.

|  | **Effect** |
| --- | --- |
| Development of diabetes | 60% lower risk |
| Fasting blood glucose | 30–60% fall |
| Glycosylated haemoglobin | 15% fall |
| Diabetes-related deaths | 30–40% fall |
| Serum cholesterol | 10% reduction |
| LDL cholesterol | 15% reduction |
| Plasma triglycerides | 30% reduction |
| HDL cholesterol | 8% rise |

HDL = high-density lipoprotein; LDL = low-density lipoprotein

## Exercise

There is a close relationship between physical exercise and CHD as well as blood pressure. These effects remain after adjustment for confounding variables including BMI. Short-term studies of a physical exercise programme demonstrated that there can be a 10% fall in mean arterial pressure, associated with a 25% fall in total peripheral resistance and a 20% rise in cardiac index.[5] It is generally held that the amount of physical exercise necessary is that which would induce a tachycardia with perspiration. Thus, occasional light exercise is not sufficient.

## Salt and hypertension

### Hypertensive patients

The topic of salt and hypertension remains controversial. Many clinicians have entrenched views, although the early international epidemiological comparisons were not conducted with sufficient rigour to satisfy present-day observers.

In the International Study of Salt and Blood Pressure (INTERSALT) project, an international collaborative study in 52 populations in 32 countries, clinical data collection and blood pressure measurement were carefully standardised. The salt intake was estimated on the basis of a single 24-hour urine collection, and all urine sodium assays were conducted in one laboratory. There was a significant positive relationship between blood pressure and salt intake in 15 of the populations, but only a weak relationship when all 52 populations were compared.[6] The relationship became nonsignificant when four primitive or tribal populations were removed from the study. By contrast, INTERSALT showed a close relationship between salt intake and the gradient of the blood pressure rise with advancing age.

Given the evidence that salt is a factor in the development of hypertension, the question arises as to whether salt restriction lowers blood pressure. Many short-term studies (some extremely short) have been conducted, but some of them examined extreme salt restriction to a level which is not feasible in clinical practice. These short-term, extreme salt restriction studies cannot give a true picture of the value of salt restriction in managing hypertensive patients. A meta-analysis of longer-term moderate salt restriction studies, however, shows that a reduction of salt intake in hypertensive patients by 78 mmol per day (4.6 g salt) results in about 5.0 mmHg and 2.7 mmHg falls in systolic and diastolic blood pressure, respectively.[7] This effect is slightly smaller than is achieved with monotherapy with antihypertensive drugs, but there is evidence of an additive effect of salt restriction in hypertensive patients when used in conjunction with drugs which block the renin-angiotensin-aldosterone system.

There is almost universal agreement that hypertensive patients should be advised to restrict their salt intake, mainly by avoiding notoriously salty foods (particularly processed foods).

*Normotensive subjects*

The value of salt restriction in normotensives is more difficult to assess. In epidemiological terms, it would be desirable to reduce the average blood pressure of the whole population, not just those with raised levels. Several trials of salt restriction in normotensives have been conducted. At first sight, the effects do not seem impressive: about 2.0 mmHg and 1.0 mmHg falls in systolic and diastolic blood pressure, respectively.[7] Again, this must seem trivial to the clinician and within the range of observer error and replicate variation. Nevertheless, in epidemiological terms, a real fall in population average systolic blood pressure by 2 mmHg would be expected to bring about a 9% fall in CHD. This again illustrates Geoffrey Rose's point about the relative effects of public health manoeuvres on populations compared with the effects on individuals.[2]

**Potassium intake**

Epidemiological studies show an inverse relationship between potassium intake and blood pressure and also the risk of stroke. A great many intervention trials have demonstrated that increasing potassium intake, given as potassium chloride tablets, brings about a significant fall in blood pressure.[8] These studies are of scientific rather than clinical interest, as it is not generally recommended that patients should take potassium chloride for the treatment of hypertension. The best way to achieve a rise in potassium intake is to increase the intake of fruit and vegetables. The beneficial effects of an increased potassium intake are usually seen pari passu with a reduction in sodium chloride intake, and there is some evidence that these two manoeuvres have an additive effect.

### The DASH and DASH-sodium studies

All the changes in dietary and lifestyle factors discussed above have been studied in isolation. In general, good effects have been seen, although the magnitude of some has been disappointing. In order to investigate the effects of these approaches in combination, a major American study (DASH) has examined the blood pressure lowering effects of:

- ☐ a diet with decreased content of dairy produce

- ☐ a diet with increased fruit and vegetable content, and

- ☐ these two diets in combination.

The first two manoeuvres had an independent effect on blood pressure, with an added effect when applied together.[9]

The DASH study was extended to investigate the effects of adding salt restriction to the other dietary changes. A small, but significant effect of salt restriction was shown in both normotensive and hypertensive individuals, with or without an increase in fruit and vegetable intake or a reduction of dairy produce. Although the DASH study is reliable, it was not long-term. Long-term dietary intervention studies with hard cardiovascular end-points are sadly lacking.

### Alcohol restriction

Many studies show a close correlation between alcohol intake and blood pressure, and some research suggests a relationship between high alcohol intake and stroke morbidity. The relationship between alcohol intake and CHD is more complex as there may be a partly preventive effect mediated by the beneficial effects of alcohol on HDL cholesterol.

The limited number of studies of alteration of alcohol intake and its effects on blood pressure have shown that moderation or cessation of alcohol intake is associated with a significant fall in both systolic and diastolic blood pressure.[10] Other studies suggest that moderation of alcohol intake can reduce the need for antihypertensive medication in certain circumstances.

Moderation of alcohol intake must be seen as one of the package of lifestyle manoeuvres which have beneficial effects on both public health and patient care. There is almost universal agreement that the average lifestyle in developed countries is not healthy, with excessive smoking, alcohol intake and animal fat and salt, coupled with insufficient intake of fruit and vegetables. Whether these adverse effects can be reversed on a national basis is open to speculation, particularly in the context of an ever rising prevalence of obesity.

## □ CONCLUSIONS

At an epidemiological level, there is no doubt that CHD, strokes, plasma lipid levels and blood pressure are all closely related to diet and other lifestyle factors. There is, however, some doubt about the reversibility of these parameters in response to changes in lifestyle, and there have been disappointing results clinically. It is likely that simple advice on change of lifestyle is not sufficient in clinical practice, and that more active measures are necessary to aid patients in altering their diet. At a public health level, a reduction of salt intake, BMI and animal fat intake should be beneficial, but the effects are relatively small in clinical terms even though they may be important if applied across the board. Thus, many clinicians are impatient with what they see as trivial changes clinically, whereas epidemiologists tend to be optimistic that small changes in population averages can have profound effects on public health. There is a shortage of long-term outcome studies of the effects of lifestyle intervention on CHD, stroke and the risk factors for these two diseases.

The natural experiment of watching the migration (usually urbanisation) of populations, with the concomitant adverse alterations in cardiovascular risk factors, supports a role for changes in lifestyle in the aetiology of vascular diseases. However, all too few studies have demonstrated a reverse effect, with an improvement in population lifestyle leading to an improvement in vascular disease or its risk factors.

The universal adoption of healthy diets will, in theory, prove advantageous at a personal and clinical level, but can be achieved only if central governments do more to persuade, first, the food industry to alter the quality of processed and convenience foods to contain less fat and salt and, secondly, the public to eat more fruit and vegetables.

## REFERENCES

1   Tang JT, Armitage JM, Lancaster T, Silagy CA *et al.* Systematic review of dietary intervention trials to lower total blood cholesterol in free-living subjects. *BMJ* 1998;**316**:1213–20.

2   Rose GA. Strategy for prevention: lessons from cardiovascular disease. *BMJ* 1981;**282**:1847–51.

3   Reisin E, Frohlich ED, Messerli FH, Dreslinski GR *et al.* Cardiovascular changes after weight reduction in obesity hypertension. *Ann Intern Med* 1983;**98**:315–9.

4   Ramsay LE, Ramsay MH, Hettiarachchi J, Davies DL, Winchester J. Weight reduction in a blood pressure clinic. *BMJ* 1978;**2**:244–5.

5   Nelson L, Jennings GL, Esler MD, Kormer PI. Effect of changing levels of physical activity on blood pressure and haemodynamics in essential hypertension. *Lancet* 1986;**ii**:473–6.

6   Intersalt: an international study of electrolyte excretion and blood pressure. Results for 24 hour urinary sodium and potassium excretion. Intersalt Cooperative Research Group. *BMJ* 1988;**297**:319–28.

7   He FJ, MacGregor GA. Effect of modest salt reduction on blood pressure: a meta-analysis of randomized trials. Implications for public health. *J Hum Hypertens* 2002;**16**:761–70.

8    He FJ, MacGregor GA. Beneficial effects of potassium. Review. *BMJ* 2001;**323**:497–501.

9    Sacks FM, Svetkey LP, Vollmes WM, Appel LJ *et al.* Effects on blood pressure of reduced dietary sodium and the Dietary Approaches to Stop Hypertension (DASH) diet. DASH-Sodium Collaborative Research Group. *N Engl J Med* 2001;**344**:3–10.

10   Potter JF, Beevers DG. Pressor effect of alcohol in hypertension. *Lancet* 1984;i:119–22.

# ☐ PREVENTION OF CORONARY ARTERY DISEASE SELF ASSESSMENT QUESTIONS

## Therapeutic intervention to prevent coronary heart disease and stroke

1  Aspirin:
   (a) Should be routinely recommended for all men over 55 years to reduce risk of cardiovascular disease (CVD)
   (b) Should be given to all hypertensives at risk of CVD
   (c) Should be given only to high cardiovascular risk patients with normal blood pressure (BP)
   (d) At low doses does not cause gastrointestinal bleeding
   (e) Can precipitate asthma

2  Antihypertensive drugs:
   (a) Newer agents (angiotensin-converting enzyme inhibitors and calcium-channel blockers) are significantly better than older drugs (diuretics and beta-blockers) at preventing coronary heart disease events
   (b) Are usually required in combination to achieve target BP (<140/90 mmHg)
   (c) In borderline hypertension should be prescribed on the basis of an estimated global cardiovascular risk of 20% over 10 years
   (d) Older drugs may increase the likelihood of development of diabetes
   (e) Are no more effective when combined with lifestyle advice (diet, exercise, etc)

3  Lipid-lowering therapy:
   (a) Does not prevent strokes
   (b) Should be considered for middle-aged men at increased risk of CVD based on global risk scores and not simply on cholesterol level
   (c) Does not benefit the elderly (over 65 years)
   (d) In conjunction with antioxidants provides greater benefit than when used alone
   (e) Has been shown in clinical trials to benefit a much greater number of people than currently recommended for its use

## Lifestyle interventions in the prevention of coronary heart disease

1  Salt restriction:
   (a) Does not lower BP in normotensive subjects
   (b) Down to about 5 g per day reduces BP in hypertensives by as much as a single hypertensive drug
   (c) Has an additive effect on BP when used with other dietary manoeuvres
   (d) In the short term, BP reduction is blunted because of the neurohumoral additive effect of the renin and sympathetic systems
   (e) To below 3 g per day is easy to achieve

2    Restriction of dairy products:
   (a)  Does not affect plasma cholesterol levels
   (b)  Does not lower BP
   (c)  Is as effective as prescribing a statin
   (d)  Is part of a package of nondrug manoeuvres which improve coronary risk factors
   (e)  Requires restriction of red meat consumption

3    Weight reduction:
   (a)  Lowers the risk of type 2 diabetes
   (b)  Of 10 kg lowers mean arterial pressure by 5 mmHg
   (c)  Requires more than just giving advice in the clinic
   (d)  Lowers serum total cholesterol
   (e)  Does not reduce triglycerides

# Croonian Lecture

# Coronary heart disease and type 2 diabetes: disorders of growth

David Barker

## ☐ INTRODUCTION

It is a paradox that, although rates of coronary heart disease (CHD) rise in populations as they become more affluent, in Britain[1] and elsewhere in Europe the highest rates occur among poorer people in the least affluent areas. It has been known for twenty years that this paradox cannot be explained by the lifestyles of people in lower socio-economic groups, though these may contribute.

Another possibility is that less affluent people are more vulnerable to the adverse effects of westernisation. If so, when might such vulnerability be acquired? Much of the structure of the body, and the setting of its physiological and metabolic systems, is complete at birth. Only a few organs such as the brain and liver continue to be plastic. Intrauterine life is therefore an obvious time during which vulnerability might develop. Early evidence to support this came from detailed studies of the distribution of deaths among newborn babies in England and Wales. In the early years of the last century neonatal death rates were considerably higher in the less affluent places – the northern industrial towns and poor rural areas in the north and west. Most of these deaths were attributable to low birthweight. Remarkably, across the country neonatal death rates in those days mapped closely to death rates from CHD 60–70 years later.[2]

To explore this geographical link between low birthweight and CHD required studies of a kind not hitherto carried out. It was necessary to identify groups of men and women now in middle to late life whose size at birth had been recorded. Their birthweight could thereby be related to the later occurrence of CHD. In Hertfordshire from 1911 onwards women in childbirth were attended by a midwife who recorded the baby's birthweight. A health visitor, who went to the baby's home at intervals throughout infancy, recorded the weight at one year. Table 1 shows the findings in the first group of people to be traced, 5,654 men born between 1911 and 1930. Standardised mortality ratios for CHD fell with increasing birthweight.[3] There were stronger trends with weight at one year. A subsequent study confirmed a similar trend with birthweight among women. In the 370 men who had glucose tolerance tests, the percentage with impaired glucose tolerance or type 2 diabetes fell steeply with increasing birthweight and weight at one year (Table 2).

The association between low birthweight and CHD has now been replicated among men and women in Europe, North America and India,[4] and that between low weight gain in infancy and CHD in men has been confirmed in Helsinki. Low birthweight has been shown to predict altered glucose tolerance in studies around the world.

**Table 1** Standardised mortality ratios for coronary heart disease according to birthweight and weight at one year in 5,654 men in Hertfordshire.

| | Birthweight (lb) | Coronary heart disease | |
| | | No. of men | SMR |
|---|---|---|---|
| Birthweight | ≤5.5 | 251 | 104 |
| | 5.6–6.5 | 752 | 77 |
| | 6.6–7.5 | 1,598 | 90 |
| | 7.6–8.5 | 1,757 | 85 |
| | 8.6–9.5 | 868 | 62 |
| | ≥10 | 428 | 81 |
| *Total* | | 5,654 | |
| One year | ≤18 | 324 | 111 |
| | 19–20 | 71 | 81 |
| | 21–22 | 1,850 | 98 |
| | 23–24 | 1,464 | 71 |
| | 25–26 | 769 | 68 |
| | ≥27 | 276 | 42 |
| *Total** | | 4,754 | 82 |

* One-year-old weights were unavailable for 900 of the men.
SMR = standardised mortality ratio.

**Table 2** Percentage of men aged 64 in the Hertfordshire cohort with impaired glucose tolerance or diabetes, according to birthweight (n = 370).

| Birthweight (lb) | No. of men | % with 2-hour glucose ≥7.8 mmol/l | Odds ratio | (95% CI) |
|---|---|---|---|---|
| ≤5.5 | 20 | 40 | 6.6 | 1.5–28 |
| 5.6–6.5 | 47 | 34 | 4.8 | 1.3–17 |
| 6.6–7.5 | 104 | 31 | 4.6 | 1.4–16 |
| 7.6–8.5 | 117 | 22 | 2.6 | 0.8–8.9 |
| 8.6–9.5 | 54 | 13 | 1.4 | 0.3–5.6 |
| >9.5 | 28 | 14 | 1.0 | – |
| *Total* | 370 | 25 | | |

*Odds ratio for 2-hour glucose concentration ≥7.8 mmol/l adjusted for body mass index ($\chi^2$ for trend = 15.4; $p <0.001$).
CI = confidence interval.

## ☐ BIOLOGICAL BASIS

### Developmental plasticity

Since McCance and Widdowson's pioneering observations in Cambridge,[5] experimentalists have repeatedly demonstrated that minor alterations to the diets of pregnant animals can produce lasting changes in their offspring's physiology and metabolism. This is not surprising because so-called 'developmental plasticity'

enables one genotype to give rise to a range of different physiological or morphological states in response to different environmental conditions during development.
Such gene-environment interactions are ubiquitous in development and can be
considered a universal quality of life. The benefit of developmental plasticity is that,
in a changing environment, it enables the production of phenotypes better matched
to their environment than would be possible by the production of the same
phenotype in all environments.

## Gene-environment interactions

Evidence of gene-environment interactions in the genesis of type 2 diabetes is
beginning to appear. The effects of a polymorphism of the peroxisome
proliferator-activated receptor-γ2 gene depend on birthweight, which serves as a
marker for intrauterine nutrition.[6] It has been suggested that the Pro12Ala
polymorphism of the gene increases tissue sensitivity to insulin and thereby protects
against type 2 diabetes. Table 3 is based on a study of 476 elderly people in Helsinki.
The Pro12Ala polymorphism influenced fasting plasma insulin concentrations only
in those men and women who had low birthweight. It has repeatedly been shown
that low birthweight is associated with raised plasma insulin concentrations,
indicating insulin resistance, but this was confined to people with the Pro12Pro
polymorphism. The Pro12Ala polymorphism protects against the effect.

**Table 3** Mean fasting insulin concentrations in 476 elderly people in Helsinki according to
peroxisome proliferator-activated receptor-γ gene polymorphism and birthweight.

| Polymorphism | Birthweight (g) | | | p for difference |
|---|---|---|---|---|
| | ≤3,000 | 3,000–3,500 | >3,500 | |
| Pro12Pro (n) | 84 (56) | 71 (161) | 65 (107) | 0.003 |
| Pro12Ala/Ala12Ala (n) | 60 (37) | 60 (67) | 65 (48) | 0.31 |
| p for difference | 0.008 | 0.02 | 0.99 | |

Figures in parentheses are number of subjects.

## Nutrients and fetal growth

The different size of newborn human babies exemplifies plasticity. The growth of
babies is constrained by the size of the mother, otherwise normal birth could not
occur. Small women have small babies; in pregnancies occurring after ovum
donation, the babies are small even if the woman donating the egg is large. Babies
may be small because their growth is constrained in this way or because they lack the
nutrients for growth. As McCance wrote long ago:

> The size attained *in utero* depends on the services which the mother is able to supply.
> These are mainly food and accommodation.[7]

Since mother's height or pelvic dimensions are generally not found to be important predictors of the baby's long-term health, research into the fetal origins of disease has focused on the nutrient supply to the baby.[6] The central concept is that, despite current levels of nutrition in Western countries, the nutrition of many fetuses and infants remains suboptimal, either because the nutrients available are unbalanced or because their delivery is constrained by the long and vulnerable fetal supply line.

## □ FETAL ORIGINS HYPOTHESIS

The fetal origins hypothesis proposes that CHD, type 2 diabetes and hypertension originate in developmental plasticity in response to undernutrition during fetal life and infancy.

**Life history theory**

Why should fetal responses to undernutrition lead to disease in later life? 'Life history theory', which embraces all living things, states that increased allocation of energy to one trait such as brain development or rapid growth of the body necessarily reduces allocation to one or more other traits. Smaller babies, who have had a lesser allocation of energy, must incur higher costs which include disease. More specifically, people small at birth have fewer cells in key organs such as the kidney. Brenner and Chertow[8] have proposed that hypertension is initiated by the reduced number of nephrons found in people who were small at birth. A reduced number of nephrons leads to increased blood flow in the remaining glomeruli. This is thought to lead to the development of glomerulosclerosis. Combined with the loss of nephrons that accompanies normal ageing, this leads to further loss of nephrons and a self-perpetuating cycle of rising blood pressure and nephron loss.

*Hormones and metabolism*

Another process by which slow fetal growth may be linked to later disease is in the setting of hormones and metabolism. An undernourished baby may establish a 'thrifty' way of handling food. Insulin resistance, which is associated with low birthweight, may be viewed as persistence of a fetal response by which blood glucose concentrations are maintained for the benefit of the brain at the expense of glucose transport into the muscles.[9]

*Vulnerability to environmental stresses*

A third link between low birthweight and later disease may be that people small at birth are more vulnerable to adverse environmental influences in later life. Observations on animals show that the environment during development permanently changes not only the body's structure and function but also its responses to environmental influences encountered in later life. The effect of low income in adult life on CHD among men in Helsinki is shown in Table 4. As

**Table 4** Hazard ratios (95% confidence intervals) for coronary heart disease in men in Helsinki according to ponderal index at birth (kg/m³) and taxable income in adult life.

| Annual household income (£ sterling) | Ponderal index | |
|---|---|---|
| | ≤26.0 (n=1,475) | >26.0 (n=2,154) |
| >15,700 | 1.00 | 1.19 (0.65–2.19) |
| 15,700 | 1.54 (0.83–2.87) | 1.42 (0.78–2.57) |
| 12,400 | 1.07 (0.51–2.22) | 1.66 (0.90–3.07) |
| 10,700 | 2.07 (1.13–3.79) | 1.44 (0.79–2.62) |
| ≤8,400 | 2.58 (1.45–4.60) | 1.37 (0.75–2.51) |
| p for trend | <0.001 | 0.75 |

expected, men with a low taxable income have higher rates of the disease. This is a major component of the social inequalities in health in western countries for which there is no agreed explanation. The effect of low income, however, is confined to men who had slow fetal growth and were thin at birth, defined by a ponderal index (birthweight/length³) of less than 26 kg/m³. Men who were not thin at birth were resilient to the effects of low income on CHD.

One explanation of these findings emphasises the psychosocial consequences of a low position in the social hierarchy, as indicated by low income and social class, and suggests that perceptions of low social status and lack of success lead to changes in neuroendocrine pathways and hence to disease. The findings in Helsinki seem consistent with this. People who are small at birth are known to have persisting alterations in responses to stress, including raised serum cortisol concentrations. It is suggested that persisting small elevations of serum cortisol over many years may have effects similar to those seen when tumours lead to more sudden, large increases in glucocorticoid concentrations. People with Cushing's syndrome are insulin resistant and have raised blood pressure.

## ☐ CHILDHOOD GROWTH AND CORONARY HEART DISEASE

The growth of 357 men from a cohort of 4,630 men born in Helsinki who were either admitted to hospital with CHD or died from it is illustrated graphically in Fig 1. Their growth is expressed as Z-scores, with the Z-score for the cohort set at zero. A boy maintaining a steady position as large or small in relation to other boys would follow a horizontal path. Boys who later developed CHD, however, were small at birth, remained small in infancy but had accelerated gain in weight and body mass index (BMI) thereafter. In contrast, their heights remained below average. As in Hertfordshire, the hazard ratios for CHD fell with increasing weight at one year, increasing height and BMI (Table 5). Small size at one year predicted CHD independently of size at birth.

Table 6 is based on 1,235 patients who were admitted to hospital or died from CHD and on 480 patients who died from the disease among people born in Helsinki from 1924–1944. Hazard ratios according to birthweight and BMI at age 11 years are

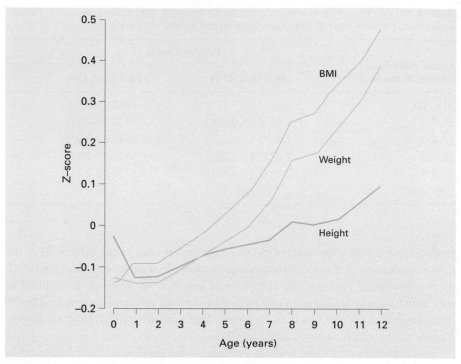

**Fig 1** Growth of 357 men who later developed coronary heart disease from a cohort of 4,630 boys born in Helsinki during 1934–1944 (BMI = body mass index)

**Table 5** Hazard ratios for coronary heart disease in men in Helsinki according to body size at one year.

| | | Hazard ratio (95% CI) | No. of men | No. of cases |
|---|---|---|---|---|
| **Weight** (kg) | ≤9 | 1.82 (1.25–2.64) | 781 | 96 |
| | 9–10 | 1.17 (0.80–1.71) | 1,126 | 85 |
| | 10–11 | 1.12 (0.77–1.64) | 1,243 | 89 |
| | 11–12 | 0.94 (0.62–1.44) | 852 | 49 |
| | >12 | 1.00 | 619 | 38 |
| *p* for trend | | <0.0001 | | |
| **Height** (cm) | ≤73 | 1.55 (1.11–2.18) | 636 | 79 |
| | 74–75 | 0.90 (0.63–1.27) | 962 | 68 |
| | 76–77 | 0.94 (0.68–1.31) | 1,210 | 87 |
| | 78–79 | 0.83 (0.58–1.18) | 1,011 | 64 |
| | >79 | 1.00 | 802 | 59 |
| *p* for trend | | 0.007 | | |
| **BMI** (kg/m²) | ≤16 | 1.83 (1.28–2.60) | 654 | 72 |
| | 16–17 | 1.61 (1.15–2.25) | 936 | 89 |
| | 17–18 | 1.29 (0.91–1.81) | 1,136 | 83 |
| | 18–19 | 1.12 (0.77–1.62) | 941 | 59 |
| | >19 | 1.00 | 954 | 54 |
| *p* for trend | | 0.0004 | | |

BMI = body mass index; CI = confidence interval.

shown. The risks of disease fell with increasing birthweight and rose with increasing BMI, with a similar pattern in men and women. In a simultaneous regression the hazard ratios for admissions and deaths were 0.80 (95% confidence interval (CI) 0.72–0.90) for each kilogram increase in birthweight and 1.06 (CI 1.03–1.10) for each kg/m² increase in BMI at age 11 years. The hazard ratios for deaths alone were 0.83 (CI 0.69–0.99) and 1.10 (CI 1.04–1.16), respectively.

**Table 6** Hazard ratios, adjusted for sex and year of birth, for coronary heart disease according to birthweight and body mass index at (BMI) 11 years (13,517 men and women born in Helsinki 1924–1944).

| | Birthweight (kg) | BMI at 11 years (kg/m²) | | | |
|---|---|---|---|---|---|
| | | ≤15.7 | 15.7–16.6 | 16.6–17.6 | >17.6 |
| Hospital admissions and | ≤3 | 1.4 | 1.6 | 1.8 | 2.1 |
| deaths (1,235) | 3.1–3.5 | 1.3 | 1.5 | 1.5 | 1.6 |
| | 3.6–4.0 | 1.3 | 1.4 | 1.3 | 1.4 |
| | >4.0 | 1.0 | 1.2 | 1.1 | 1.0 |
| Deaths (480) | ≤3 | 1.4 | 1.8 | 2.1 | 3.0 |
| | 3.1–3.5 | 1.4 | 1.9 | 2.2 | 2.7 |
| | 3.6–4.0 | 1.9 | 1.8 | 1.7 | 1.6 |
| | >4.0 | 1.0 | 1.4 | 1.6 | 1.3 |

The growth of 8,760 men and women born in Helsinki is shown in Fig 2. The 290 children who later developed type 2 diabetes had below average body size at birth and at one year, after which their weights and BMIs rose progressively to exceed the average. After the age of two years the degree of obesity in young children as measured by BMI decreases to a minimum at around six years of age, then increases again: the so-called 'adiposity rebound'. Early adiposity rebound is strongly related to a high BMI in childhood and also predicts an increased incidence of type 2 diabetes (Table 7).[10]

An early adiposity rebound was associated with thinness at birth and at one year, and with low weight gain during infancy. It is therefore the thin one- or two-year olds who are at risk of type 2 diabetes, not the overweight ones. One possible explanation for the association between small body size at birth, early adiposity rebound and later type 2 diabetes is that there are persisting alterations in body composition. Babies who are small and thin at birth lack muscle; this deficiency will persist because the critical period for muscle growth occurs *in utero* and there is little cell replication after birth. If they develop a high body mass during childhood, children may have a disproportionately high fat mass in relation to lean body mass, which will lead to insulin resistance.

## ☐ PATHWAYS OF DEVELOPMENT

New studies, especially those of the two exceptionally well documented cohorts in Helsinki, increasingly suggest that CHD and the disorders related to it develop through a series of interactions:

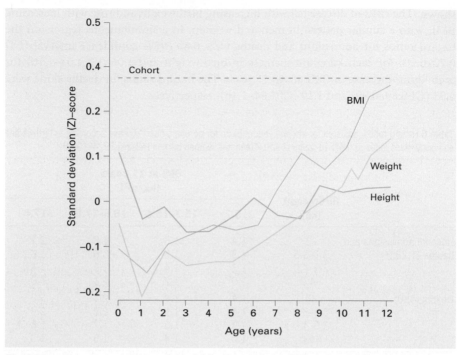

**Fig 2** Mean Z-scores for height, weight and body mass index (BMI) during childhood in 290 people born in Helsinki during 1934-1944 who later developed type 2 diabetes in a cohort of 8,760 men and women. At any age, the mean Z-score and standard deviation for the cohort are set at 0 and 1, respectively.

**Table 7** Body mass index (BMI) at 12 years of age and cumulative incidence of type 2 diabetes according to age at adiposity rebound in 8,760 men and women in Helsinki.

| Age at adiposity rebound (years) | Mean BMI at age 12 (kg/m²) All | % Cumulative incidence of diabetes | | |
|---|---|---|---|---|
| | | Men | Women | All |
| ≤4 | 20.1 | 8.1 (86) | 8.9 (112) | 8.6 (198) |
| 5 | 17.9 | 6.2 (904) | 2.5 (864) | 4.4 (1,768) |
| 6 | 17.2 | 3.7 (1,861) | 2.5 (1,456) | 3.2 (3,317) |
| 7 | 17.1 | 2.4 (249) | 2.1 (243) | 2.2 (492) |
| ≥8 | 16.9 | 3.0 (135) | 0.7 (150) | 1.8 (285) |
| p for trend | <0.001 | <0.001 | 0.002 | <0.001 |

Figures in parentheses are numbers of subjects.

☐ the effects of genes are conditioned by fetal growth

☐ the effects of small body size at birth are conditioned by growth during childhood and by living conditions in childhood and adult life.

Any one influence, such as low income, does not have a single quantifiable risk associated with it. Its risk to an individual is conditioned by events at earlier critical stages of development. This embodies the concept of developmental 'switches' triggered by the environment.

Fetal life is an important phase in branching paths of development. The branchings are triggered by the environment and determine the vulnerability of each individual to what lies ahead. Birthweight, though a convenient marker in epidemiological studies, is an inadequate description of the phenotypic characteristics of a baby that determine its long-term health. The wartime famine in Holland produced lifelong insulin resistance in babies *in utero* at the time, with little alteration in birthweight. In babies, as in children, slowing of growth is a response to a poor environment but does not describe the morphological and physiological consequences. The same birthweight can be attained by many different paths of fetal growth, each of which is likely to be accompanied by different gene-environment interactions.

## ☐ CONCLUSIONS

The associations between slow fetal, infant and childhood growth and later CHD are strong and graded. In Helsinki, boys who at birth had a ponderal index above 26 kg/m³ and at one year of age were above the cohort average for BMI (17.7 kg/m²) and height (76.2 cm) had half the risk of developing CHD before the age of 65 years when compared with all other boys. Such findings confirm the close relation between early growth and later disease.

The principal determinant of growth rates in early life is the availability of nutrition. As yet, the impact of maternal nutrition on fetal nutrition is not known. It is becoming clear, however, that the concept of maternal nutrition must be extended beyond mother's diet in pregnancy to include her body composition and metabolism both during pregnancy and at the time of conception. Moreover, a more sophisticated view of optimal fetal development is needed which takes account of the long-term sequelae of fetal responses to undernutrition.

## REFERENCES

1 Acheson D. *Independent inquiry into inequalities in health.* London: The Stationery Office, 1998.
2 Barker DJ, Osmond C. Infant mortality, childhood nutrition, and ischaemic heart disease in England and Wales. *Lancet* 1986;i:1077–81.
3 Barker DJ. *Mothers, babies and health in later life.* Churchill Livingstone: Edinburgh,1998.
4 Barker DJ. Fetal programming of coronary heart disease. Review. *Trends Endocrinol Metab* 2002;**13**:364–8.
5 Widdowson EM, McCance RA. The effect of finite periods of undernutrition at different ages on the composition and subsequent development of the rat. *Proc R Soc Lond B Biol Sci* 1963; **158**:329–42.
6 Harding J. The nutritional basis of the fetal origins of adult disease. Review. *Int J Epidemiol* 2001;**30**:15–23.
7 McCance RA. Food, growth and time. *Lancet* 1962;ii:621–6, 671–5.
8 Brenner BM, Chertow GM. Congenital oligonephropathy and the etiology of adult hypertension and progressive renal injury. Review. *Am J Kidney Dis* 1994;**23**:171–5.
9 Phillips DI. Insulin resistance as a programmed response to fetal undernutrition. Review. *Diabetologia* 1996;**39**:1119–22.
10 Eriksson JG, Forsén T, Tuomilehto J, Osmond C, Barker DJ. Early adiposity rebound in childhood and risk of Type 2 diabetes in adult life. *Diabetologia* 2003;**46**:190–4.

# Lumleian Lecture

# Immunology as taught by Darwin

Rodney Phillips

## ☐ INTRODUCTION

In 1859 Charles Darwin published the *Origin of Species* in which he enunciated ideas which revolutionised biology. With the publication of this book he launched an enduring way of thinking about biological questions. My purpose here is to persuade the reader of the continuing importance of Darwin's legacy to medicine and biology.

After the publication of the *Origin of Species* Darwin was racked by illness which is now believed to be psychosomatic. He had been under fire from clerics and from the creationists since the book appeared, although he had stout defenders of course in Hooker and Huxley. Wilberforce, Bishop of Oxford, denigrated Darwin on several occasions and, despite Huxley's defence, Oxford did not judge Darwin well in those early days. So, in a small part, but as a representative of Oxford, I would hope to make a tiny recompense for Wilberforce's attack on Darwin.

It is my hope to express convincingly that the operation of Darwinian ideas, which he thought would operate over the millennia, can work much faster – within weeks or even days. The example that will be used to illustrate this rapid evolution and natural selection is the cause of a modern plague, the AIDS virus.

The overwhelming importance of natural selection and survival of the fittest was clearly expounded by Darwin:

> What limit can be put to this power acting during long ages and rigidly scrutinising the whole constitution, structure and habits of each creature, favouring the good and rejecting the bad?

Darwin knew no genetics. Although Mendel had already performed his original experiments, it was not until about 1900 that Mendel's ideas were rediscovered.

Natural selection is described to today's Oxford undergraduates in the following way:

> All species produce more offspring than can possibly survive and reproduce. Organisms differ in their ability to survive and reproduce, in part due to differences in genotypes. The genetic variation generates the populations against which selection operates. In every generation, those genotypes which promote survival in the current environment are present in excess at the reproductive age, and therefore contribute disproportionately to the offspring of the next generation.

Thus, reproductive success is the essence of survival. For natural selection to operate, there must be heritable variation of the traits that are correlated with reproductive success.

After Darwin's enunciation of his ideas and their promotion, particularly by Huxley, people started looking at plant and animal variation in the light of Darwin's ideas. There were many false trails but the notions stimulated a new era of natural history exploration.

It could be argued that it was not until the appearance of a paper in *Nature* on 25 April 1953, 50 years ago this year – arguably the most famous paper ever published in *Nature* – that Darwin's ideas began to be interpreted through the analysis of the biochemicals responsible for encoding genetic information. This paper by Watson and Crick postulated a structure for DNA as a double helix. It proved to be correct, and so provided a basis for understanding both genetic variation and mutation. One sentence in this paper continues to resonate:

> It has not escaped our notice that the specific pairing we have postulated immediately suggests a possible copying mechanism for genetic material.

The speculation implied that the two strands of DNA could be unwound and then copied. More than that, the structure suggested that the alignment of the base pairs could provide a coding mechanism. That insight proved to be absolutely true. After this initial speculation, clever ideas about how DNA could code for protein sequence and how that code might be translated were also proposed. This research was difficult and slow and it took some years to elucidate how the code worked.

Using modern genomic techniques to look at the frequency with which mutation occurs, DNA turns out to be very stable, but there is a measurable mutation rate per nucleotide site per year. By contrast, for an organism like HIV composed of ribonucleic acid (RNA) (a much more unstable genome for reasons discussed later), the mutation rate is a million times faster than that of human DNA; in other words, the AIDS virus could evolve a million times faster than humans.

Important progress towards solving how the code worked was the discovery by Marshall Nurenberg (at the National Institutes of Health, Washington) whose elegant experiments showed that a string of U's translated as phenylalanine. Thus he produced the first clues that indeed the coding was specific for amino acids. Later it became clear that there is some degeneracy at the third coding position in the triplet code. The result of this is that changes at the third site in some triplets, however generated, would not produce a change in the amino acid encoded and would therefore be a synonymous change.

In the case of proline, there is tolerance for all four nucleotides, but with histidine there are only two possible versions, so with a slip from C to A there is a change in the amino acid. When a novel amino acid is substituted as a result of mutation, there is potential for the protein that bears that amino acid to become faulty or functionless. The change might sometimes confer an advantage in some way. By analysing this type of sequence variation, we begin to get measures of selection.

The ratio of changes productive of a different amino acid (non-synonymous) to those that produce no change (synonymous) provides one measure of selection in genetics. This tool, together with phylogenetics, enables the concept of change, variation and selection to begin to be unravelled. For example, an enzyme absolutely crucial for the function of a cell will be under intense negative selection because, as soon as an amino acid changes, particularly in places like the active site, the enzyme will not work. These genes will be under negative selection, which is the situation for many in the human genome.

Genes that have been knocked out because changes in the past have made them functionless have random, neutral sorts of changes. Those loci where change and improvement are under selection will have a ratio greater than 1; for those places under intense selection it can be as high as 15. An analysis of this type can provide evidence of true positive or negative selection.

## ☐ HUMAN IMMUNODEFICIENCY VIRUS

### Basic genetic set up

HIV has two pieces of nucleic acid (RNA, not DNA). It is copied by an enzyme, reverse transcriptase, a type of RNA polymerase which makes mistakes. It cannot proof read, so cannot look back to see if it has made an error of nucleotide incorporation. This is unlike a DNA polymerase which has elegant mechanisms of checking the accuracy of nucleotide incorporation, so ensuring that copies reflect the original sequence with a high level of fidelity. This feature of DNA-copying enzymes is responsible, in part, for the much lower mutation rate in DNA-bearing organisms.

HIV is enormously variable, both because of the error prone qualities of its polymerase and also because there is a very high turnover of the virus in untreated patients. How high this turnover is was shown six or seven years ago by Ho in New York and Shaw and others at Birmingham, Alabama. HIV has an enormous generation rate and it also recombines, so those two strands of RNA can cross over, recombine and form chimaeric viruses. Indeed, as more extensive sequencing is performed worldwide, evidence of chimaeric viruses has become apparent, so the concept of strictly defined subtypes is beginning to collapse.

### Origin

The origin of HIV has engendered immense controversy. Phylogenetic analysis has now mapped HIV on to its many simian derived relatives, the simian immunodeficiency viruses (SIV). This work has shown that HIV is virtually indistinguishable from SIV from chimpanzees. Some African viruses called HIV-2 are much less common than HIV-1; these viruses cluster closely with SIV isolated from the macaque. When we look at the place of HIV-1 and HIV-2 against accumulating sequences from monkey-derived viruses, it is clear that AIDS is a zoonosis, and the controversy contained in many books has been largely settled.

### Subtypes

The spectrum of variation in HIV worldwide is represented by subtypes. Surveys show, for example, that subtype B is very common. This virus spread across the US and

Europe and is the dominant variant in those countries. Subtype E is a Thai virus. Subtype C is an intrusive virus now in southern Africa and driving the hideous epidemic in that part of the world where more than five million people are already infected. Arraying the variation represented by 197 isolates from the Congo shows that they map to all the known subtypes. Viruses can be found in the Congo that carry and represent sequence forms from across the world epidemic; there is a much more restricted pattern of variation in other places such as Russia, Europe or North America.

What is the significance of this? A reasonable start would be to say that the Congo is where the epidemic may have been launched as a human infection. This frightening pattern of variation must also give us a most sobering message. How could any vaccine, no matter how well designed, possibly cope with this staggering amount of diversity? These facts make me very pessimistic. I believe that current vaccines in development will have no utility in the field where HIV variation is staggering. I am also unconvinced that vaccines which might elicit some immunity against limited strain variation will work in practice. Challenges to this immunity by novel variants will probably lead to the selection of vaccine escape mutants. More Darwinism!

## ☐ CONTROL OF THE VIRUS IN HUMANS

How is the virus controlled when it infects human beings? After about 12 years of rather controversial work it is fairly clear now that the virus does not rapidly destroy human beings because of the presence of an intense, effective immune response; this controls the viraemia, but fails to eradicate the virus.

A crucial controlling part of this effective immune response is the T cells which bear T cell receptors (TCRs). These TCRs, discovered by Mark Davis at Stanford and Tak Mak in Toronto many years ago, are crucial for the recognition of antigens. A molecule, CD8, defines a subset of T cells that can kill. These cells survey the surface of other cells to look for 'foreignness' – that is, the presence of infection or unwanted mutation within the cell. The question of what is the marker of 'foreignness' was unknown for many years. In 1976, Rolf Zinkernagel and Peter Doherty, working at the Australian National University, discovered that the recognition event depended on two things: a self-encoded protein and something derived from the infecting agent. In the case of viruses, there is a virus-derived peptide antigen; the host genetic component is a molecule encoded in the so-called 'histocompatibility complex'. For this discovery, now called 'major histocompatibility complex (MHC) restriction', they won the Nobel Prize 20 years later.

When the T cell recognises the 'foreignness' or infected qualities of a cell, it kills it by punching a hole in the cell membrane and pouring in an unpleasant mix of lethal enzymes — hence their name, cytolytic T cells (CTCs) or killer T cells. These cells are believed to be crucial in the control of HIV.

Human CTCs recognise an HLA class I molecule on the infected cell surface. HLA A2 is the commonest class I molecule in Caucasians (about 44% carry it). The way MHC restriction operated was not clear until the late Don Wylie at Harvard, together with Pam Bjorkman, crystallised these molecules. Using X-ray crystallography, they showed that the self-component is a claw-shaped molecule which holds the peptide derived from the virus on the cell surface where it is displayed to the passing T cells. These short fragments of viral peptide are usually 8–10 amino acids in length and form the antigen for T cells of this type. The rest of the molecular structure is derived from self, as is the beta2-microglobulin.

These HLA molecules are encoded at a site which is the most polymorphic in man, and which has been under Darwinian selection pressure for a long time. The Darwinian pressure arises because the possession of HLA molecules with the capacity to bind disparate antigens improves the host's capacity to respond to different pathogens. Over time, different infections have been plaguing us, so different HLA molecules have been more or less useful, depending on the prevailing infections. The diversity has also been generated by gene duplication, followed by further selection.

Using the DN:DS concept (the ratio of nucleotide changes which alter amino acid to those which do not) to analyse variation in class II molecules, the antigen binding site is seen to be under intense positive selection, whereas the structural parts of the protein have largely synonymous nucleotide changes and are not under selection. In fact, there is a strong pressure to preserve the general framework of the molecule, but also a strong pressure for variation within the groove so that different types of peptide can be presented.

## ☐ EVIDENCE THAT T CELLS CONTROL RETROVIRUSES

How good is the evidence that those T cells actually control a retrovirus? In the early, acute phase of infection the viral load goes up to several millions per millilitre of plasma. There is then a quenching of that viraemia over a few weeks. When this early storm is over a pseudo-steady state of 'set-point' viraemia (as it is called) is reached. In this period, the virus is apparently under good immunological control. The term 'pseudo' is used advisedly because the situation is hardly steady – there is still an enormous amount of virus turnover and, in turn, much destruction of CD4-positive lymphocytes. Some patients do not settle down in this way and have a rapid decline, with escalating viraemia and early death. The set-point level correlates closely with when AIDS will be reached. The specific T cells that attack HIV are detected some time after the appearance of the virus in the blood. They are then present in very high numbers and peak at the time that the virus load is controlled. This close relationship between the presence of these cells and the successful control of the virus is good, if indirect, evidence of their role in controlling the infection.

However, the best evidence comes from a simian model. If a monkey is challenged with an SIV (a very similar virus to HIV) and all the CD8 lymphocytes are depleted with an efficient antibody which sweeps them out of the blood of the monkey, the viraemia is not controlled. These experiments have probably convinced the doubters that the CD8 cells are important. There is, however, no question that other types of T cells and antibodies are also crucial in the control of this infection.

If the virus is under intense pressure from these T cells, why does it persist and why does it win the race? All pathogens which persist in the host have methods of evading immunity, some of which are exquisitely effective. HIV is a highly accomplished immune escape artist. One mechanism is antigenic variation. In the case of HLA class I-dependent immunity, changes in the bound peptide can foil the T cell response. This happens if:

☐   the peptide can no longer bind to the class I molecule

☐   it is so different that the TCR can no longer see it

☐   the peptide has some perverse qualities of twisting the TCR, or

☐   if the protein from which the peptide is derived is never broken down because it is resistant to degradation.

HIV will escape T-cell mediated immunity if it encodes antigens of that type. If the viral antigen is not loaded on to the MHC because it cannot bind that molecule, the immune escape mechanism is clear. The viruses that bear this variant antigen survive attack, so those viruses escape and proliferate. The consequence of this idea is that, if there is failure of the antigen to be presented and failure of the killer T cell to kill, these sorts of viruses should be detectable, particularly using powerful molecular techniques.

## ☐ SELECTION BY IMMUNITY DIRECTED TOWARDS HIV

The high replication rate of the virus produces a myriad of mutations. Consequently, every individual with HIV is infected with a swarm of variants. Some of these mutations will be deleterious, the virus will be left less fit and there will be a dying off, 'extinction', of those sorts of changes. Other mutations will lead to increased fitness because of evasion of immunity or the promotion of better replication; those viruses will go on to survive.

If there is further mutation of a particularly fit surviving virus (the reverse transcriptase continues to make mistakes in the replication of new viruses), the fit variant will, in turn, acquire new mutations. Some of these will eliminate the advantage and there will be extinction, while others will be more fit and survive. These dual mutations are of particular interest because they are found in the real world.

The concept of extinction is of course fundamental to Darwinian thought:

> Extinction has only separated groups; it has by no means made them. If every form which has ever been were suddenly to reappear, all would blend together by steps as fine as those between the finest existing varieties.

In other words, those myriad variants that appeared because of the high replication and mutation of the virus existed, at least transiently, but died off leaving only the small set of fit viral forms. The missing links, or predecessors, are not around.

### Rhesus macaque monkey model

Rhesus macaque monkeys have turned out to be an extraordinary model for SIV and HIV research, probably one of the best animal models of all time. These monkeys can be infected with the virus, and the natural history, although abbreviated, closely resembles the natural history of AIDS.

My colleague, David Watkins, at the University of Wisconsin at Madison, has set up a number of experiments to look at the concepts described above using a model system and powerful molecular techniques which he can control. He has identified five distinct antigens in SIV, a virus with a complex structure but a similar genetic layout to HIV. When these monkeys are challenged with the virus, T cells and virus clash in ways similar to that seen in human infection. The monkeys are challenged with a molecular clone, which means that it is genetically homogeneous because it starts as a DNA construct before the RNA is made. The inoculums are checked by sequencing. In known, well characterised antigenic loci the peptide sequence is always the same as the prototype DNA.

During acute infection, antigens are derived from the virus from different sites. As sequencing is performed over time, mutations appear within these antigens, sometimes early but sometimes quite late. The lateness of these changes is thought to be because other changes in the protein flanking this area are necessary for the protein correctly to form so-called 'compensatory' mutations. The time course is different, but there are many mutations. Using special assays to look for the ability of the T cells to recognise these variants, Watkins found that, compared with the wild-type, some variants are not recognised at all. These variant viruses encode peptides that do not bind to the MHC molecules and do not get to the cell surface. Others are recognised to some extent, but less well, still giving the virus a survival advantage.

What is the evidence that selection operates in this system? Is the T cell providing a selective force or are these sorts of mutants appearing by random change only – a sort of chaos across the whole genome? Watkins performed a variety of analyses to examine whether selection operated at these antigenic loci, and found overwhelming evidence. He subjected his data to careful selection analysis using the tools I have described. Those sites in the viral genome to which an immune response was directed had clear evidence for positive selection, but where a monkey lacked the appropriate MHC molecule and could not mount a response to the site there was no evidence of positive selection. Across this genome, therefore, Darwinian selection operates in a matter of weeks to select out escape mutants.

## ☐ SUMMARY OF BACKGROUND

Antiretrovirus T lymphocytes recognise peptide antigens dictated by – bound to – MHC molecules. These peptides are presented to T cells when they arrive on the cell surface. Genetic variants of the virus can alter or even abolish recognition of infected targets if all the mutants produce peptides that do not bind or do not allow TCR recognition. Even a virus possessing some of these escape changes, but not at all loci, should have a survival advantage, given that a small genetic change in a fast running virus should produce genetic advantage. Escape mutants, as demonstrated in the monkey system, seem to grow out at different rates.

## ☐ THE HUMAN SYSTEM

Despite the effective publicity about the risks of acquisition of HIV, there is no doubt that in the US and in Europe new infections continue to be seen in a number of groups in the population. It is my privilege to collaborate with Jonathan Weber and Philippa Easterbrook (now at King's College) to study acute HIV infection in humans.

I want to present a small piece of data from what has been a large programme. An individual was admitted to hospital with an illness reminiscent of aseptic meningitis. A good history was taken, from which it was clear that he was a gay man and potentially had a high-risk exposure to HIV. His antibody test was negative on 10 October 1995, but antigen was present in his blood so there was yet to be an antibody response. There was evidence of virus, confirmed by a highly specific polymerase chain reaction experiment.

Blood was received from this patient nine days after he was found to be ELISA-negative and he had this acute illness. Therefore, he was studied nine days after the appearance of symptoms, but probably slightly longer after acquisition of the virus.

On assaying his T cells, he was found to have made a single response focused on a single peptide antigen, instead of making an array of responses across the whole genome which is seen in some cases. This was an antigen derived from *nef*, a somewhat interesting molecule in a retrovirus because it is not absolutely essential for viral replication but is essential for pathogenicity. This peptide, which bound to HLA B8, was the sole response that could be found in this individual soon after the time he acquired HIV. There is immense variability of the peptide sequences from the peptides that can be found to bind to B8 molecules, but positions 3 and 5 are highly conserved because these amino acids are crucial for anchoring the peptide into the groove of the HLA molecule. Knowing no more than this, it can be predicted that change at that site could lead to loss of binding of the peptide, while changes at other sites might affect the way the TCR recognises the peptides.

David Price sequenced this patient's proviral DNA. At the time the first blood sample was obtained there was no sequence variation at that site. Quite a few clones were sampled and the locus encoding this single nef-derived peptide was completely monomorphic. However, by the next month there was evidence both of mutation and that the epitope had been dropped off by the acquisition of stop codons upstream of the sequence. Six months after the original clinical presentation of acute HIV infection there was a large array of variants, including sequences with two amino acid changes, including position 5 which is an anchor residue. The virus with epitope deletion persisted in the patient's blood. T cell assays were then performed simply to look for the ability of the patient's T cells to recognise the variant antigens that had arisen in his blood.

Antigenic variation detected within patients' HIV was often well recognised by T cells which could cope with this variation. As old-school immunology would have predicted, as new antigens appear, new T cell clones will expand to cope with these novel antigens. The enormous diversity in HIV produces changes in antigens which cannot be met by appropriate T cell response. Some variants are not seen well, and some have no recognition even at the quite unphysiological concentrations in this particular type of *in vitro* assay. The mutants that are not recognised are mutated at position 5; in binding assays, those peptides do not bind to HLA class I and so never reach the cell surface. It is a fundamental way to escape immunity: never show the antigen. Thus, the patient's immune system is driving out variants which cannot be seen by the T cells. This is a result similar to the monkey experiment in which selection operates where the immune response operates.

## ☐ POPULATIONS

### Vertical transmission

If the immune escape variants discussed above arise in individual patients, do they have an impact on the epidemic and do these viruses have anything to do with the diversity seen in populations? For example, does the separation of subtypes have anything to do with a selection force coming from the immune response?

The first step in such a demonstration is to show transmission. The problem with transmission is that both the transmitting virus and the recipient virus are needed. It is difficult to obtain the appropriate material in human infections transmitted sexually, but vertical transmission of the virus is tragically still easy to study in Africa. Vertical transmission can occur *in utero*, at the time of delivery of the child and during breast-feeding. Trials currently underway in Africa are attempting to show how risky breast-feeding is – but, of course, to stop these African mothers breast-feeding might in any case result in the death of the child. My Oxford colleague, Philip Goulder, a Wellcome Senior Fellow, has been studying vertical transmission, first in the US and more recently in Durban and KwaZulu-Natal in South Africa.

The questions being asked are fundamental to the issue of whether viruses that are beginning to make trouble for the immune system can spread into the population. This is rather reminiscent of the way in which drug-resistant viruses arise and are transmissible to naïve populations.

First, a couple of quite straightforward concepts need to be understood. Children can inherit a class I molecule which has dictated an immune response in the mother. For example, if the mother possesses HLA B27 and passes it on to the child, both have the requisite molecule to evoke the same immune response. However, the child could inherit the molecule not from the mother but from the father. Thus, when the maternal immune response selects escape mutants can she transmit them? If they arrive in the child, does that help propagate the viraemia because the transmitted viruses are pre-adapted to evade the immunity dictated by the shared HLA B27 molecule?

A child who inherits HLA B27 from the mother will begin to try to mount a response to whatever viruses come across from the mother, developed or – if you like – evolved against this particular molecule. If, however, the HLA B27 is inherited from the father, the mother will never have mounted a response to the locus dictated by this molecule. This could be a mess as an experiment, save for one rather useful fact in the case of HLA B27 in man. It tends to dictate a response to a particular 10-amino acid in the p24 gag protein of HIV. There is little responsiveness to antigens elsewhere in the genome; T cell immune responses are almost all focused on this particular site in HLA B27-bearing individuals. It is also interesting to immunologists and vaccinologists because it is one of the most invariant parts of a quite invariant molecule. When this particular peptide binds to HLA B27, it has a crucial position for anchoring the peptide to the B27 molecule: position 2.

This antigen is located on a helical component of the gag subunit and forms an interface where these crucial interactions hold the subcomponents together – hence the sequence conservation. Even minor changes here would disrupt the interface crucial for these subunits coming together, and would therefore disrupt the function of the virus.

A number of things can be learnt if individuals who make responses to this peptide are sequenced. If adults are sequenced, whether or not pregnant women, an array of variants is found in individuals mounting a strong, focused immunodominant response. There is variation in position 2 and also further down in the peptide. When changes occur outside position 2 there is no change in recognition – the T cells keep up – but with anchor position mutants, particularly a threonine to arginine change, there is effectively no recognition and no binding. Despite the intense sequence conservation at this site, variants arise which can escape. If this is the sole response to the virus, those individuals will have trouble containing the virus.

Studying the ability of children who bear HLA B27 molecules to respond to that particular peptide gives interesting results. For example, of children who possess HLA B27, those who receives virus from a B27-negative mother, but who inherit the B27 from the father, make a good response to the wild-type peptide. However, children who receive B27 from their mother do not respond to the wild-type peptide. This means that the B27-negative mother did not select an escape mutant and passed on the standard peptide.

To investigate this and to clarify these questions, four children were studied. A child who inherited HLA B27 from its father was able to make a response, but three children who inherited HLA B27 from their mother were infected with an escape mutant where the anchor position was knocked out in a 'pre-evolved' form of HIV. Thus, there is clear evidence in the vertical transmission studies that escape mutants can be transmitted across the placenta or through breast milk.

### Are these mutants found in populations?

The next step is to find out whether these mutants appear or are detectable in population studies. They are transmissible vertically, and there is preliminary evidence that they are transmissible sexually, so an essential requirement for the dissemination of these HLA related mutations exists.

Simon Mallal and his colleagues in Perth, Western Australia, have sequenced over 400 individuals who, because of Perth's relative isolation, do not move much out of Western Australia: they have been captive, to some extent, because of the clinical structure in Perth. These individuals are infected largely with subtype B, so have a relatively similar virus despite the large number of people in this cohort.

Mallal's hypothesis, based on some of the ideas discussed here, is that T cells, working under the dictates of HLA class I, operate to imprint mutations on the virus population. They should be detectable, and these CTC epitope changes should be linked with the possession of a given HLA molecule. With the sequence capacity that he has available, Mallal has shown that this is true. This is evidence that the sequences I have shown are in populations and are linked with HLA. He is sequencing reverse transcriptase, partly because he is interested in drug resistance but also because he is finding polymorphisms of amino acids, some of which are seen only in individuals who possess a given HLA molecule – B37 in one case, B5 in another. There are similar findings along other parts of the reading frame encoding reverse transcriptase. This is an intensively conserved locus. The changes detected are often stereotypic; in other words, there is a favoured amino acid, and some of those favoured changes are in anchor residues. Selection is operating to knock out the amino acid capacity to bind specifically to HLA; many of these changes are linked to quite common HLA molecules.

## □ THE FUTURE

Intense efforts have been made to try to control HIV worldwide. We lack a vaccine and, if we are honest, we lack good ideas for a vaccine. There have been intense prevention programmes, highly successful in parts of the US and Europe, but in other parts of the world there has been total ignorance of the potential epidemic qualities of this infection.

Figures from the UK from early in the epidemic until 2001 show a continuing, steady new infection rate amongst homosexual men. Heterosexual transmission of HIV in the UK also has a steady rise. From talking to my colleagues, I believe this is in large measure among people coming from Africa.

Finally, some statistics demonstrating that this situation is much worse than is probably understood. Data from the US Census Bureau world population profile show a prediction of a population structure in Botswana, which has one of the highest HIV prevalence rates in the world. Obviously, as would be expected, there is a steady attrition towards old age. With the onset of AIDS, and it playing as an epidemic through that population, there is a 'coring out' in particular age group strata. Only about 30% of children are vertically infected, so there are a lot of survivors in early childhood, but there are a lot of deaths later. Many of the children are orphans, their parents are dead and the elderly are looking after those orphans.

An estimate can be made of the risk of dying of HIV for a 15-year-old boy living in Botswana. If the existing prevalence rate risk is maintained there, a boy of 15 has something like a 90% chance of dying of HIV. If a vaccine of limited efficacy of the type being strongly promoted by colleagues of mine produced a reduction, but not absolute protection from the ability to acquire the virus so that it dropped it by half, that 15-year-old would still have an 80% chance of dying of HIV.

I hope I have convinced you that Charles Darwin made a contribution to science that will live on for ever, that his contribution to our understanding not just of the evolution of the animal species and of plants, but also of microorganisms like viruses, has been fundamental. If we are ever to understand the true basis of HIV infection it will only be in the light of Darwin's thoughts.

# Answers to self assessment questions

## ☐ RENAL

### Chronic kidney failure: advances in understanding and treatment

| 1a True | 2a True | 3a False | 4a False | 5a True |
|---------|---------|----------|----------|---------|
| b True | b True | b False | b False | b False |
| c True | c False | c True | c True | c False |
| d True | d False | d False | d True | d True |
| e True | e True | e False | e False | e True |

### Treatment of glomerulonephritis

| 1a False | 2a False | 3a True | 4a True | 5a True |
|----------|----------|---------|---------|---------|
| b True | b False | b True | b False | b True |
| c False | c True | c True | c False | c True |
| d True | d False | d False | d True | d True |
| e False | e True | e False | e True | e True |

### Selection of dialysis modality

| 1a True | 2a False | 3a True |
|---------|----------|---------|
| b False | b True | b False |
| c False | c True | c True |
| d False | d False | d False |
| e True | e False | e True |

## ☐ INTERNATIONAL HEALTH

### The emerging threat of multidrug resistant tuberculosis

| 1a False | 2a False | 3a True |
|----------|----------|---------|
| b True | b False | b True |
| c False | c True | c False |
| d False | d False | d True |
| e True | e False | e True |

### Malaria for the physician

| 1a False | 2a False | 3a True |
|----------|----------|---------|
| b True | b True | b True |
| c False | c True | c True |
| d False | d False | d True |
| e True | e True | e False |

## ☐ NEUROLOGY

### Multiple sclerosis

| | | |
|---|---|---|
| 1a False | 2a True | 3a False |
| b False | b True | b True |
| c False | c True | c True |
| d False | d True | d True |
| e True | e False | e True |

### Investigation and management of headache

| | | |
|---|---|---|
| 1a True | 2a False | 3a True |
| b False | b False | b True |
| c True | c True | c False |
| d False | d False | d False |
| e True | e True | e True |

## ☐ NUTRITION AND PATIENTS: A DOCTOR'S RESPONSIBILITY

### Why the metabolic syndrome?

| | | | |
|---|---|---|---|
| 1a True | 2a False | 3a True | 4a True |
| b False | b True | b True | b False |
| c True | c True | c False | c True |
| d False | d False | d True | d True |
| e True | e False | e False | e True |

### Clinical nutrition in a district general hospital

| | | | | |
|---|---|---|---|---|
| 1a True | 2a False | 3a True | 4a False | 5a False |
| b True | b False | b False | b False | b False |
| c False | c False | c True | c False | c True |
| d False | d True | d False | d False | d False |
| e True | e False | e False | e True | e True |

### Nutrition in the intensive care unit

| | | | |
|---|---|---|---|
| 1a False | 2a False | 3a True | 4a True |
| b True | b True | b False | b False |
| c False | c False | c False | c True |
| d True | d True | d True | d True |
| e True | e True | e True | e False |

## ☐ IMAGING

### Interventional magnetic resonance imaging

| | | | | |
|---|---|---|---|---|
| 1a False | 2a True | 3a True | 4a True | 5a True |
| b False | b True | b False | b True | b False |
| c True | c True | c True | c False | c False |
| d True | d False | d False | d False | d False |
| e True | e False | e True | e False | e False |

## ☐ INFECTION: THE ANTIVIRAL REVOLUTION

### Treatment of HIV infection

| | | |
|---|---|---|
| 1a False | 2a True | 3a True |
| b False | b False | b False |
| c True | c False | c True |
| d True | d True | d False |
| e False | e True | e True |

### Treatment of respiratory viruses

| | | | | |
|---|---|---|---|---|
| 1a False | 2a True | 3a True | 4a False | 5a False |
| b False | b False | b True | b False | b True |
| c True | c True | c True | c False | c False |
| d True | d False | d False | d False | d False |
| e False | e False | e True | e True | e True |

### Current issues in the treatment of genital herpes virus infections

| | | |
|---|---|---|
| 1a True | 2a False | 3a True |
| b True | b True | b False |
| c False | c False | c True |
| d True | d False | d True |
| e True | e True | e False |

### Immunotherapy for Epstein-Barr virus-associated lymphoma

| | | |
|---|---|---|
| 1a True | 2a True | 3a False |
| b False | b False | b True |
| c True | c True | c True |
| d True | d False | d True |
| e True | e True | e True |

## ☐ RHEUMATOLOGY

### Glucocorticoids in rheumatoid arthritis

| | | | | |
|---|---|---|---|---|
| 1a True | 2a True | 3a False | 4a False | 5a True |
| b False | b False | b True | b False | b True |
| c False | c True | c True | c False | c False |
| d True | d True | d True | d True | d False |
| e True | e True | e False | e False | e True |

### Primary systemic vasculitis

| | | | |
|---|---|---|---|
| 1a False | 2a False | 3a True | 4a False |
| b False | b True | b False | b False |
| c True | c False | c True | c True |
| d False | d True | d True | d True |
| e False | e True | e False | e True |

### Joint replacement in rheumatoid arthritis

| | | |
|---|---|---|
| 1a False | 2a False | 3a True |
| b True | b True | b False |
| c True | c False | c True |
| d False | d False | d False |
| e False | e True | e False |

## ☐ RESPIRATORY MEDICINE

### Chronic obstructive pulmonary disease

| | | |
|---|---|---|
| 1a False | 2a True | 3a False |
| b True | b False | b False |
| c False | c True | c True |
| d False | d True | d True |
| e True | e False | e False |

### Sleep apnoea

| | | | | |
|---|---|---|---|---|
| 1a True | 2a True | 3a False | 4a True | 5a False |
| b False | b True | b True | b False | b True |
| c True | c True | c True | c True | c True |
| d False | d True | d False | d False | d True |
| e False | e True | e True | e True | e False |

## ☐ GASTROENTEROLOGY

### *Helicobacter pylori*

| | | |
|---|---|---|
| 1a True | 2a True | 3a True |
| b False | b False | b False |
| c True | c True | c False |
| d False | d False | d False |
| e False | e True | e True |

### Medically unexplained gastrointestinal symptoms

| | | |
|---|---|---|
| 1a False | 2a False | 3a True |
| b False | b True | b False |
| c True | c False | c False |
| d False | d True | d True |
| e False | e False | e False |

### Advances in inflammatory bowel disease

| | | |
|---|---|---|
| 1a True | 2a True | 3a True |
| b True | b True | b True |
| c False | c False | c False |
| d True | d True | d True |
| e False | e False | e False |

## ☐ PREVENTION OF CORONARY ARTERY DISEASE

### Therapeutic intervention to prevent coronary heart disease and stroke

| | | |
|---|---|---|
| 1a False | 2a False | 3a False |
| b False | b True | b True |
| c True | c True | c False |
| d False | d True | d False |
| e True | e False | e True |

### Lifestyle interventions in the prevention of coronary heart disease

| | | |
|---|---|---|
| 1a False | 2a False | 3a True |
| b True | b False | b False |
| c True | c False | c True |
| d True | d True | d True |
| e False | e False | e False |